Months of Morphemes

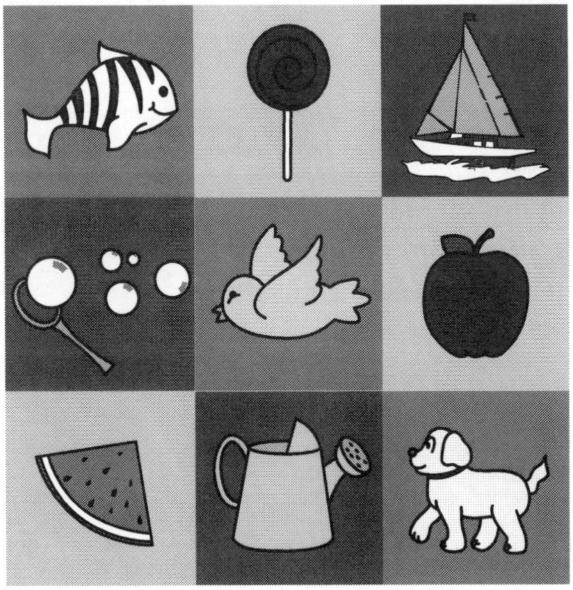

A Theme-Based Cycles Approach

Allison M. Haskill, MS, CCC-SLP

Ann A. Tyler, PhD, CCC-SLP

Leslie C. Tolbert, MS, CCC-SLP

Thinking Publications • Eau Claire, Wisconsin

09 08 07 06 05 04 03 02 01 9 8 7 6 5 4 3 2 1

Libary of Congress Cataloging-in-Publication Data

Haskill, Allison M., date.

Months of morphemes : a theme-based cycles approach / Allison, M. Haskill, Ann A. Tyler, Leslie C. Tolbert.

p. cm.

Includes bibliographical references.

ISBN 1-888222-73-5 (pbk.)

1. Speech therapy for children—Handbooks, manuals, etc. 2. Language disorders in children—Handbooks, manuals, etc. 3. Activity programs in education—Handbooks, manuals, etc. I. Tyler, Ann A., date. II. Tolbert, Leslie C., date. III. Title.

LB3454 .H29 2001

371.91'42—dc21

2001027733

Printed in the United States of America

Cover design by Debbie Olson

THINKING PUBLICATIONS®

a division of McKinley Companies, Inc.

424 Galloway Street • Eau Claire, WI 54703

(715) 832-2488 • FAX (715) 832-9082

Email: custserv@ThinkingPublications.com

COMMUNICATION SOLUTIONS THAT CHANGE LIVES®

To the children and families
in the Washoe County School District who participated
in the study on which this program was based

ABOUT THE AUTHORS

Allison Haskill is a doctoral candidate in the Department of Speech Pathology and Audiology at the University of Nevada, Reno. Ms. Haskill is interested in studying and providing intervention to young children with phonological and language impairments. Specifically, she is interested in the areas of morphosyntax and early literacy. In addition to her coursework, Ms. Haskill has worked as a speech-language pathologist both in private practice and in the local school district.

Dr. Ann Tyler is a fellow of ASHA and a professor at the University of Nevada, Reno, where she teaches courses in phonological intervention, experimental phonetics, and clinical assessment. She previously taught at Syracuse University, where she received her PhD, and the State University of New York at Cortland. Dr. Tyler's clinical interests focus on efficient interventions for children with phonological or language impairments. Similarly, Dr. Tyler's research currently focuses on different treatment strategies for children with both phonological and language impairments. Her research in treatment efficacy has lead to the development of unique intervention protocols for targeting phonological and language goals in preschoolers enrolled in her local school district's early-childhood programs. These protocols were developed as part of a treatment evaluation study ("Speech and Language Goal Attack Strategies," DC03358) funded by the National Institute on Deafness and Other Communication Disorders (NIDCD). She has made over 50 presentations on original research and issues in clinical phonology and has published scientific papers in a variety of professional journals, such as the *Journal of Speech and Hearing Disorders, Journal of Speech and Hearing Research, Journal of Child Language, Clinical Linguistics and Phonetics,* and *Topics in Language Disorders.*

Leslie Tolbert is a doctoral candidate in speech-language pathology at the University of Nevada, Reno. Her interests are in phonological and language disorders in infants and toddlers, early social-emotional development, and family-focused service delivery models. Ms. Tolbert also provides consultative intervention services for Nevada's early intervention programs, Head Start, and Special Children's Clinic. She coordinates speech and language screenings for children ages 0–5 who attend Head Start and local preschools. In addition to providing direct services, Ms. Tolbert is also employed as a speech-language consultant by the Nevada Bureau of Disability Adjudication.

CONTENTS

Cycle 2: Animals, Cloze Task

Cycle 3: Food, Preparatory Set

PREFACE

Months of Morphemes: A Theme-Based Cycles Approach resulted from a study funded by the National Institute on Deafness and Other Communication Disorders (NIDCD) entitled "Speech and Language Goal Attack Strategies" (DC03358). This study involved examining the effects of different strategies of targeting both speech and language goals in preschool-age children who had co-occurring speech and language disorders. The children involved in this study were to receive both phonological (speech) and language intervention for one academic year. As we planned the project, we realized that we would need a clear, detailed language intervention program that would uphold theoretical and empirical evidence regarding language intervention and that would target aspects of language with which children are documented to (and that our experience verified) have the most difficulty.

The end result of the study planning and implementation is this resource. *Months of Morphemes* is a theme-based language intervention program that includes detailed scripts that have an emphasis on morphological goals. The scripts in this program arose from the need to have an intervention program implemented in the same manner by several different graduate-student clinicians. Over the course of the two-year study on which this program was based, there were 15 graduate-student clinicians and 4 speech-language pathologists (SLPs) who provided parts of the same interventions. We believed that if lessons were planned, materials were provided, and scripts were made (to be followed for the "talk" of the intervention sessions), there would be a greater likelihood that the program would be implemented in a similar manner across settings and clinicians.

We chose to include naturalistic, focused stimulation activities and direct-elicitation techniques in the production activities because the language intervention literature reports the efficacy of all the activity types and, moreover, because our combined experiences suggested that children benefit from a combination of instructional techniques across the continuum from least to most natural. We chose to include children's literature as a basis for many of the activities within lessons because of the importance of emergent literacy experiences for children with speech and language disorders and because literacy activities are enjoyable for all involved.

Finally, we chose to focus on finite morphemes that reflect tense and agreement because they are an area of considerable vulnerability for children with specific language impairment (SLI) and because we could find no commercially available program that focused on these morphemes. Since the development of *Months of Morphemes,* we have become even more convinced of the importance of targeting this group of morphemes given recent reports of their protracted development in comparison to other aspects of language in children with SLI (Goffman and Leonard, 2000; Rice, Wexler, and Hershberger, 1998).

Our decision to publish *Months of Morphemes* stemmed from the presentation of our cycles approach at the 1999 convention of the American Speech-Language-Hearing Association (ASHA) in San Francisco, California, where we received many enthusiastic responses to the language intervention program. We also received very positive responses from the public school speech-language pathologists who used the scripts and materials. Consequently, we were encouraged to make the program available to a wider audience. Thus, we hope that a variety of educational professionals will be able to use the scripts and materials provided in *Months of Morphemes.* We further hope that the children and families who use the program will see a long-term improvement in communicative functioning similar to what we saw in so many of the children involved in the development of this resource.

ACKNOWLEDGMENTS

Our ideas for *Months of Morphemes* came from many combined years of experience working with and supervising graduate students as they worked with young children with language impairments. We are thankful for the opportunities we had to experiment with different intervention approaches, different levels of instructional support, and different activities and to watch students experiment with these same items during their intervention sessions. From these experiences, we were able to formulate our ideas about intervention and about what we envisioned worked best for our immediate goals.

We wish to express special appreciation to the graduate students at the University of Nevada, Reno, who, as part of their clinical externships, implemented the language intervention program in *Months of Morphemes* and provided valuable feedback about their experiences: Holly Anderson, Amy Cocanour, Pennie Iannicionni, Angela Johnson, Pam Katzorke, Melissa Ogilvie, Kellie Paul, Veronica Spurlock, Rebecca Torres, and Peter Wolf.

We also sincerely appreciate the efforts of the four speech-language pathologists (SLPs) we worked with during the two-year study for which this program was developed: Heather Cook, Sandra Martin, Tanna Rader, and June Rosta. Their feedback about the intervention program and their supervision of our graduate-student externs was invaluable, as was their willingness to work cooperatively and share the preschoolers on their caseload with us.

We are indebted to Joy Erickson, who helped coordinate and promote the project with SLPs in the Washoe County School District.

We also want to thank the parents who so willingly allowed their children to participate in the study and supported it with their efforts at home, reviewing and reinforcing the language intervention program's targets and activities.

We wish to thank our reviewers—Becca Jarzynski, Margot Kelman, Peg Nechkash, and Nancy Nicolin—for their time and insights.

Introduction

Overview

Months of Morphemes: A Theme-Based Cycles Approach is a language intervention program designed to be used by educators to improve the grammatical morpheme usage of young children with speech and language disorders. Three one-month cycles are included; each cycle uses a different theme and can be used with individuals or groups. Cycles are arranged hierarchically, with decreasing levels of educator support.

This theme-based language intervention program is unique in that it includes detailed scripts for naturalistic, focused stimulation activities and direct-elicitation techniques. These scripts are organized in easy-to-use cycles with interesting, multimodality activities. Letters and resources to encourage family participation in the language intervention process and suggestions for measuring progress are included.

Months of Morphemes offers complete intervention scripts for eight frequently targeted grammatical morphemes (see Table 1). The four primary targets of the language intervention program (i.e., primary morphemes) are regular third person singular, irregular past tense, regular past tense, and copula *be.* Scripts are also included for four supplementary targets (i.e., supplemental morphemes): regular plurals, possessives, pronouns, and auxiliary *be.*

Table 1 **Grammatical Morpheme Targets**

Grammatical Morpheme	Example
Regular third person singular	The dog **barks.**
Irregular past tense	The dog **ran.**
Regular past tense	The dog **barked.**
Copula *be* (contractible and uncontractible)	He **is** my dog.
Regular plurals *	I have two **dogs.**
Possessives *	It is **dad's** dog.
Pronouns * (nominative, objective, and possessive)	**He** is **her** dog.
Auxiliary *be* * (contractible and uncontractible)	The dog **is** barking.

* Indicates "supplemental" targets, the scripts for which are found in Part II.

The scripts were designed to improve the morphological performance of children with speech and language disorders, with an emphasis on finite morphemes that reflect tense and agreement. However, this language intervention program inherently targets other important language skills as well. Functional, age-appropriate, theme-related vocabulary concepts, and direction-following tasks are incorporated into each activity. Although some activities are more structured and contrived than others, there are many opportunities for naturalistic models of appropriate discourse and pragmatics in each session. Age-appropriate pragmatic and discourse skills are practiced and modeled in the context of story retelling, dramatic play, art, science, gross motor, and snack activities.

Goals

This language intervention program has four primary goals:

1. Improve the morphosyntactic performance of children aged 3–6 who present with speech and language disorders. The program is hierarchically organized to decrease the levels of support given to children, allowing them to accurately use a variety of grammatical morphemes and facilitating carryover of new skills.

2. Provide educators with a structured and thorough language program that uses a cycles approach and a variety of elicitation and modeling techniques (see "Types of Activities" on page 8).

3. Include families in the intervention process by providing weekly family letters that describe suggested follow-up activities, books to read to encourage morphological improvement, and ways family members can work on improving their child's morphological skills at home.

4. Provide children with speech and language disorders with thematically related, meaningful activities to encourage language development and maximum child participation. The program focuses on pragmatic language skills in that there are numerous opportunities for turn taking, contingent responding, and topic maintenance. Although the activities in *Months of Morphemes* focus on facilitating language improvement, they also require using skills in other modalities. Fine-motor skills are developed through the completion of art activities. Problem-solving skills are used in simple science experiments. Gross-motor activities include playing physical games, such as hide-and-seek. Dramatic play is encouraged through use of puppet shows, retelling stories using felt boards, and dress-up activities. Snack time activities provide opportunities for practicing social skills, such as sharing and turn taking. All focused stimulation and elicited production activity scripts include a Skills Used section that captures key focus areas beyond morphological development.

Target Users

The goals and activities emphasized in this language intervention program are directed at 3- to 6-year-old children with impaired language who have a mean length of utterance of at least 2.0. However, many activities may also be appropriate for use with other populations of children with morphological deficits (e.g., older children with global developmental delays and older children who are learning

English as a second language). Although this intervention program was initially developed for English-speaking children with morphosyntactically based language disorders, it has been used successfully with children from a variety of ethnically and economically diverse backgrounds.

Months of Morphemes is designed to be used primarily by educators who have the challenge of managing large caseloads comprised of children with a variety of language needs. This language intervention program can be readily implemented by educators who work with children who could benefit from improved language stimulation. Specifically, trained speech-language pathologists, students of speech-language pathology, or early-childhood special education teachers who want to facilitate language improvement should be able to follow the scripts included in this program without difficulty.

This language intervention program is designed to be used in the following settings: regular and special preschool and kindergarten classrooms; programs for at-risk children (e.g., Head Start); university speech, language, and hearing clinics; and home-based daycare facilities.

Background

Development of *Months of Morphemes*

The scripts included in *Months of Morphemes* were initially used to provide language intervention to a group of preschoolers with impaired language and phonology who were participants in a study of the effects of different types of intervention strategies. The speech-language pathologists who administered this language intervention program reported that they appreciated its creative aspects and stated that they enjoyed the incorporation of both structured and naturalistic activities. Teachers of the study's participants commented on how they liked that the intervention contained the types of themes typically used in their classrooms. Several family members of the children in the study reported that they noticed improvement in their child's language skills at home. They also appreciated receiving family letters, which described what was taking place during intervention sessions and gave suggestions on how they could continue to work on their child's language at home.

Finite morphemes were selected as priority targets for this language intervention program for two main reasons: (1) participants in the study this program was based on performed more poorly on these morphemes than on other targets and (2) results of recent studies and reports (Goffman and Leonard, 2000; Rice, 2000) indicated that deficits in finite morpheme usage are likely to persist longer than deficits in other areas of language for children with specific language impairments.

Months of Morphemes uses a cycles approach for targeting language goals. Hodson and Paden (1983, 1991) originally applied the cycles time-based approach to structuring phonology intervention. Under this approach, various targets are addressed for a prespecified period of time and then "recycled." During each phase of recycling, the level of difficulty gradually increases. The main goal of this approach is for the child to focus on numerous individual phonemes, each for a short period of time. This approach has the appeal of providing a manageable way for educators to target multiple goals. Although cycles are typically associated with phonology intervention, they are also very appropriate for use with language intervention, particularly for use with morphological goals (Fey, Cleave, Long, and Hughes, 1993).

Results from the first year of the study indicated that the implementation of this language intervention program resulted in significantly improved morphological performance as measured after all three cycles had been completed (Tyler, Lewis, Haskill, and Tolbert, 2001). The 10 children who received the intervention described in this book had an average 15.7% increase in their finite morpheme composite (FMC) score after 12 weeks of intervention (pre-treatment = 40.2; post-treatment = 55.90). In comparison, a group of 7 children who did not receive the intervention had an average increase of only 2.75% in their FMC score (pre-treatment= 50.95; post-treatment= 53.70) (see Figure 1). In addition to improvement in FMCs, increases in mean length of utterance were observed for most participants.

Figure 1 **Finite Morpheme Composite (FMC) Improvement**

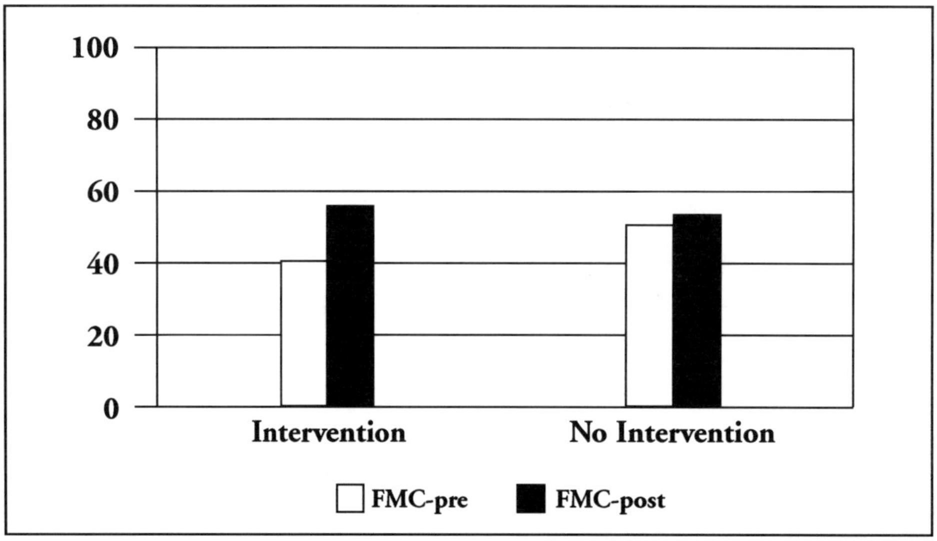

NOTE: Finite morpheme composites (FMCs) (see Bedore and Leonard, 1998) were the indices used in this study to indicate morphological improvement. This composite measure is derived from language sample data and reflects the number of correct productions divided by the total number of obligatory contexts for the following finite morphemes: regular third person singular, regular past tense, contractible and uncontractible *be*, and contractible and uncontractible auxiliary *be*. The rationale for emphasizing finite morphemes is explained in detail in the "Finite Morphemes" section (see page 7).

Finite Morphemes

Although children with language disorders might present with difficulties in a variety of language domains, it has been well documented that the domain of grammatical morphology, and more specifically that of finite morphology, is particularly problematic (Leonard, 1998; Rice, 2000; Rice and Wexler, 1996; Rice, Wexler, and Cleave, 1995). Whereas other areas of language, such as lexical diversity, may improve with age for children with language disorders, finite morpheme deficits frequently persist for a much longer period of time (Goffman and Leonard, 2000). *Finite morphemes* are those that reflect tense and agreement. For example, in the clause *she runs,* the suffix *-s* is finite because it reflects both tense (present) and agreement (third person: she). Finite morphemes addressed in this resource are listed in Table 2.

Table 2 **Finite Morphemes**

Finite Morpheme	Example
Regular third person singular ***-s***	She **runs**.
Regular past tense ***-ed***	She **skipped**.
Copula ***be*** (contractible and uncontractible) is, am, are, was, were (main verb)	**She's** happy He **was** happy.
Auxiliary ***be*** (contractible and uncontractible) is, am, are, was, were (helping verb)	**He's** running. He **was** running.

Because of this well-documented vulnerability for finite morphemes and because the 40 children in the study this language intervention program was developed around had particular difficulty with these forms, they are a major focus of this program. Further, there is some preliminary indication that not only will finite morpheme productions be improved when they are targeted, but nonfinite morphemes that are not directly targeted will also be improved. Therefore, when selecting targets, the highest priority should be given to finite forms.

Three of the four morphemes targeted in Part I of *Months of Morphemes* are finite morphemes. Scripts for nonfinite morphemes (i.e., irregular past tense, regular plurals, possessives, and pronouns) are also included (see irregular past tense in Part I and all morphemes in Part II). Note that scripts for one finite morpheme, auxiliary *be,* were included in Part II, not Part I. Although auxiliary *be* is a finite form, it was not included as a priority target because results of a recent study by Tyler, Haskill, and Paul (2001) indicated that when copula *be* was an intervention target, generalization occurred with auxiliary *be.* That is, for the overwhelming majority of children in their study who received intervention for copula *be,* untreated auxiliary *be* also improved. Thus, when prioritizing during the target selection process, it may be more efficient to choose either copula or auxiliary *be* as an intervention target instead of treating these two *be* forms simultaneously.

Morpheme targets and exemplars included in *Months of Morphemes* were selected based on several factors: (1) finiteness; (2) familiar, age-appropriate vocabulary; (3) relation to the central theme; (4) frequency of occurrence in the language; and (5) pragmatic appropriateness. In *Months of Morphemes,* four morphemes are treated in the 12-week period. The choice to focus on four morphemes was made because it was thought that more than four might be too confusing and demanding for children whereas fewer than four might not have resulted in as much systemwide improvement. In addition, four targets adhered nicely to a month-long cycle. Morphemes in Part II are generally taught after the Part I cycles are completed.

Types of Activities

Months of Morphemes includes naturalistic, child-centered focused stimulation activities and educator-directed elicited production tasks that provide children with opportunities to practice using the targeted morphemes. The intervention procedures involve auditory-awareness activities, focused stimulation activities, and elicited production activities (Camarata, Nelson, and Camarata, 1994; Cleave and Fey, 1997; Fey, et al., 1993; Nelson, 1989).

Auditory-Awareness Activities

Auditory-awareness activities are designed to heighten children's awareness of morphological targets. In *Months of Morphemes,* auditory awareness is accomplished by reading books and singing songs that contain multiple exemplars of target morphemes. A detailed description of these activities is in the "Books and Songs" section (see page 16).

Focused Stimulation Activities

Focused stimulation activities are designed to provide children with multiple models of target structures in natural communicative contexts. They involve expansions and recasts of children's utterances. Educators use *expansions* to respond to what children say, making utterances grammatically correct by "expanding" them (e.g., Child: "Mommy shoe"; Educator: "That's mommy's shoe!"). *Recasts* are used to expand children's utterances using a different sentence type (e.g., Child: "That mommy shoe" *[statement];* Educator: "Is that mommy's shoe?" *[question]).* The educator's role in focused stimulation activities is to emphasize, as naturally as possible, the morpheme that children are supposed to direct their attention to. In these activities, children are not required to produce the targets, though pragmatically appropriate opportunities for their use may arise. The educator may ask questions but should not expect or wait for a child's response. An example of a regular past tense focused stimulation activity script follows.

EDUCATOR: Let's talk about what we did to make our drink. First we **poured** the water in the pitcher. Remember what happened next? Some of the water **spilled** out. Then we **scooped** up the drink mix and **poured** it in the water. Next Bobby **stirred** the drink with his straw. Then we **sipped** our drink and **cleaned** up.

In these activities, the educator's task is to focus attention on the target morpheme by producing the form more frequently than children would be exposed to in normal conversation. In keeping with the cycles philosophy, consistency in the educator's use of the target is crucial. Therefore, during focused stimulation activities, the educator should not provide models or examples of contrasting forms. Instead, the educator is challenged to use only the morpheme children are to focus on. For example, the educator would not say, "Bobby **stirs** the drink" *[Pause]* See, he **stirred** it," if the target form is regular third person singular present tense *(stirs).* The educator's use of focused stimulation should make it abundantly clear to children which form is being targeted.

Elicited Production Activities

Elicited production activities provide children with structured opportunities to practice producing the targets in a variety of communicative contexts. These activities are arranged hierarchically in increasing difficulty from Cycle 1 to 3. In Cycle 1, the educator provides the greatest amount of support by eliciting morphemes using a forced choice format. As children progress to Cycles 2 and 3, the educator lessens the amount of support and children are provided with more opportunities for independent production of the targets by using cloze procedures and preparatory sets. It is extremely important for educators to realize that individual children may require flexibility with regard to levels of support. Some children may be able to progress from Cycle 1 to 3 with the levels of support explained below whereas other children may continue to require maximum support (i.e., forced choice) in Cycle 3. The levels of support recommended for the three cycles are merely guidelines; individual children and individual morphemes may require the educator to adapt his or her support level as appropriate.

In Cycle 1, the forced choice technique is used. *Forced choice* is a technique that obligates the use of morphological structures by providing a child with two possible responses, both of which include the target morpheme. For example, to elicit the regular past tense morpheme, the educator might provide the child with this choice: "Tell me what the boy in the story did. He **jumped** or he **skipped?"** If the child does not correctly use the morpheme, the educator might choose to repeat the choices using the same format or might simply recast the child's production, providing indirect corrective feedback (e.g., "Oh, the boy **jumped").**

In Cycle 2, the educator decreases the level of support to that of cloze tasks. *Cloze tasks* use a "fill-in-the-blank" format. For this level of support, the educator begins an utterance and then pauses when a child is asked to complete the utterance. For example, a cloze task item targeting uncontractible auxiliary *be* forms might be, "Look who **is** running. The boy *[Pause for child to supply target]*." If the child does not use the target form, the educator has the option of re-eliciting the form or recasting for the child.

The level of support for Cycle 3 is decreased even further to that of preparatory sets. *Preparatory sets* provide a child with the basic syntactic organization of the concept or morpheme expressed. The educator indirectly demonstrates how to use the target forms and then provides the child with an opportunity to engage in similar discourse by following the educator's initial model. For example, to elicit uncontractible copula *be* while playing with toy figures, the educator might use the following preparatory set: "Sister, **are** you hungry? Now have mommy ask the baby if she is hungry." This will obligate the child to say, "Baby, **are** you hungry?"

Children may not be successful using the target morpheme when given little educator support, as in preparatory sets. In these cases, the educator should increase support (i.e., use cloze tasks or forced choice) until children successfully produce the morpheme.

How to Use the Program

Organization of Sessions

Part I of *Months of Morphemes* (primary morphemes) includes activities for 12 weeks of treatment with two sessions per week. Part II (supplementary morphemes) includes activities for an additional 12 weeks, although most children will not present with deficits across all morphological targets included in *Months of Morphemes*. This language intervention program can be used for group or individual language intervention sessions. The program works ideally if there is one 30-minute individual session and one 45-minute group session per week; however, it is also possible to have two 45-minute group sessions or two 30-minute individual sessions per week. The scripts for each week were designed in such a way that both can be used for individual or group sessions. It should be noted that scripts for three particular morphemes—regular third person singular, possessives, and pronouns—are implemented more readily in group sessions. In an effort to help educators adapt the existing scripts for these morphemes for individual sessions, suggested elicitation formats are listed in the "Instructions" for each activity (see page 25 for an example).

Groups generally function best if they are comprised of two to four children with similar goals. However, these activities have been used successfully for circle time in preschool classes with up to seven children participating. Many of the activities in this program lend themselves to circle-time-type activities because they are similar to those that are normally completed in preschools. Examples include science experiments that involve sinking and floating objects, snack time routines that include decorating and eating gingerbread person cookies, and activities that include retelling familiar stories using puppets.

Supplementary Morphemes

The targets of regular third person singular, irregular past tense, regular past tense, and copula *be* were selected to be the main focus of *Months of Morphemes* because the children in the study this language intervention program is based on overwhelmingly had difficulty with these forms. However, some children may need intervention for different morphemes. Part II contains activities for three cycles that have the same general structure, themes, materials, and books as the activities found in Part I. The targets in Part II are regular plurals, possessives, pronouns, and auxiliary *be*. The supplemental scripts serve two functions: they illustrate how to adapt existing activities to target different morphemes and they can also be used in place of the morphemes targeted in Part I.

As an example, suppose that 4-year-old Jane's language sample performance indicated that she needed to work on the following morphemes: regular third person singular, regular past tense, copula *be*, and pronouns. In this scenario, the educator could use activity scripts from Part I for regular third person singular, regular past tense, and copula *be* beginning on pages 21, 44, and 54. Instead of using the scripts for irregular past tense, which Jane does not need to work on, the educator could use the supplemental script from Part II for pronouns beginning on page 166. Once core activities are established, the educator can easily modify activities and books to target a variety of morphemes. It is the authors' experience that because children will most likely have goals for finite morphemes (Part I), it is unlikely that children would repeat activities while targeting different morphemes. For example, Cycle 1 activities for regular third person singular (Part I) and regular plurals (Part II) are very similar, but it is unlikely that a child would work on both goals.

If *Months of Morphemes* does not include a script for a particular morpheme a child has difficulty with, educators can create their own scripts using the guide found in Appendix A. Further, if a particular child needs to work on two morphemes for which *Months of Morphemes* uses similar activities (e.g., the Part I script for regular third person singular and the Part II script for regular plurals), the educator may choose to create new activities for one of the morphemes to avoid repetition.

Choosing Treatment Targets for Intervention

Treatment targets should be selected according to individual needs as much as possible. However, in this age of increasing caseload sizes and limited funding for speech and language services, it is frequently the case that children with diverse goals must be grouped together. The educator should try to choose goals for groups that will benefit the most children while at the same time benefit the children whose systems are the most negatively impacted. Treatment targets can be selected in several different ways, including language sample analysis, direct-elicitation probes, and language assessment tests. Each of these methods should yield similar information about a child's morphological system.

Language Sample Analysis

The most ideal, though time-consuming, method for selecting targets for intervention is through language sample analysis. A 100–200 utterance language sample can be elicited using supplementary semistructured elicitation methods to ensure that a child has sufficient opportunities to produce the morphological targets. Appendix B shows examples of how the educator can create obligatory contexts for various morphemes in a language sample. Although many children with language disorders have difficulty with finite morphemes, other morphosyntactic structures may also be problematic. Thus, language sampling offers a natural, conversational format for capturing a child's entire language system. Once the sample has been elicited and transcribed, percent correct usage for each morpheme should be derived. This is accomplished by dividing the number of correct productions by the total number of obligatory contexts for each morpheme. For example, if a 5-year-old child with a language disorder produced the following utterances in which regular past tense *–ed* verbs were obligatory, he or she would have a percent correct usage of 25 percent.

1. Yesterday the dog jump(*ed).
2. I watch(*ed) TV after school.
3. I colored my picture.
4. Me grab(*ed) it.

(*) indicates omitted forms.

Although there are no standard percentage cutoffs for choosing treatment targets, the educator might choose to target morphemes that a child produced with the least amount of accuracy. In the study for which *Months of Morphemes* was developed, morphemes that a child used with less than 30 percent accuracy were given the highest priority. Morphemes that were used with less than 50 percent accuracy were of secondary priority. Morphemes used with greater than 60 percent accuracy were considered "emerging" in the child's system and, thus, generally were not targeted. It is important to consider developmental expectations when choosing targets. For example, you would not choose a morpheme for which the expected age of mastery is 5 years old for a child who is 3 years old. Table 3 presents developmental data for Brown's (1973) 14 grammatical morphemes. Note that Brown did not include pronouns in his data, but other researchers have recognized their importance and documented the emergence of pronouns (e.g., Haas and Owens, 1985; Wells, 1985).

Direct-Elicitation Probes

An alternative to language sample analyses to determine language targets is to use direct-elicitation probes. An example elicitation procedure might include setting up 5–10 opportunities for a child to produce selected morphemes. For example, to elicit regular third person singular *-s,* the educator might show pictures of people completing various actions and elicit the target from the child by saying, "This boy is walking to school. Every day he ___." The child would be obligated to reply **"walks."** Percent correct usage for each morpheme can be derived in a manner similar to that described for language sample analysis (see above). The number of correct usages of each morpheme would be divided by the total number of obligatory contexts.

Table 3 **Ages of Mastery of Brown's (1973) 14 Grammatical Morphemes**

Grammatical Morpheme	Example	Age of Mastery (>90% correct usage in obligatory contexts)
Present progressive ***-ing****	Dog **barking.**	19–28 mo.
Preposition ***in****	Go **in** house.	27–30 mo.
Preposition ***on****	Dog **on** chair.	27–30 mo.
Regular plural ***-s***	Two **dogs.**	23–33 mo.
Irregular past tense	She **ran.**	25–46 mo.
Possessive ***'s***	**Dog's** house.	26–40 mo.
Uncontractible copula ***be*** is, am, are, was, were (main verb)	She **was** mad.	27–39 mo.
Articles ***a, an, the****	There's **a** dog.	28–46 mo.
Regular past tense ***-ed***	The dog **barked.**	26–48 mo.
Regular third person singular ***-s***	The dog **barks.**	26–46 mo.
Irregular third person * has, says, does	She **has** a dog.	28–50 mo.
Uncontractible auxiliary ***be*** is, am, are, was, were (helping verb)	He **was** barking.	29–48 mo.
Contractible copula ***be*** is, am, are, was, were (main verb)	The **dog's** big.	29–49 mo.
Contractible auxiliary ***be*** is, am, are, was, were (helping verb)	The **dog's** barking.	30–50 mo.

Sources: Brown (1973); Miller and Chapman (1981)

* Indicates items not included in this resource.

Language Assessment Tests

A frequently used method for determining levels of morphosyntactic functioning includes analyzing results of standardized and/or criterion-referenced commercially available tests. There are numerous language assessment tests that include subtests that assess a child's morphological performance. Table 4 (see page 14) includes a list of tests that are frequently used in clinical settings to assess expressive morphological performance in young children.

Language samples, direct-elicitation probes, and language assessment test results should all yield similar information about a child's morphological system. Language samples have the advantage of reflecting how a child uses morphemes in natural communicative contexts. Because direct-elicitation probes and standardized language assessment tests use structured situations to elicit morphemes, children could use morphemes with greater accuracy on these measures than they do in conversation (as reflected in a language sample).

Table 4 Tests for Morphosyntactic Performance			
Test	**Subtest(s)**	**Author(s) & Copyright Date**	**Age Range**
Clinical Evaluation of Language Fundamentals, 3rd ed. (CELF–3)	Recalling Sentences (RS) & Word Structure (WS)	Semel, Wiig, and Secord, 1995	RS: 6+ WS: 6–8
Clinical Evaluation of Language Fundamentals–Preschool (CELF–P)	Recalling Sentences in Context (RS) & Word Structure (WS)	Wiig, Secord, and Semel, 1992	RS & WS: 3;0–6;11
Comprehensive Assessment of Spoken Language (CASL)	Syntax Construction	Carrow and Woolfolk, 1999	3–6
Structured Photographic Expressive Language Test–II (SPELT–II)	Not applicable	O'Hara Werner and Dawson Kresheck, 1983	4+
Structured Photo Expressive Language Tests–Preschool (SPELT–P)	Not applicable	O'Hara Werner and Dawson Kresheck, 1983	3;0–5;11
Test for Examining Expressive Morphology (TEEM)	Not applicable	Shipley, Stone, and Sue, 1983	3;0–7;11
Test of Language Development–Primary, 3rd ed. (TOLD–P)	Grammatical Completion & Sentence Imitation	Newcomer and Hammill, 1997	4;0–8;11

Organizing Targets within Cycles

Months of Morphemes uses a cycles approach modified from Hodson and Paden's (1983, 1991) original description of a 12–14 week cycle. *Months of Morphemes* uses a four-week cycle to address four morpheme targets in Part I. Four additional supplementary target morphemes are also available in Part II. For this language intervention program, each target is focused on for one week during two sessions. Four different targets (i.e., four weeks) compose a cycle that is part of a series of three theme-based cycles. Thus, a child works on each target for a total of three weeks (one week per cycle), devoting approximately 3 hours and 45 minutes to each morpheme. Figure 2 illustrates the modified cycles approach used in this program. After four morpheme targets have been selected, the next step for implementation is to determine their sequence (e.g., week 1: regular third person singular; week 2:

Figure 2 **Modified Cycles Approach Used in *Months of Morphemes***

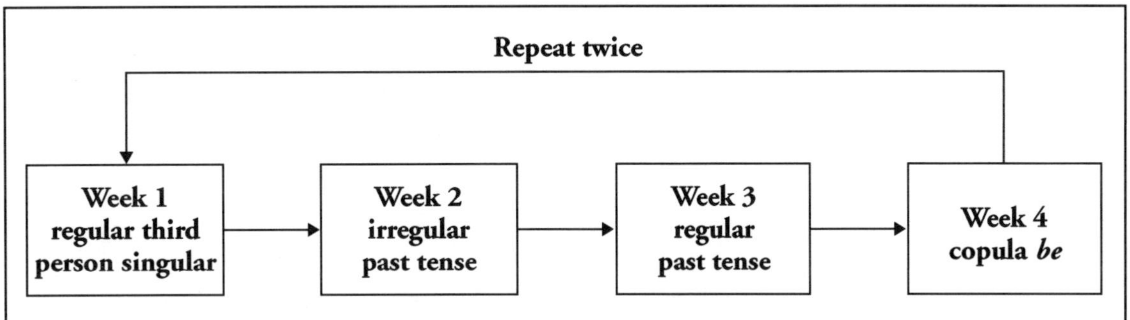

Example targets: regular third person singular, irregular past tense, regular past tense, copula *be*

irregular past tense; week 3: regular past tense; and week 4: copula *be).* Note that morphemes do not need to be used in the order presented in this resource.

Family Letters and Family Involvement

Family involvement is critical to the success of this and any other language intervention program (Crais, 1991; Donahue-Kilburg, 1992, 1993). An important way in which *Months of Morphemes* involves families in the intervention process is by providing weekly family letters. The *Introductory Family Letter* (Appendix C) should be sent home before implementing the program. Weekly family letters (preceding activities in each cycle) should be sent home each week before each morpheme is targeted. Family letters explain the theme, target morpheme, book, song, activities, and follow-up home practice. Educators who wish to create their own letters or adapt existing letters can use the *Weekly Family Letter* template provided in Appendix D.

Family letters are organized and worded in a way that is easy to understand for most family members who are readers. For families with nonreaders or for families whose primary language is not English, the educator (or a speaker of the family's primary language) should explain orally, either in person or over the telephone, the information contained in the family letters.

Activity Components

Themes

Activities in each 4-week cycle are related to one of three major themes: water, animals, or food. The three themes in this language intervention program were selected because they are frequently found in popular preschool children's literature, they reflect age-appropriate vocabulary and concepts, and they are often encountered in preschool classrooms. Cycle 1's theme is water. Some activities in the water theme include sinking and floating objects in water, creating bubbles with water, and making beverages using water. The theme of Cycle 2 is animals, and the activities in this theme revolve around making animal art projects and reading stories about various animals. Food is the theme of Cycle 3, and activities in this very popular theme include making gingerbread cookies and completing a series of activities associated with stories about hungry animals and people such as *The Very Hungry Caterpillar* (Carle, 1987) and *There Was an Old Lady Who Swallowed a Fly* (Adams, 1997).

Scripts

Months of Morphemes includes a collection of detailed scripts that create an integrated cycles approach to language intervention with an emphasis on morphological goals. This approach includes three different elicitation techniques (see "Types of Activities" on page 8) in the context of interesting, communicatively stimulating hands-on activities. The scripts serve as a framework from which to structure intervention for young children with speech and language disorders. The scripts are highlighted in gray boxes within each of the activities. They are labeled "Example Script" because the dialogue between the educator and children will approximate the oral exchange proposed in the script, but it will not be identical. (Remember, children do not see the script.)

Books and Songs

A key feature of *Months of Morphemes* is auditory awareness of the target morphemes. Similar to focused stimulation, auditory-awareness activities are designed to provide children with multiple examples of the target morphemes. In *Months of Morphemes,* auditory awareness is completed through reading popular children's literature and singing common children's songs adapted to contain multiple examples of target morphemes.

Each session begins with the educator reading a theme-related book chosen specifically because of its frequent use of the target morpheme. When such a book was unavailable, popular stories were adapted so as to provide multiple exemplars of the target. Suggestions on how to discuss existing stories are included in the scripts as appropriate. The use of books serves the double purpose of providing auditory awareness of the targets while at the same time encouraging the following preliteracy skills:

- Knowledge of narratives
- Knowledge of the functions of print
- Concept of word (i.e., the knowledge that spoken and written sentences are made up of individual words)

Through weekly family letters, families are informed about which books will be read so that they can read or discuss the books at home if they choose. For families with members who are nonreaders, educators might suggest that pictures in the weekly stories be discussed instead of reading the stories. This procedure should be demonstrated by the educator.

The same book is read during both sessions in each week of intervention. Books are read twice in an effort to better familiarize children with the stories to increase the likelihood of child participation. During the study this language intervention program was based on, it was observed that as a result of reading the same book during both weekly sessions, children were very interactive and produced numerous target morphemes spontaneously. In addition, supplemental theme-related books are listed in the event that the educator would like to extend the activity by including related stories. Full bibliographic references for weekly reading selections and supplemental books are found in the Bibliography.

Each session concludes with the singing of a theme-related song created to provide further auditory awareness in a festive manner. These songs are sung to the tune of popular songs such as "Twinkle, Twinkle, Little Star." Songs provide children with an opportunity to both hear and produce examples of the week's target morpheme. As is the case with the weekly book, the same song is used in both weekly sessions. The song may be repeated at the end of each session for the benefit of children's growing auditory awareness. For the book reading and song activities, there are no direct demands for children to produce the target morpheme; however, in many cases it is pragmatically appropriate for them to do so. The educator should review books and songs one week before implementation to become familiar with the content of the story and the song's lyrics.

Materials

Materials for activities are generally common household and/or school items (e.g., art supplies, soap, and food). Materials lists are included on the first page of each session's script. Some activities require that items be made or prepared by the educator prior to the activities. In such cases, templates and directions are included in Appendix E. A worksheet for planning each week's sessions is located in Appendix F. The most important preparation the educator should do before each session is to gather materials, review the session's scripts, and practice applicable elicitation techniques.

Educator's and Children's Roles in Intervention

During auditory-awareness activities (book and song) and focused stimulation activities, it is the educator's job to make it clear to children what morpheme is being targeted. This is accomplished by the educator using targets with increasing frequency and emphasizing them in as natural a way as possible. Throughout the scripts, target morphemes are in bold and underlined type. Children's role in these activities is to listen and participate. Remember that children are not required to talk during these activities. However, if children use the target during these activities, the educator should respond naturally. If children misuse or omit the target in obligatory contexts during these activities, the educator should recast children's productions and continue to provide models of the correct usage.

In elicited production activities, the educator's task is to set up meaningful situations in which children have opportunities to practice using the morphemes. It is important to note that child utterances included in the scripts are merely an example of what children might say given the context. It is entirely likely that other utterances may be grammatically and pragmatically appropriate.

Measuring Progress

Progress for each session can be recorded on data sheets (Appendix G) that should be prepared before each session. A completed data sheet for a hypothetical child can be found in Appendix G. The goal of each session is for a child to have at least 20–30 opportunities to use the target morpheme throughout the session's activities (e.g., 15 opportunities in the elicited production activity and 5 in the focused stimulation and auditory-awareness activities). Perhaps the most efficient method for recording data is a +/- system in which a (+) indicates that the child produced the target morpheme correctly and a (-) indicates that the target morpheme was used incorrectly or omitted in an obligatory context. Percent correct usage is calculated by dividing the number of correct productions by the total number of obligatory contexts for the target. For example, if a child used regular past tense *-ed* forms correctly on 10 occasions within a total of 30 obligatory contexts, his or her percent correct usage for *-ed* would be 33 percent.

As noted above, incorrect productions are in the form of omissions (e.g., the child said "jump" for the obligatory *jumped)* or errors (e.g., the child said "eated" for the obligatory *ate).* In some circumstances, the educator may choose to take more detailed data than that which results from a +/- system. For example, what the child says might be recorded (e.g., instead of recording a (-) for irregular past tense, the educator may transcribe the child's error, *eated).* If educators are unable to keep data for every session, pre-intervention and post-intervention testing using language-sample or morpheme-probe data can also be used to document progress.

Part I:

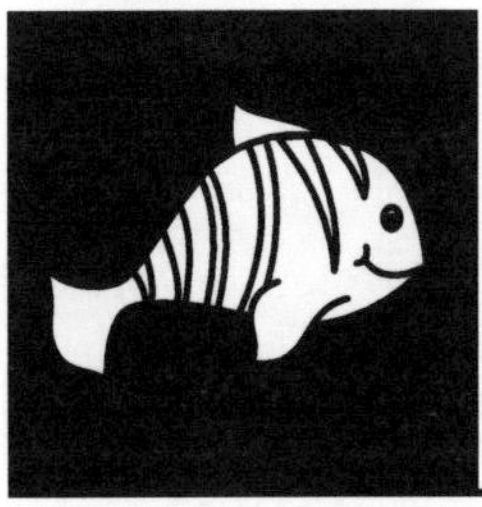

Primary Morphemes

Weekly Family Letter

For: ______________________________ **Date:** ____________

Theme

Our theme for language intervention this week is *water.*

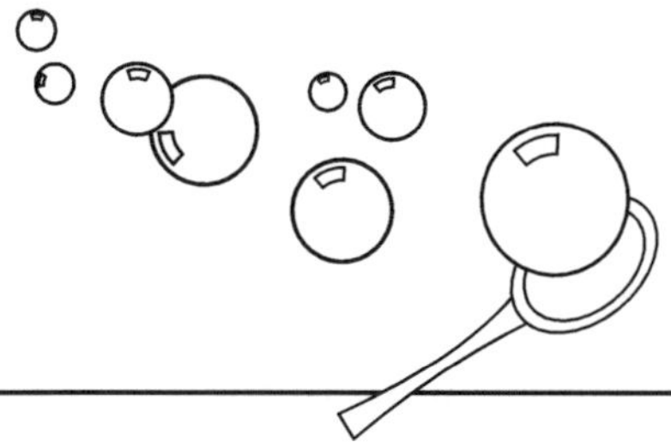

Target

Our target language structures are *regular third person singular verbs.* These verbs indicate actions by a single person or object and have a regular *-s* ending. Examples include:

- She **eats** the cake.
- The dog **jumps** over the fence.
- Mommy **kisses** the baby.

Book

Our book for the week is *Bubble Trouble* by Mary Packard and Elena Kucharik (illustrator).

Here are some related books you could read at home: *Bubble Bubble* by Mercer Mayer and *Clifford Counts Bubbles* by Norman Bridwell.

Song

This Is the Way We Blow Our Bubbles
(Tune: "This Is the Way We...")

This is the way Jane **blows** her bubbles,
blows her bubbles, **blows** her bubbles.

This is the way Jane **blows** her bubbles
early in the morning!

(Repeat using the regular third person singular verbs **stomps, pops,** and **pokes;** sing using your child's name.)

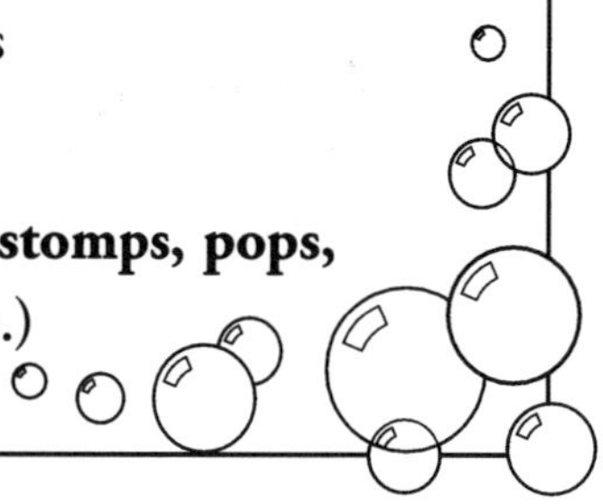

Activities

Our planned activities for the week include:

- Blowing bubbles using bubble blowers made from pipe cleaners and strawberry baskets
- Making colored bubbles in a jar
- Creating a picture using colored bubble soap

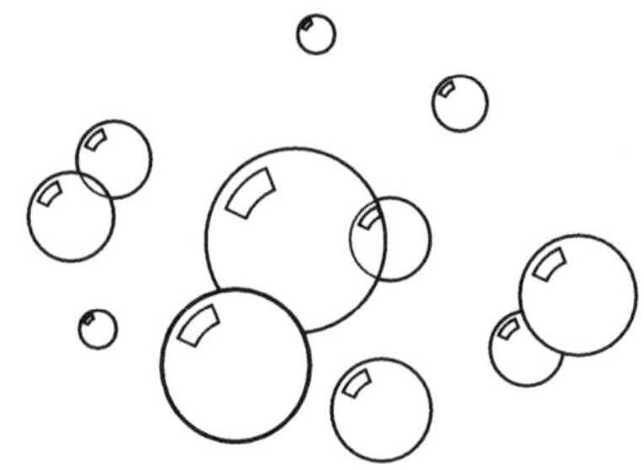

Follow-Up

Suggested follow-up activities for home include:

- Find bubbles around the house. They can be found in the kitchen sink, in bubble baths, and other places.
- As you explore bubbles with your child, provide him or her with many examples of regular third person singular verbs. Examples include:

  Daddy **pops** the bubbles.

  Mom **turns** the water on and **makes** bubbles.

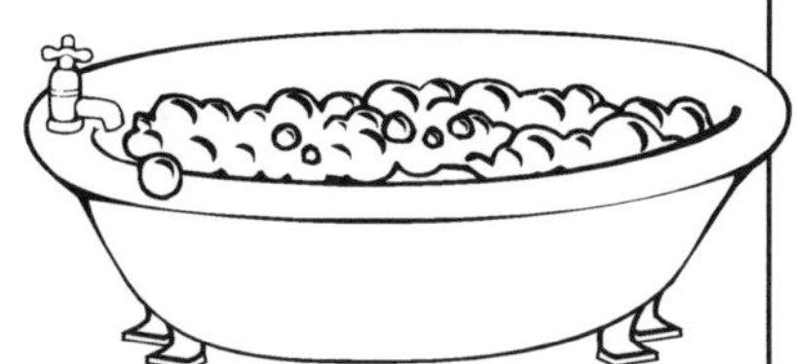

Thank You Very Much for your participation!

Phone Number

Email

Signature

Regular Third Person Singular

Cycle 1, Session 1

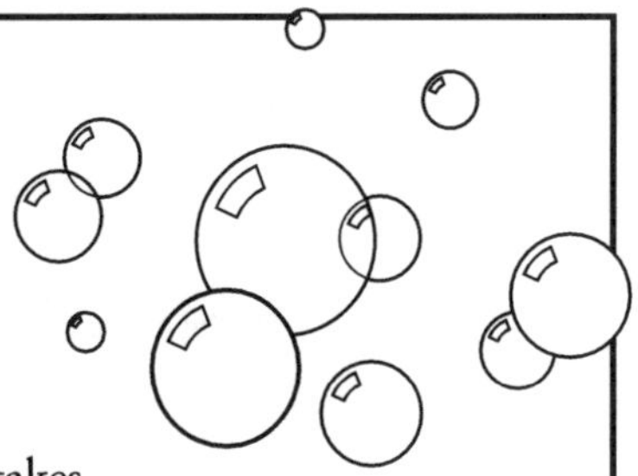

Theme: Water

Description: Creating bubbles

Exemplars: blows, drops, eats, grabs, finds, likes, makes, needs, picks, pokes, pops, pours, puts, sees, spills, stomps, takes

Materials:

Bubble Trouble by Mary Packard and Elena Kucharik (illustrator)
Plastic bubble wands
Bubble soap materials (see page 271 for recipe and directions)
Plastic pint-size strawberry baskets
Plate (not paper)

INTRODUCTION TO THEME

EDUCATOR: We are going to talk about water today. We use water every day. We use water when we take a bath, and we drink water when we are thirsty. There are lots of different things we can do with water. One thing people do with water is make bubbles. Bubbles are made of water. Who **likes** to play with bubbles? *[Allow children to respond]* You do? Me too! Well, today we are going to read a book about bubbles and we are going to do a special activity with bubbles. Are you ready? *[Allow children to respond]* Let's read our bubble book.

BOOK ACTIVITY

Book: *Bubble Trouble* by Mary Packard and Elena Kucharik (illustrator)

Instructions: Read the book with children. Comment on the story using regular third person singular verbs.

Suggested Theme-Related Supplemental Books:
Bubble Bubble by Mercer Mayer
Clifford Counts Bubbles by Norman Bridwell

Transition

Educator: The animals in our story made lots of bubbles in their bathtub! Now we are going to make lots of bubbles too!

FOCUSED STIMULATION ACTIVITY

Description: Discussing the steps and materials for making bubbles

Skills Used: Prediction, sequencing, and conversation

Instructions: Comment on actions as they occur to provide natural models of regular third person singular verbs. For sessions with an individual child, use objects as the subjects of utterances instead of people (e.g., "The cup **looks** big," "Sugar **tastes** sweet," and "The water **feels** cold").

Example Script

Educator: Today I brought some things we can use to make bubbles. Let's see what we have.

Educator: *[Present bag full of items to do bubble project]* Let's see what we need to make our bubbles. Jane, could you please see what's in my bag?

Educator: Jane **grabs** the cup.

Educator: I wonder if there's anything in the bag that we can use to make bubble soap. John, can you look in the bag? John **finds** some soap.

Educator: Look! Now he **sees** some sugar. This white stuff is called sugar.

Educator: Who can tell me what you can do with sugar?

Child: Eat it!

Educator: Jane **eats** sugar! I bet she **eats** it on her cereal!

Educator: We aren't going to eat sugar today. We are going to put sugar in our bubble soap! Sugar **makes** bubbles strong so that they won't pop too fast!

Educator: Let's see if there's anything else in the bag. Look what Jane does to the baskets. She **takes** them out of the bag.

[Continue in a similar manner until numerous models of regular third person singular verbs have been provided.]

Transition

EDUCATOR: Now that we have found all the things to make bubbles, let's have fun and blow some bubbles!

ELICITED PRODUCTION ACTIVITY

Description: Making bubbles

Skills Used: Direction following and fine motor

Goal: 10 productions of regular third person singular verbs per child

Level of Educator Support: Forced choice

Instructions: Comment on actions as they occur to provide natural models of regular third person singular verbs. For sessions with an individual child, use objects as the subjects of utterances instead of people (e.g., "The water **spills** or **falls?"** "It **feels** cold or it **tastes** cold?" "The soap **makes** bubbles or **breaks** bubbles?").

Example Script

EDUCATOR: I'm ready to make some bubbles! First, we need to make our bubble soap. John, will you help me? Please pour the water *[1/2 cup]* into the bowl.

EDUCATOR: John **pours** the water or **spills** the water?

CHILD: He **pours** it!

EDUCATOR: I wonder what John **needs** to add to make the water soapy.

CHILD: Soap!

EDUCATOR: *[Instruct a child to pour in 3 tablespoons of dish soap into the water]* Yes! He **pours** the soap or **eats** the soap?

CHILD: He **pours** the soap.

EDUCATOR: Yes, he **pours** the soap. John **needs** to add something that's white and grainy to the soap and water. *[Hint to children that they need to add sugar]*

CHILD: This stuff!

EDUCATOR: What a good idea! John **needs** to put sugar in the soap and water. Sugar **makes** bubbles stronger. Jane, please put two spoons of sugar into the water.

EDUCATOR: Watch what Jane does. She **pours** sugar or she **drops** sugar?

CHILD: She **pours** it!

Continued on next page

Example Script—*Continued*

EDUCATOR: Now that we have our bubble soap made, we can blow some bubbles. Which one of these things should we use first? *[Present strawberry baskets and bubble wands]*

CHILD: *[Chooses strawberry basket]*

EDUCATOR: Jane **picks** a basket or **drops** a basket?

CHILD: She **picks** it.

EDUCATOR: The basket has lots of holes in it. We need to get soap into those holes. Let's pour some of our bubble soap on a plate so that we can get the soap into the holes. *[Proceed after soap is poured]*

EDUCATOR: John can go first. Watch what he does.

EDUCATOR: He **puts** soap on or he **takes** it off?

CHILD: He **puts** it on.

EDUCATOR: Yes, he **puts** soap on the basket.

EDUCATOR: Watch what he does now. *[Instruct a child to blow a bubble]*

EDUCATOR: He **blows** bubbles or **pops** bubbles?

CHILD: **Blows** bubbles!

EDUCATOR: Yes, he **blows** bubbles!

[Continue in a similar manner until each child has had at least 10 opportunities to use regular third person singular verbs.]

Transition

EDUCATOR: Wow, that was fun! Let's clean up now and get ready to sing our bubble song.

SONG ACTIVITY

Instructions: Sing to the tune of "This Is the Way We…," emphasizing regular third person singular forms. Use a different child's name for each verse. (When using the song with an individual child, use his or her name.) Encourage children to take turns performing gestures for the regular third person singular verbs as they occur in the song. For example, as Jane sings, Jake can perform gestures.

This Is the Way We Blow Our Bubbles

This is the way Jane **blows** her bubbles,
blows her bubbles, **blows** her bubbles.
This is the way Jane **blows** her bubbles
early in the morning!

(Repeat using the regular third person singular verbs **stomps, pops,** and **pokes.**)

Regular Third Person Singular

Cycle 1, Session 2

Theme: Water

Description: Creating bubbles

Exemplars: blows, breaks, drinks, eats, finds, happens, hits, likes, jumps, looks, makes, needs, picks, pokes, pops, pours, puts, remembers, rolls, shakes, spills, stirs, stomps, thinks, uses, wants

Materials:

Bubble Trouble by Mary Packard and Elena Kucharik (illustrator)
Bubble soap materials (see page 271 for recipe and instructions)
Baby food jars with lids (1 or more per color)
Food coloring (3–4 colors)
Bubble wands
White construction paper

BOOK ACTIVITY

Book: *Bubble Trouble* by Mary Packard and Elena Kucharik (illustrator)

Instructions: Reread the book with children. Comment on the story using regular third person singular verbs.

Suggested Theme-Related Supplemental Books: *Bubble Bubble* by Mercer Mayer
Clifford Counts Bubbles by Norman Bridwell

Transition

EDUCATOR: There were lots of bubbles in our story! Remember last time you were here when we made lots of bubbles? Well, that was so much fun that we are going to make even more bubbles today!

FOCUSED STIMULATION ACTIVITY

Description: Making and shaking colored bubbles in jars

Skills Used: Fine motor, gross motor, direction following, sharing, and sequencing

Instructions: Comment on actions as they occur to provide natural models of regular third person singular verbs. For sessions with an individual child, use objects as the subjects of utterances instead of people (e.g., "The bubble **pops,**" "The water **spills,**" "The lid **goes** on tightly").

Example Script

EDUCATOR: We have been playing with bubbles. Last time we used different kinds of bubble blowers. Today we are going to make lots of little bubbles in jars.

EDUCATOR: Before we make our bubbles, we need to make bubble soap. Do you remember how we made our bubble soap last time? Here are the things we need. *[Present materials]* Let's see who **remembers** what we need to do.

EDUCATOR: First, John **finds** a mixing bowl.

EDUCATOR: Then he **pours** in the water using a measuring cup.

EDUCATOR: See how he **pours** in the water. He **needs** lots of water. *[Use 1/2 cup]*

EDUCATOR: Look what he does now.

CHILD: He **uses** a measuring spoon.

EDUCATOR: Let's see what he does now. It looks like he **pours** in the soap.

EDUCATOR: He **pours** in three spoons of soap.

EDUCATOR: It **looks** like our soap and water mixture **needs** something. It **needs** something to make the bubbles stronger. Who **remembers** what we used last time to make our bubbles strong?

CHILD: *[Indicates sugar]*

EDUCATOR: Maria **thinks** we need sugar to make our bubbles strong.

EDUCATOR: Now Maria **needs** to pour two spoons of sugar in the bubble soap.

EDUCATOR: John **stirs** it up.

EDUCATOR: Now let's put our soap and water mixture into one of these jars. You do it, John.

EDUCATOR: See how John **pours** it?

Continued on next page

Example Script—*Continued*

EDUCATOR:	I thought it would be nice if we made our bubbles different colors. What color should we use? *[Present food coloring]*
CHILD:	*[Selects a color]*
EDUCATOR:	Jane **picks** green.
EDUCATOR:	She **puts** in lots of color. [*Repeat this exemplar for each child]*
EDUCATOR:	If we want to make lots of little bubbles, we need to put the top on our jar and shake. Who **wants** to go first?
EDUCATOR:	Jane **wants** to go.
EDUCATOR:	Watch what Jane does to the lid. She **puts** it on.
EDUCATOR:	Now she **shakes** the jar.
EDUCATOR:	Wow, Jane **makes** lots of bubbles!

[Continue in a similar manner until numerous models of regular third person singular verbs have been provided.]

Transition

EDUCATOR: That sure was fun. Now we are going to use the bubbles in our jars to make a picture.

ELICITED PRODUCTION ACTIVITY

Description: Making pictures with colored bubbles

Skills Used: Fine motor, oral motor, and describing

Goal: 10 productions of regular third person singular forms per child

Level of Educator Support: Forced choice

Instructions: To begin, give each child a piece of paper. For sessions with an individual child, use objects as the subjects of the utterances instead of people (e.g., "What does the bubble do? It **pops** or **breaks?**" "What does the soap do? It **makes** bubbles or it **uses** bubbles?").

Example Script

EDUCATOR: You did such a good job making all those colors in your jars. I thought we could make pictures with your colored bubbles. We need our bubble soap in the jars.

EDUCATOR: Miguel, use this bubble wand and blow a bubble at the paper.

EDUCATOR: What does he do? He **blows** it or **drinks** it?

CHILD: He **blows** it!

EDUCATOR: Jane, now it's your turn. What does she do? She **blows** or **pops** a bubble?

CHILD: She **blows** a bubble!

EDUCATOR: *[Repeat this exemplar for each child]*

EDUCATOR: Look at the bubble. What does it do when it **hits** the paper? It **pops** or **jumps?**

CHILD: It **pops!**

EDUCATOR: When it **pops**, what **happens?** It **makes** a picture or it **spills?**

CHILD: It **makes** a picture.

EDUCATOR: Yes, it **makes** a very pretty picture!

EDUCATOR: Look what **happens** when we blow a green bubble. It **makes** a green spot or it **breaks?**

CHILD: It **makes** a green spot.

EDUCATOR: Yes, and a red bubble **makes** a red spot.

EDUCATOR: What does Jane do? She **blows** bubbles or she **drops** bubbles?

CHILD: She **blows** bubbles.

EDUCATOR: What does this bubble do when it **hits** the paper? It **pops** or it **rolls?**

CHILD: It **pops.**

EDUCATOR: John, which color do you like? *[If the child does not know color names, the educator can label the choices for the child]*

CHILD: Red.

EDUCATOR: John **likes** red or he **eats** red?

CHILD: He **likes** red!

EDUCATOR: Yes, he **likes** the red bubbles.

[Continue in a similar manner until each child has had at least 10 opportunities to use regular third person singular verbs.]

Transition

Educator: I had fun shaking up the bubbles and making bubble pictures. Now it's time to clean up and sing our bubble song!

SONG ACTIVITY

Instructions: Sing to the tune of "This Is the Way We…," emphasizing regular third person singular forms. Use a different child's name for each verse. (When using the song with an individual child, use his or her name.) Encourage children to take turns performing gestures for the regular third person singular verbs as they occur in the song. For example, as Jane sings, Jake can perform gestures.

This Is the Way We Blow Our Bubbles

This is the way Jane **blows** her bubbles,
blows her bubbles, **blows** her bubbles.
This is the way Jane **blows** her bubbles
early in the morning!

(Repeat using the regular third person singular verbs **stomps, pops,** and **pokes.)**

Weekly Family Letter

For: ______________________________ **Date:** ______________

Theme

Our theme for language intervention this week is *water.*

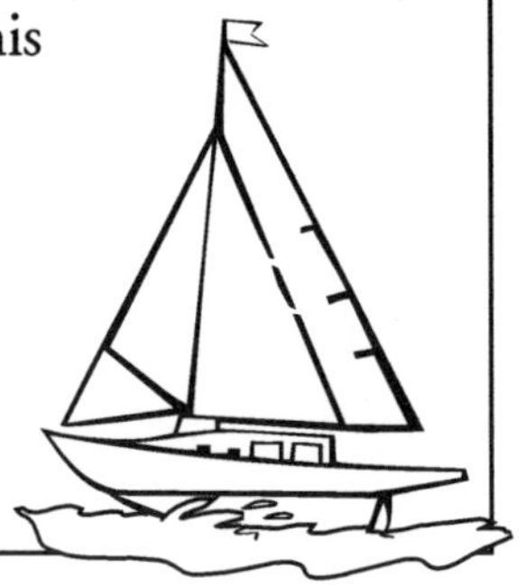

Target

Our target language structures are *irregular past tense verbs.* These verbs indicate past actions, but they do not have the regular *-ed* ending. Examples include:

- She **ate** the cake.
- The dog **ran** through the field.
- Mommy **sang** to the baby.

Book

Our book for the week is *At the Beach* by Anne Rockwell and Harlow Rockwell.

Here are some related books you could read at home: *Curious George Goes to the Beach* by Margret Rey and H.A. Rey and *For Sand Castles or Seashells* by Gail Hartman and Ellen Weiss (illustrator).

Song

Down by the Seashore
(Tune: "Little Bunny Foo Foo")

Down by the seashore, early in the morning,
I **saw** the children. They played in the sun.

I **saw** all the mommies. They **spread** out the blankets.
I **saw** all the children. They **ran** to the water.
I **saw** the children. They **had** so much fun!

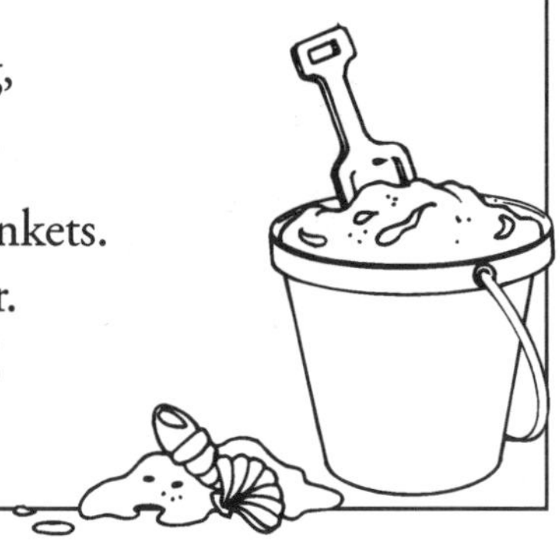

Activities

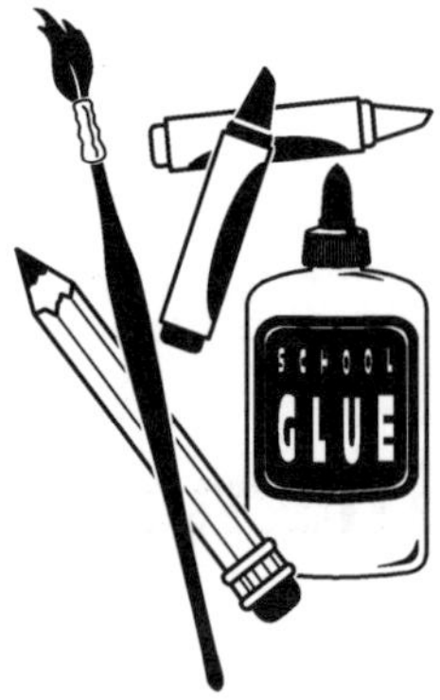

Our planned activities for the week include:

- Sinking and floating objects in water
- Discussing events in the book using irregular past tense verbs
- Making a milk carton sailboat
- Having a boat race with index card boats

Follow-Up

Suggested follow-up activities for home include:

- Read one of your child's books (preferably one dealing with the beach or the water), and discuss what happened in the story using irregular past tense verbs, for example:

  The girl **saw** a seashell.

  They **made** a sandcastle.

  He **ran** on the beach.

- Ask your child to tell you how he or she made a sailboat in language intervention, for example:

  I **stuck** the stick in the foam.

  I **made** a sail.

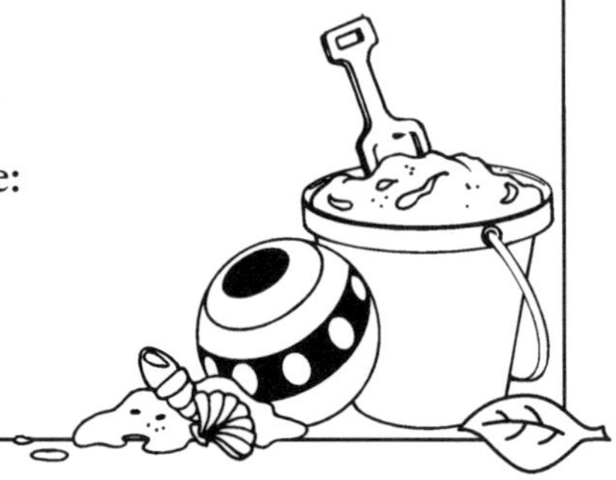

Thank You Very Much *for your participation!*

Phone Number

Email

Signature

Irregular Past Tense

Cycle 1, Session 1

Theme: Water

Description: Discussing places with water; floating and sinking objects

Exemplars: ate, broke, built, did, fell, found, got, had, made, ran, sank, saw, slept, spread, swam, thought, threw, took, went

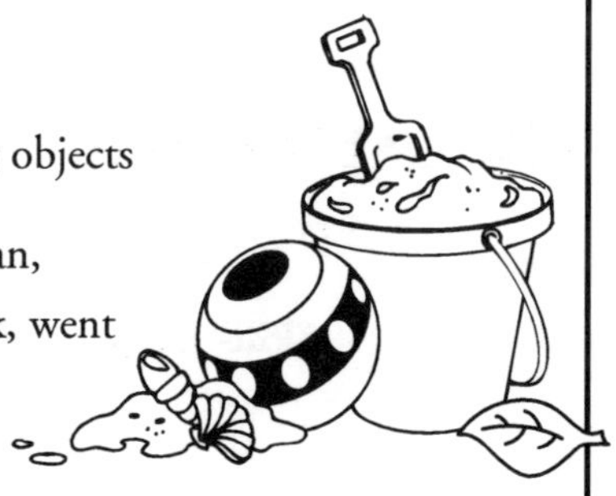

Materials:

At the Beach by Anne Rockwell and Harlow Rockwell
Bag filled with objects that sink (e.g., rocks and seashells) and objects that float (e.g., sponges and feathers)
Container filled with water

INTRODUCTION TO THEME

EDUCATOR: Remember how we **made** bubbles with water last week? Well, this week we are going to talk about something else we can do with water. We are going to talk about things to do with water at the beach. *[Ask children if they have been to the beach and discuss what they have done there]* There are lots of fun things we can do in the water when we go to the beach.

BOOK ACTIVITY

Book: *At the Beach* by Anne Rockwell and Harlow Rockwell

Instructions: Read the book with children, emphasizing irregular past tense verbs. For places in the story where these forms do not occur naturally, use them while discussing the pictures (e.g., "See, the girl **found** a shell" and "She **saw** a shovel").

Suggested Theme-Related Supplemental Books:
Curious George Goes to the Beach by Margret Rey and H.A. Rey
For Sand Castles or Seashells by Gail Hartman and Ellen Weiss (illustrator)

Transition

EDUCATOR: The girl in our book **went** to the beach and played in the water. Now we are going to do something fun with water too!

FOCUSED STIMULATION ACTIVITY

Description: Sinking and floating items in water

Skills Used: Fine motor and direction following

Example Script

EDUCATOR: *[Show children the bag with items that sink or float inside]* Let's look and see what's in our bag. *[Child and educator look at items in the bag but do not take them out yet]*

EDUCATOR: We **saw** a seashell, a rock, a sponge, and a feather.

EDUCATOR: Who else wants a turn to look in our bag? *[Allow children to take turns looking]*

EDUCATOR: I wonder what you **saw?**

CHILD: I **saw** a seashell!

EDUCATOR: Jake **saw** a penny just like I **did**! *[Allow other children to comment on what they saw]*

EDUCATOR: Now we can take the things out of our bag. Jane, please take these things out.

EDUCATOR: Jane **took** out a penny. Then she **took** out a seashell.

EDUCATOR: Next Jake **took** some sponges. *[Continue in a similar manner for remaining items]*

EDUCATOR: Let's do something fun with these things. Watch this! *[Take the penny and drop it into the water]* Look what happened! The penny **fell** in the water and it **sank!**

EDUCATOR: Now watch what happens when I put this rock in the water. *[Put the rock in the water]*

EDUCATOR: Look at that!

CHILD: It **sank** and **got** wet.

EDUCATOR: Yes, the rock **sank** and **got** wet. *[Throw a rock in water]*

EDUCATOR: Look what I **did!**

Example Script—*Continued*

CHILD:	You **threw** the rock.
EDUCATOR:	Yes, I **threw** the rock in the water.
EDUCATOR:	Look, the rock **sank** to the bottom of the container.
EDUCATOR:	Now let's see what happens when we put a feather in the water. Jane, it's your turn.
EDUCATOR:	Look, Jane **made** it float!
EDUCATOR:	The rock **sank** but we **saw** the feather float! *[Continue until all items have been used]*
EDUCATOR:	Now we need to take everything out of the water.
EDUCATOR:	Look, Jane **found** a penny.
EDUCATOR:	John **took** out the rock.

[Continue in a similar manner until all items have been pulled out of the water and numerous models of irregular past tense verbs have been provided.]

Transition

EDUCATOR: I **had** fun sinking and floating things in the water! Now I **thought** we could look at our story again and talk about what happened in it.

ELICITED PRODUCTION ACTIVITY

Description: Discussing the story using irregular past tense verbs

Skills Used: Narrative and describing

Goal: 10 productions of irregular past tense verbs per child

Level of Educator Support: Forced choice

Example Script

EDUCATOR:	Jane, look at this picture. Tell me about the girl. She **ran** or she **ate?**
CHILD:	She **ran.**
EDUCATOR:	What happened here? She **found** a shell or she **ate** a shell?
CHILD:	She **found** a shell.
EDUCATOR:	What happened next? She **made** a sandcastle or she **saw** a sandcastle?
CHILD:	She **made** a sandcastle.
EDUCATOR:	What happened here? He **built** a river or **broke** a river?
CHILD:	**Built** a river!
EDUCATOR:	What did the fish do? They **swam** or **slept?**
CHILD:	They **swam!**

[Continue in a similar manner until each child has had at least 10 opportunities to use irregular past tense verbs.]

Transition

EDUCATOR: We talked about our beach story, and now it's time to sing our beach song!

SONG ACTIVITY

Instructions: Sing to the tune of "Little Bunny Foo Foo," emphasizing irregular past tense verbs.

Down by the Seashore

Down by the seashore, early in the morning,
I **saw** the children. They played in the sun.

I **saw** all the mommies. They **spread** out the blankets.
I **saw** all the children. They **ran** to the water.
I **saw** the children. They **had** so much fun!

Irregular Past Tense

Cycle 1, Session 2

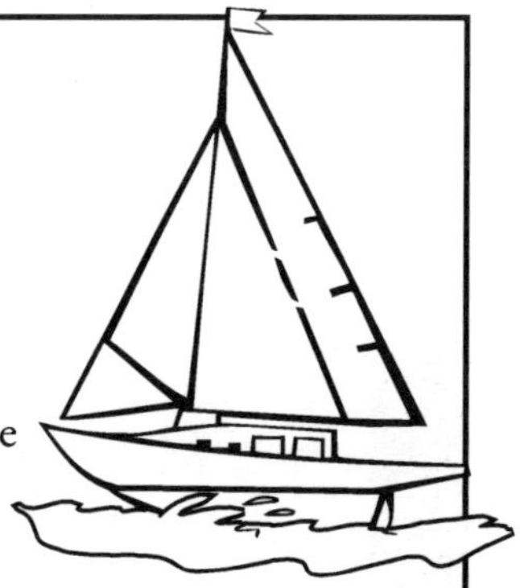

Theme: Water

Description: Completing activities relating to boats

Exemplars: ate, broke, blew, built, cut, did, drew, found, had, lost, made, won, ran, saw, spread, stuck, took, went, won, wrote

Materials:

At the Beach by Anne Rockwell and Harlow Rockwell

Bag containing:

- Milk cartons (cut in half lengthwise; 1 half per child)
- Tape
- Styrofoam (cut in 1 square inch pieces; 1 piece per child)
- Craft sticks
- Completed sailboat (see page 272 for directions)
- Child-safe scissors
- Boat sails (see page 272 for directions; 2 per child)
- Glue
- Decorative stickers
- Crayons and markers

Index cards (1 per child)

Pencils or pens

Container filled with water

Puppet (for individual sessions only)

BOOK ACTIVITY

Book: *At the Beach* by Anne Rockwell and Harlow Rockwell

Instructions: Reread the book with children, emphasizing irregular past tense verbs. For places in the story where these forms do not occur naturally, use them while discussing the pictures (e.g., "See, the girl **found** a shell" and "She **saw** a shovel").

Suggested Theme-Related Supplemental Books: *Curious George Goes to the Beach* by Margret Rey and H.A. Rey
For Sand Castles or Seashells by Gail Hartman and Ellen Weiss (illustrator)

Transition

Educator: The girl in our book played with a boat when she **went** to the beach. Today we are going to make some boats too!

FOCUSED STIMULATION ACTIVITY

Description: Making milk carton sailboats

Skills Used: Fine motor and direction following

Instructions: Prepare a sailboat prior to the activity to serve as a model.

Example Script

EDUCATOR:	Let's see what's in our bag. Let's watch Jane. Let's see what she does with all this stuff.
EDUCATOR:	Oh, Maria **found** a milk carton. She also **found** the tape, the Styrofoam, the sticks, and the paper. She **took** all these things out of the bag.
EDUCATOR:	I think I **saw** Maria take out a sailboat. Wouldn't it be fun to make a boat like this today?
EDUCATOR:	Let's see how this boat was **built**. *[Present model; narrate after children complete actions]*
EDUCATOR:	I think this part of the boat was **made** from a milk carton.
EDUCATOR:	I wonder if we have milk cartons in our bag. Please look for us, John.
EDUCATOR:	Look, John **found** milk cartons.
EDUCATOR:	Let's see what else we need to make our boat. Please look in the bag, John.
EDUCATOR:	Now John **found** some Styrofoam.
EDUCATOR:	Look at this boat. *[Present model]* This white stuff is called Styrofoam. The Styrofoam gets glued in the bottom of the milk carton. Let's do that.
EDUCATOR:	Maria **stuck** some Styrofoam in a milk carton.
EDUCATOR:	Let's look at this boat again. *[Present model]* Somebody **stuck** a craft stick in the Styrofoam. Let's do that.
EDUCATOR:	Let's see what Sally **did.**
CHILD:	She **stuck** the stick in here.
EDUCATOR:	That's right, Sally **stuck** it in the Styrofoam.
EDUCATOR:	Now John needs a stick.
EDUCATOR:	You **found** a big stick!
EDUCATOR:	Look, Maria **stuck** the stick in the Styrofoam.

Example Script—*Continued*

EDUCATOR:	Somebody **made** this boat with a sail. *[Present model]* Let's put sails on our boats too. Let's use these. *[Present boat sails]*
EDUCATOR:	I think the sails were **stuck** on with glue.
EDUCATOR:	John **cut** out a sail and **stuck** it on the stick.
EDUCATOR:	Somebody **made** this sail very pretty. *[Present model]* I wonder what we could use to make our sails pretty too?
CHILD:	Stickers, crayons, and markers!
EDUCATOR:	Let's use these things to decorate our sails. *[Present stickers, crayons, and markers]*
EDUCATOR:	Sally **stuck** stickers on her sail.
EDUCATOR:	Maria **made** a green sail. John **made** a red sail. Miguel **drew** a smile on his sail.

[Continue in a similar manner until the sailboats have been completed and numerous models of irregular past tense verbs have been provided.]

Transition

EDUCATOR: The girl in our story liked to do things in the water. She **went** to the beach and **made** sandcastles. Another fun thing to do in water is ride on boats. We just **made** some boats. Now we are going to make boats and have a race in water to see whose boat is the fastest!

ELICITED PRODUCTION ACTIVITY

Description: Having a boat race

Skills Used: Fine motor, turn taking, and oral motor

Goal: 10 productions of irregular past tense verbs per child

Level of Educator Support: Forced choice

Instructions: Cut a boat shape out of each child's index card. Children may choose to decorate their boats. Children's names should be written on their boats. Then laminate the boats. Using the container, have children, two at a time, race their boats by blowing on them. For sessions with an individual child, wear a puppet and have the puppet race a boat.

Example Script

EDUCATOR: We are going to use these for our boats. *[Present index card boats]*

EDUCATOR: Look what somebody **did**! *[Present names written on boats]* What **did** they do to your boats? They **wrote** on them or **broke** them?

CHILD: They **wrote** on them!

EDUCATOR: Yes, somebody **wrote** your names on them.

EDUCATOR: Now we will know whose boats these are. *[Distribute boats]*

EDUCATOR: Now that everyone has a boat, we are going to have a race.

EDUCATOR: Let's have our race here in this water.

EDUCATOR: Jane and Jake, you go first. Put your boats in the water. We are going to start on this end. If you want your boats to move, you have to blow on them like this. *[Demonstrate]* Are you ready? Go!

EDUCATOR: What **did** they do to their boats? They **blew** on them or they **ate** them?

CHILD: They **blew** on them.

EDUCATOR: When they **blew** on them, what happened? They **went** or they **broke**?

CHILD: They **went!**

EDUCATOR: Tell me what happened to Jake. He **won** or he **lost**?

CHILD: He **lost**.

EDUCATOR: Tell me what happened to Jane. She **won** or she **lost**?

CHILD: She **won**! *[Repeat these elicitations for other children]*

[Continue in a similar manner until each child has had at least 10 opportunities to use irregular past tense verbs.]

Transition

EDUCATOR: We had fun sailing our boats. Let's finish up by singing our beach song!

SONG ACTIVITY

Instructions: Sing to the tune of "Little Bunny Foo Foo," emphasizing past tense irregular verbs.

Down by the Seashore

Down by the seashore, early in the morning,
I **saw** the children. They played in the sun.

I **saw** all the mommies. They **spread** out the blankets.
I **saw** all the children. They **ran** to the water.
I **saw** the children. They **had** so much fun!

Weekly Family Letter

For: ______________________________ **Date:** ______________

Theme

Our theme for language intervention this week is *water.*

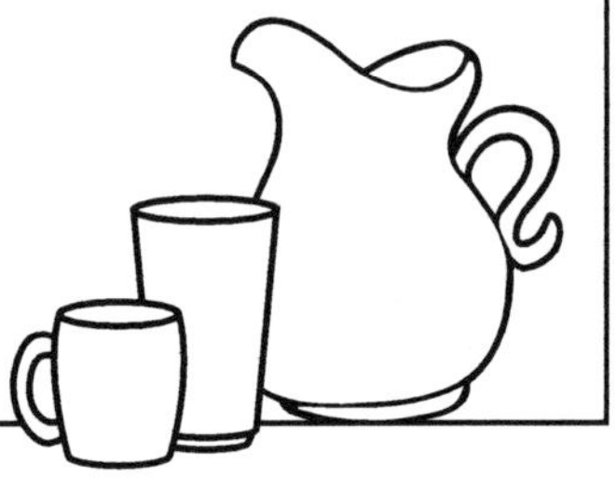

Target

Our target language structures are *regular past tense verbs.* These are verbs that indicate past actions and have the regular *-ed* ending. Examples include:

- She **frosted** the cake.
- The dog **jumped** through the window.
- Mommy **tickled** the baby.

Book

Our book for the week is *Miss Spider's Tea Party* by David Kirk.

Here is a related book you could read at home: *Let's Have a Tea Party* by Emilie Barnes and Michal Sparks and Sue Junker (illustrators).

Song

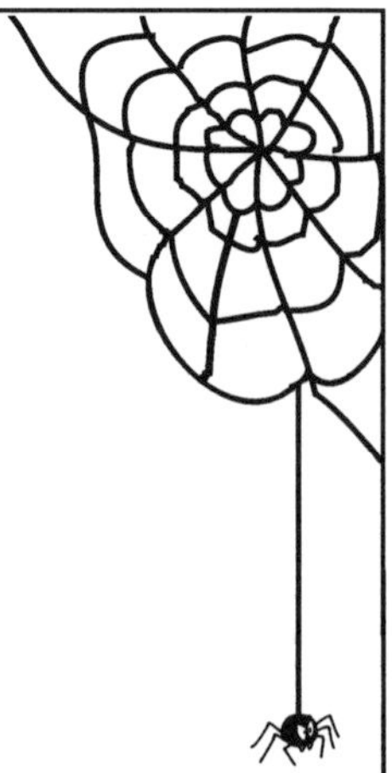

The Itsy Bitsy Spider
(Traditional)

The Itsy Bitsy spider **climbed** up the waterspout.
Down came the rain and **washed** the spider out!
Out came the sun and **dried** up all the rain, and
the Itsy Bitsy spider **climbed** up the spout again!

(Include hand motions if desired.)

Activities

Our planned activities for the week include:

- Making a drink with sugar, water, and drink mix
- Drawing a sequence picture of making a drink
- Having a pretend tea party
- Smelling tea bags

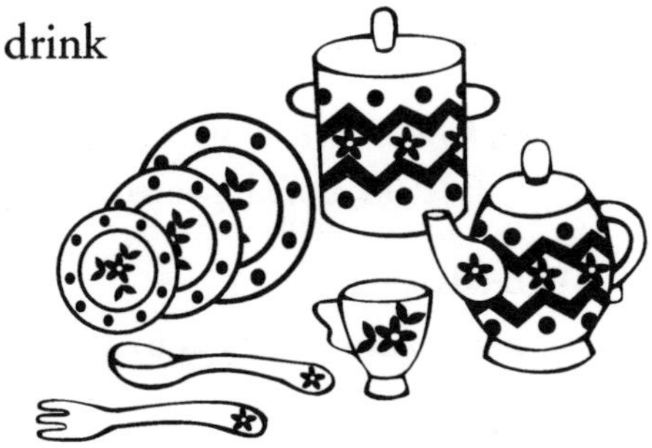

Follow-Up

Suggested follow-up activities for home include:

- Have your child tell you about the tea party he or she had
- Reenact the tea party
- Ask your child to explain to you (using regular past tense verbs) how he or she made a drink, for example:

  We **poured** water in a cup.

  I **stirred** the drink.

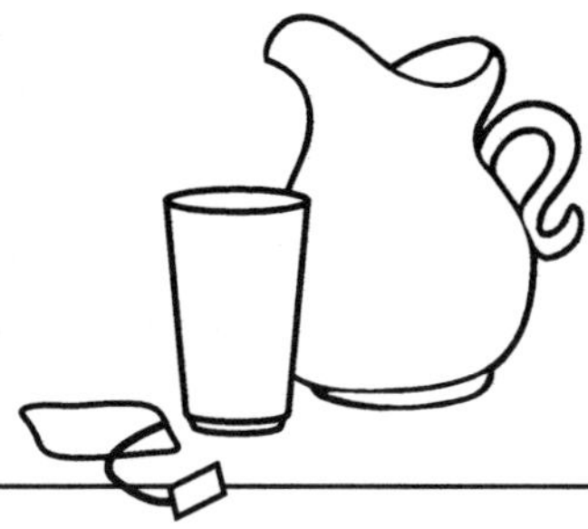

Thank You Very Much for your participation!

Phone Number

Email

Signature

Regular Past Tense

Cycle 1, Session 1

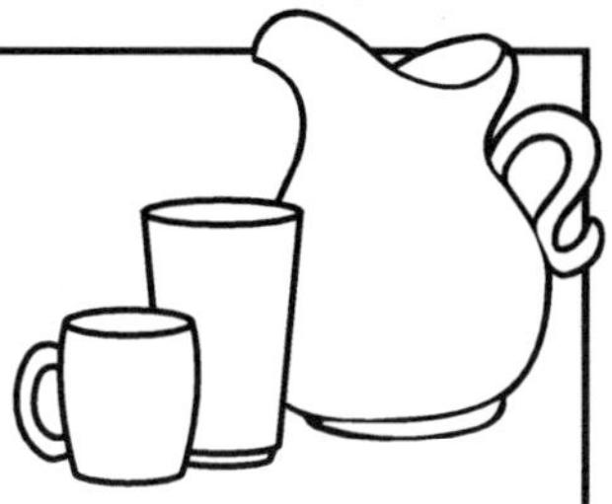

Theme: Water

Description: Making beverages with water

Exemplars: added, climbed, dried, floated, grabbed, licked, looked, measured, poured, scooped, sipped, spilled, stirred, talked, tasted, washed, wiped

Materials:

Miss Spider's Tea Party by David Kirk
Wet paper towels
Cups (1 per child; 1 for educator)
Tablespoons and teaspoons (1 each per child; 1 each for educator)
Drink mix (sweetened or unsweetened)
Sugar (if using unsweetened drink mix)
Water
Paper
Crayons or markers

INTRODUCTION TO THEME

EDUCATOR: We have been doing lots of interesting things with water. We made bubbles with water. We **talked** about places where we can find water, like the beach. We sank and **floated** things in water. There are other things we can do with water too. Can anyone tell me something else we can do with water? *[If children do not generate the response "drink it," provide a gestural or other type of cue]* That's right! We can drink water. Sometimes we drink water all by itself and sometimes we put things in water to make yummy drinks. Let's read our story and find out what Miss Spider likes to drink.

BOOK ACTIVITY

Book: *Miss Spider's Tea Party* by David Kirk

Instructions: Read the book with children, emphasizing regular past tense verbs.

Suggested Theme-Related Supplemental Book: *Let's Have a Tea Party* by Emilie Barnes and Michal Sparks and Sue Junker (illustrators)

Transition

EDUCATOR: Miss Spider had a nice tea party with her friends. Today we are going to have a tea party like hers.

FOCUSED STIMULATION ACTIVITY

Description: Making drinks

Skills Used: Sharing, direction following, and turn taking

Instructions: For the following script, use the product name in place of "drink mix."

Example Script

EDUCATOR: We are going to have a tea party like Miss Spider. We are going to have drink mix at our tea party and pretend that it is tea.

EDUCATOR: Let's sit at the table and I will show you how to make our "tea." *[Wash or wipe hands with a wet paper towel]*

EDUCATOR: I **washed** my hands. *[Take out a cup, some water, the drink mix, and a teaspoon; fill the cup with water]*

EDUCATOR: I **looked** for my spoon. I **looked** for the drink mix and I **poured** some water into my cup. *[Scoop 1 teaspoon of drink mix and pour it into the cup]*

EDUCATOR: I **scooped** out some drink mix and **poured** it into my cup. *[Scoop sugar into drink mix if necessary; then stir and take a sip]*

EDUCATOR: I **stirred** and **stirred**. Then I **sipped** my drink.

EDUCATOR: OK, now it's your turn to make a drink.

EDUCATOR: First, let's wash our hands. *[Distribute wet paper towels]*

EDUCATOR: Good, you all **washed** your hands, so now you can mix your drink. *[Pass out a tablespoon, a teaspoon, and a cup to each child]*

EDUCATOR: Oh, John **grabbed** his spoons and Jane **grabbed** her spoons. Here is some water.

EDUCATOR: John **poured** water into his cup. He **measured** the drink mix. Then he **poured** in the drink mix.

EDUCATOR: Oops, John **spilled** drink mix on the table, and then I **wiped** it up!

EDUCATOR: Look, Jane **scooped** up some drink mix.

Continued on next page

Example Script—*Continued*

EDUCATOR:	Do you remember what I did next?
CHILD:	You **stirred** it.
EDUCATOR:	That's right, I **stirred** the drink mix into my water.
EDUCATOR:	After I **stirred** the drink mix, what did I get to do?
CHILD:	You **added** sugar and **tasted**.
EDUCATOR:	That's right, I **added** sugar and then I **tasted** my pretend tea.

[Continue in a similar manner until numerous models of regular past tense verbs have been provided.]

Transition

EDUCATOR: Now that we have made drinks, we are going to draw a picture to show what we did today. Then we can take the picture home to show our families what we made.

ELICITED PRODUCTION ACTIVITY

Description: Drawing sequence pictures of making drinks

Skills Used: Sequencing and fine motor

Goal: 10 productions of regular past tense verbs per child

Level of Educator Support: Forced choice

Instructions: For the following script, use the product name in place of "drink mix." If children are unable or not interested in drawing all pictures of the sequence, they can draw a picture of one aspect of the project or, as a group, discuss the steps and the educator can draw a picture.

Example Script

EDUCATOR:	We are going to draw a picture of what we did today.
EDUCATOR:	Jane, what did we do first? We **washed** our hands or we **poured** water?
CHILD:	**Washed** our hands.
EDUCATOR:	Then what did we do? We **poured** the water or **spilled** the water?
CHILD:	We **poured** the water.

Example Script—*Continued*

EDUCATOR:	John, then what did we do? **<u>Scooped</u>** drink mix or **<u>poured</u>** water? *[Hold up items for a cue if children do not remember the order]*
CHILD:	**<u>Scooped</u>** drink mix.
EDUCATOR:	Yes, that's right. We **<u>scooped</u>** some drink mix.
EDUCATOR:	Let's draw a picture of that.
EDUCATOR:	Then what did we do? We **<u>added</u>** sugar or we **<u>added</u>** water?
CHILD:	**<u>Added</u>** sugar.
EDUCATOR:	Yes, we **<u>added</u>** the sugar.
EDUCATOR:	Then what? We **<u>stirred</u>** it or **<u>spilled</u>** it?
CHILD:	**<u>Stirred</u>** it.
EDUCATOR:	Then we did the best thing of all! What was that? We **<u>tasted</u>** it or **<u>licked</u>** it?
CHILD:	We **<u>tasted</u>** it!
EDUCATOR:	Let's draw a picture of us tasting our drinks!

[Continue in a similar manner until pictures have been drawn and each child has had at least 10 opportunities to use regular past tense verbs.]

Transition

EDUCATOR: It was fun to taste our drinks, kind of like how Miss Spider **sipped** her tea! Our pictures look great too! Now let's clean up and sing our spider song!

SONG ACTIVITY

Instructions: Sing to the traditional tune, emphasizing regular past tense verbs.

The Itsy Bitsy Spider

The Itsy Bitsy spider **climbed** up the waterspout.
Down came the rain and **washed** the spider out!
Out came the sun and **dried** up all the rain, and
the Itsy Bitsy spider **climbed** up the spout again!

(Include hand motions if desired.)

Regular Past Tense

Cycle 1, Session 2

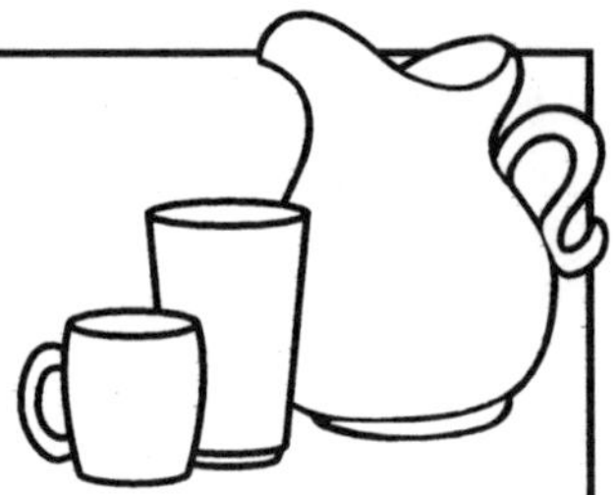

Theme: Water

Description: Making beverages with water

Exemplars: cleaned, climbed, closed, dried, grabbed, licked, looked, noticed, opened, passed, placed, poured, pulled, ripped, scooped, smelled, spilled, stirred, talked, tasted, tickled, washed

Materials:

Miss Spider's Tea Party by David Kirk

Bag containing:

- Cups, spoons, and small paper plates OR child's tea set
- Hot water (in insulated container)
- Tea bags in a variety of flavors
- Sugar
- Cookies

BOOK ACTIVITY

Book: *Miss Spider's Tea Party* by David Kirk

Instructions: Reread the book with children, emphasizing regular past tense verbs.

Suggested Theme-Related Supplemental Book: *Let's Have a Tea Party* by Emilie Barnes and Michal Sparks and Sue Junker (illustrators)

Transition

Educator: Miss Spider had such a good time at her party, so I thought today we could have a tea party too!

FOCUSED STIMULATION ACTIVITY

Description: Having a tea party

Skill Used: Dramatic play

Example Script

EDUCATOR: Let's have a tea party like Miss Spider.

EDUCATOR: Let's see, I have everything we need to set our table. You can take what we need out of this bag.

CHILD: *[Removes items from bag]*

EDUCATOR: You **pulled** out a cup.

EDUCATOR: Now you **grabbed** a spoon.

EDUCATOR: I wonder what Jane will pull out next.

EDUCATOR: Jane **pulled** out another cup.

EDUCATOR: Remember our story? What did Miss Spider do after she set her table? *[Consult pictures in the story if necessary]*

CHILD: **Poured** tea.

EDUCATOR: You think she **poured** some tea. I think she **poured** tea too.

EDUCATOR: Let's make some tea. We need some hot water and some tea bags.

EDUCATOR: Oh good, Jane **pulled** out some water and some tea bags. *[Open the tea bag]*

EDUCATOR: I **ripped** open the tea and I **placed** it into my cup. *[Pour water into cup]*

EDUCATOR: Then I **poured** some hot water on it. *[Stir tea]*

EDUCATOR: I **stirred** my tea. *[Scoop up sugar and pour it into tea]*

EDUCATOR: I **scooped** up some sugar and **poured** it into my tea.

EDUCATOR: Now let's find our snack. John **looked** for the cookies. *[Have child pass out cookies]*

EDUCATOR: Sally **passed** out the cookies.

EDUCATOR: Jane **tasted** her cookies.

[Continue in a similar manner until numerous models of regular past tense verbs have been provided.]

Transition

EDUCATOR: When we **opened** our tea bags, I **noticed** that the tea **smelled** really good. These tea bags are different. Different flavors of tea smell differently. I thought it would be fun if we **smelled** our tea bags and **talked** about them.

ELICITED PRODUCTION ACTIVITY

Description: Smelling tea bags

Skills Used: Sensory exploration and describing

Goal: 10 productions of regular past tense verbs per child

Level of Educator Support: Forced choice

Example Script

EDUCATOR:	Look, I have some tea bags in here. I'll take one out. *[Take one out and smell it]*
EDUCATOR:	Tell Jane what I did. I **smelled** it or I **licked** it?
CHILD:	**Smelled** it.
EDUCATOR:	Here, it's your turn.
EDUCATOR:	You **smelled** it or you **tasted** it?
CHILD:	I **smelled** it. *[Rip open a tea bag]*
EDUCATOR:	What did I do? I **ripped** it or I **tickled** it?
CHILD:	You **ripped** it!
EDUCATOR:	Right, I **ripped** open the bag.
EDUCATOR:	Here's a bag for you. Go ahead and open it.
EDUCATOR:	What did Sally do? She **opened** it or she **closed** it?
CHILD:	She **opened** it.
EDUCATOR:	*[Open a bag and spill some tea]* Oh no! What happened? I **poured** it or I **spilled** it?
CHILD:	You **spilled** it. *[Educator and children clean up]*
EDUCATOR:	What did we do to the tea? We **cleaned** it up or we **spilled** it?
CHILD:	**Cleaned** it up.

[Continue in a similar manner until each child has had at least 10 opportunities to use regular past tense verbs.]

Transition

EDUCATOR: We had a busy day. First we had a tea party like Miss Spider's, and then we **smelled** some delicious tea! Before we go, let's sing our spider song!

SONG ACTIVITY

Instructions: Sing to the traditional tune, emphasizing regular past tense verbs.

The Itsy Bitsy Spider

The Itsy Bitsy spider **climbed** up the waterspout.
Down came the rain and **washed** the spider out!
Out came the sun and **dried** up all the rain, and
the Itsy Bitsy spider **climbed** up the spout again!

(Include hand motions if desired.)

Weekly Family Letter

For: ______________________________ **Date:** ______________

Theme

Our theme for language intervention this week is *water.*

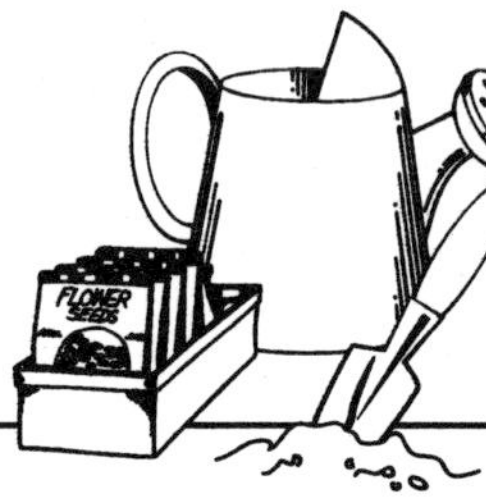

Target

Our target language structures are *copula* be *verbs.* These include the verbs *am ('m), are ('re),* and *is ('s)* when used as the only verb in a sentence. Examples include:

- She **is** happy. OR She**'s** happy.
- They **are** hungry. OR They**'re** hungry.
- I **am** sleepy. OR I**'m** sleepy.

Book

Our book for the week is *This Is Your Garden* by Maggie Smith.

Here is a related book you could read at home: *The Tiny Seed* by Eric Carle.

Song

Little Seed
(Tune: "Mary Had a Little Lamb")

Here **is** a little seed, little seed, little seed.
Here **is** a little seed. Soon it will grow.

Here **is** a little plant, little plant, little plant.
Here **is** a little plant, see how it grows.

Here **is** a big plant, big plant, big plant.
Here **is** a big plant. It **is** all grown.

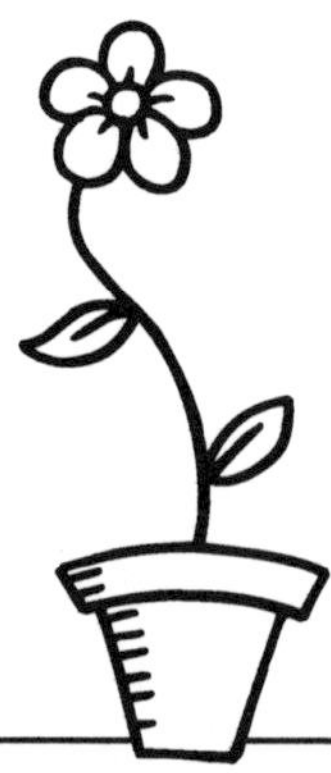

Activities

Our planned activities for the week include:

- Decorating a flower pot
- Planting seeds
- Drawing a sequence picture of planting seeds

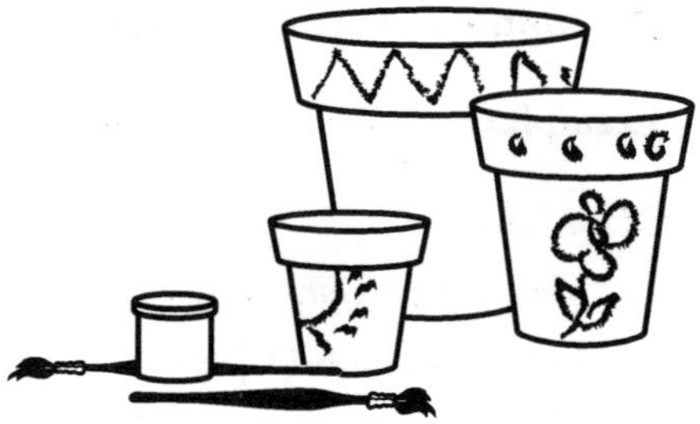

Follow-Up

Suggested follow-up activities for home include:

- Have your child describe different types of plants to you using copula *be* verbs, for example:

  This **is** a green plant.

  This **is** a flower.

  These plants **are** big.

- Pretend to have your house plants talk, for example:

  I **am** hot.

  I'm thirsty.

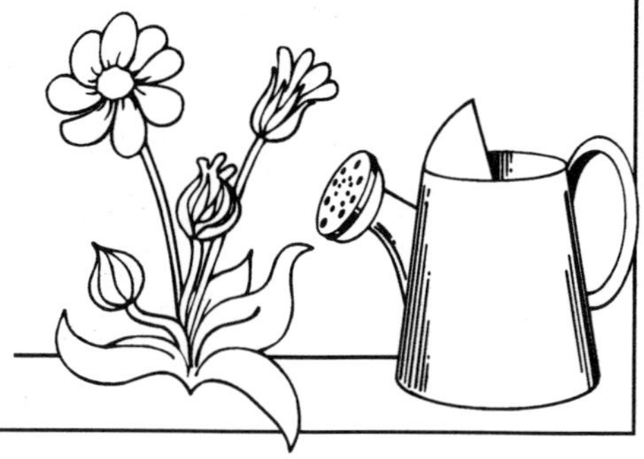

Thank You Very Much for your participation!

Phone Number

Email

Signature

Copula *be*

Cycle 1, Session 1

Theme: Water

Description: Decorating a flower pot

Exemplars: am ('m), are ('re), is ('s)

Materials:

This Is Your Garden by Maggie Smith
Styrofoam cups (1 per child)
Facial features (see page 273 for directions and patterns; 1 set per child)
Child-safe scissors
Glue

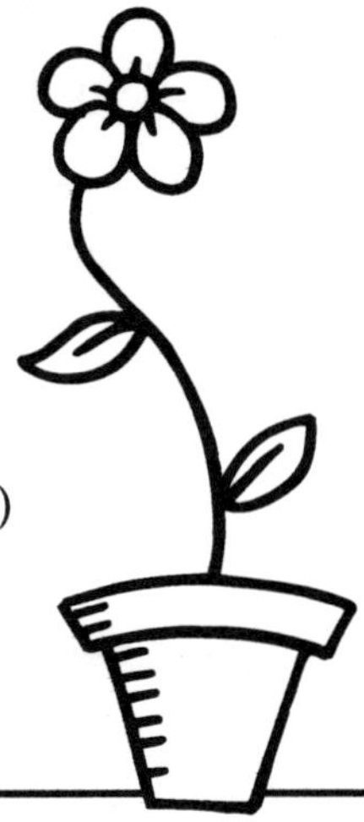

INTRODUCTION TO THEME

Educator: We have been talking about many different things we can do with water. Who remembers what we used water for last week? *[Allow children to guess/respond]* That**'s** right! We used water to make yummy things for us to drink. People like to drink water. There **is** something that needs water to grow. I will give you some hints about what it might be. The thing I am thinking about needs sunlight. It grows in the ground and it **is** very pretty. Can you guess what it **is**? *[Children may choose to guess what it is]* That**'s** right! I'm talking about flowers and plants.

BOOK ACTIVITY

Book: *This Is Your Garden* by Maggie Smith

Instructions: Read the book with children, emphasizing copula *be* verbs.

Suggested Theme-Related Supplemental Book: *The Tiny Seed* by Eric Carle

Transition

EDUCATOR: The girl in our story planted a whole garden. We can plant seeds and give them water too. If we want to plant seeds, we'll need something to put them in. Look at this. *[Present cup]* It **is** a white cup. We are going to put these things on it. *[Present facial features]*

FOCUSED STIMULATION ACTIVITY

Description: Preparing items for flower pots, which will be made in the elicited production activity

Skills Used: Prediction and planning

Example Script

EDUCATOR: *[Spread out the facial features]* Look at these mouths. This one**'s** happy. This mouth **is** sad.

EDUCATOR: Here **are** some eyes for the cup. They **are** little but this nose **is** big.

EDUCATOR: These eyes **are** blue. Look, Jane's eyes **are** blue too.

EDUCATOR: Hmmm, I wonder what this **is**. I think this **is** the nose.

EDUCATOR: This nose **is** little but this one**'s** big.

EDUCATOR: I like the mouth Sally has. It **is** pink. Miguel's mouth**'s** red.

EDUCATOR: What do we need to use to cut out all these things?

CHILD: Scissors.

EDUCATOR: I have some scissors here. They **are** sharp.

EDUCATOR: I think my cup **is** a girl.

CHILD: Mine**'s** a boy.

[Continue in a similar manner until numerous models of copula be *verbs have been provided.]*

Transition

EDUCATOR: We are going to have very pretty cups to grow our seeds in! Let's get started!

ELICITED PRODUCTION ACTIVITY

Description: Decorating flower pots

Skill Used: Fine motor

Goal: 10 productions of copula *be* forms per child

Level of Educator Support: Forced choice

Instructions: Remember that contracted (e.g., He**'s** happy) and uncontracted (e.g., This **is** your garden) copula *be* verbs are acceptable.

Example Script

EDUCATOR: Now we are ready to put our eyes, noses, and mouths on our cups.

EDUCATOR: First, we need our glue. Which of these things **is** the glue? These **are** *[point to scissors]* or this **is** *[point to glue]*?

CHILD: This **is**. *[Points to glue]*

EDUCATOR: Yes, this **is**.

EDUCATOR: *[Have children glue eyes on their cups]* OK, which eyes **are** on the cup? The green eyes **are** or the blue eyes **are**?

CHILD: The green eyes **are**.

EDUCATOR: *[Have children glue noses on their cups]* Now what **is** on the cup? The nose **is** or the eyes **are**?

CHILD: The nose **is**.

EDUCATOR: What **is** big? The nose **is** or the eyes **are**?

CHILD: The nose **is**.

EDUCATOR: *[Have children glue ears on their cups]* Sally, what **is** yellow? The ears **are** or the nose **is**?

CHILD: The ears **are**.

EDUCATOR: My cup **is** happy. Tell me about your cup, Miguel. Tell me, **is** your cup happy or **is** your cup sad?

CHILD: My cup **is** happy.

[Continue in a similar manner until each child has had at least 10 opportunities to use copula be *verbs.]*

Transition

Educator: Our flower pots look great! Let's clean up and sing our song about the little seed.

SONG ACTIVITY

Instructions: Sing to the tune of "Mary Had a Little Lamb," emphasizing copula *be* verbs.

Little Seed

Here **is** a little seed, little seed, little seed.
Here **is** a little seed. Soon it will grow.

Here **is** a little plant, little plant, little plant.
Here **is** a little plant, see how it grows.

Here **is** a big plant, big plant, big plant.
Here **is** a big plant. It **is** all grown.

Copula *be*

Cycle 1, Session 2

Theme: Water

Description: Using water to grow plants

Exemplars: am ('m), are ('re), is ('s)

Materials:

This Is Your Garden by Maggie Smith
Styrofoam cups (decorated in previous session)
Potting soil
Spoon
Seeds (grass or wheat grass seeds work best)
Water
Paper and markers OR dry erase board and markers

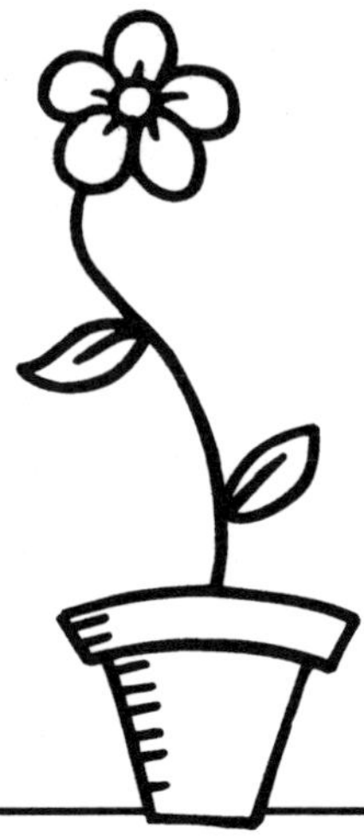

BOOK ACTIVITY

Book: *This Is Your Garden* by Maggie Smith

Instructions: Reread the book with children, emphasizing copula *be* verbs. Encourage children to comment on the book, but do not explicitly demand specific productions.

Suggested Theme-Related Supplemental Book: *The Tiny Seed* by Eric Carle

Transition

EDUCATOR: Remember how we made our face cups last time? Well, today we are going to use our cups. We are going to do something like the girl in the story. We are going to put dirt, seeds, and water in our cups and grow grass!

FOCUSED STIMULATION ACTIVITY

Description: Planting seeds

Skills Used: Direction following and fine motor

Example Script

EDUCATOR:	Here **are** the cups we made last time. I wonder whose cup this **is**?
CHILD:	It**'s** mine!
EDUCATOR:	OK, this **is** Sally's cup and this **is** Jane's cup.
EDUCATOR:	The face on this cup **is** happy and this one **is** sad.
EDUCATOR:	Well, we are going to put something inside this cup.
EDUCATOR:	Look in this cup. It**'s** empty. We need to fill it up.
EDUCATOR:	What **is** this? *[Present dirt]*
CHILD:	Dirt!
EDUCATOR:	Yes, it **is** dirt. It **is** black dirt.
EDUCATOR:	This dirt**'s** outside the cup. We want to get it inside the cup. This **is** something we can use to put the dirt in the cup. It **is** a spoon. A spoon **is** for putting dirt in the cup. *[Fill each cup with dirt]*
EDUCATOR:	Now our cups **are** not empty. They **are** full of dirt.
EDUCATOR:	I **am** happy that we got our cups filled with dirt, but we forgot something that **is** very important. We forgot these. *[Present seeds]* These **are** seeds.
EDUCATOR:	Let's put the seeds in the dirt. *[Have children mix their seeds into the dirt]*
EDUCATOR:	Now they **are** all in the dirt.
EDUCATOR:	Now, what do we need to do? Our seeds need something else. They need water. Here **is** the water. Pour some water in the cup. Feel the dirt. Now the dirt **is** wet.

[Continue in a similar manner until numerous models copula be *verbs have been provided.]*

Transition

EDUCATOR: We had fun planting our seeds. If we give them water and sunshine, they will grow in a few days. Then our cups will have hair! Let's draw a picture of what we did with our seeds.

ELICITED PRODUCTION ACTIVITY

Description: Drawing sequence pictures of planting seeds

Skills Used: Sequencing and fine motor

Goal: 10 productions of copula *be* verbs per child

Level of Educator Support: Forced choice

Instructions: If children are unable or not interested in drawing all pictures of the sequence, they can draw a picture of one aspect of the project or, as a group, discuss the steps and the educator can draw a picture.

Example Script

EDUCATOR: You draw a picture and I'll draw a picture. *[Educator and children draw pictures]*

EDUCATOR: Let's look at my picture. This **is** my cup or this **is** my seed? *[Point to cup]*

CHILD: This **is** your cup.

EDUCATOR: Yes. But tell me about this seed. *[Draw a single seed speck on your picture]* The seed **is** little or the seed **is** big?

CHILD: The seed **is** little.

EDUCATOR: Where **is** the seed? *[Draw the seed being put in a cup of dirt]* The seed **is** in the cup or the seed **is** under the cup?

CHILD: The seed **is** in the cup.

EDUCATOR: I like this cup's face. Jane, tell Sally about this funny cup. The face on the cup **is** happy or **is** sad?

CHILD: It'**s** happy!

EDUCATOR: Yes it **is**! This **is** a pretty cup. *[Point to one of the children's pictures]* John, tell us about your cup. **Is** your cup happy or **is** your cup sad?

CHILD: My cup **is** sad.

EDUCATOR: Look at this picture. *[Point to own picture]* Tell me about this. My cup **is** full or my cup **is** empty?

CHILD: The cup **is** full.

Example Script—*Continued*

EDUCATOR: Yes, here my cup **is** full of dirt.

EDUCATOR: Look at this picture. After my cup **is** full of dirt, what **is** put in the cup next? Water **is** in the cup, or seeds **are** in the cup?

CHILD: Seeds **are** put in the cup.

EDUCATOR: Yes, seeds **are** put in the cup.

EDUCATOR: Now look at my last picture. Tell me about this, Jane. Water **is** in the cup or milk **is** in the cup?

CHILD: Water **is**!

EDUCATOR: Yes, water **is** in the cup. Water **is** in the cup so the seeds will grow!

[Continue in a similar manner until each child has had at least 10 opportunities to use copula be *verbs.]*

Transition

EDUCATOR: We all planted seeds and soon they will grow into plants. Then we drew pictures of planting seeds. That reminds me of our little seed song. Let's sing it now!

SONG ACTIVITY

Instructions: Sing to the tune of "Mary Had a Little Lamb," emphasizing copula *be* verbs.

Little Seed

Here **is** a little seed, little seed, little seed.
Here **is** a little seed. Soon it will grow.

Here **is** a little plant, little plant, little plant.
Here **is** a little plant, see how it grows.

Here **is** a big plant, big plant, big plant.
Here **is** a big plant. It **is** all grown.

Weekly Family Letter

For: ______________________________ **Date:** ____________

Theme

Our theme for language intervention this week is *animals.*

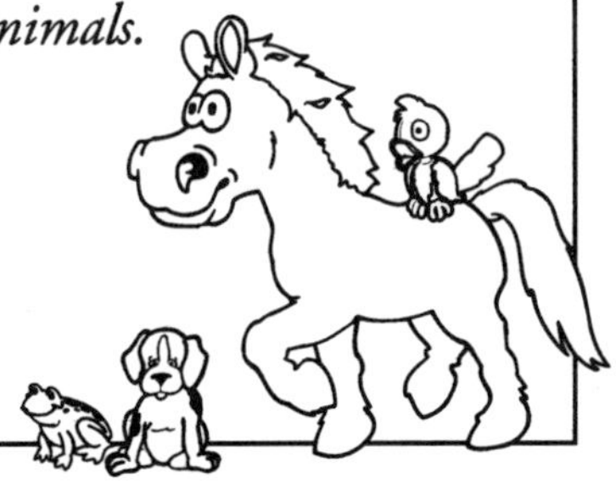

Target

Our target language structures are *regular third person singular verbs.* These verbs indicate actions by a single person or object and have a regular *-s* ending. Examples include:

- She **feels** happy.
- The dog **jumps** high.
- Mom **sleeps** in the bed.

Book

Our book for the week is *Brown Bear, Brown Bear, What Do You See?* by Bill Martin Jr. and Eric Carle (illustrator).

Here are some related books you could read at home: *Polar Bear, Polar Bear, What Do You Hear?* by Bill Martin Jr. and Eric Carle (illustrator) and *Mouse Creeps* by Peter Harris and Rey Cartwright (illustrator).

Song

Brown Bear Sees All His Friends
(Tune: "Mary Had a Little Lamb")

Brown Bear **sees** all his friends, **sees** all his friends, **sees** all his friends.
Brown Bear **sees** all his friends. He **sees** them every day.

Brown Bear **likes** all his friends, **likes** all his friends, **likes** all his friends.
Brown Bear **likes** all his friends.
He **likes** them every way!

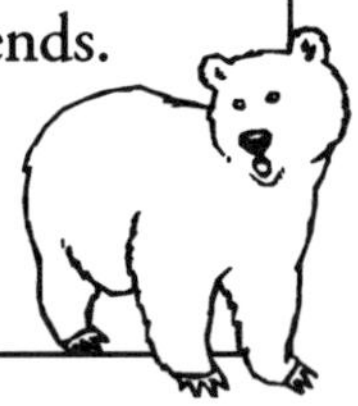

Activities

Our planned activities for the week include:

- Decorating felt animals
- Reenacting the story *Brown Bear, Brown Bear, What Do You See?*
- Making a Brown Bear stick puppet
- Playing I Spy using various animals hidden around a room

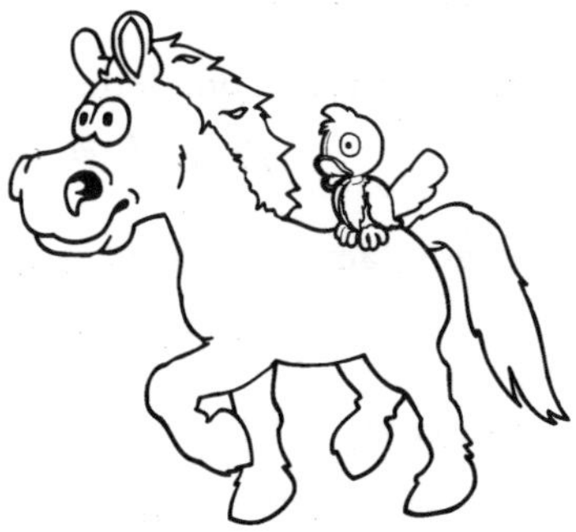

Follow-Up

Suggested follow-up activities for home include:

- Ask your child to tell you the story of the *Brown Bear* using regular third person singular verbs (see examples below).
- Use the animals made in language intervention and ask your child to give you a puppet show using third person singular verbs, for example:

  Brown Bear **sees** a horse.

  Brown Bear **sees** a dog.

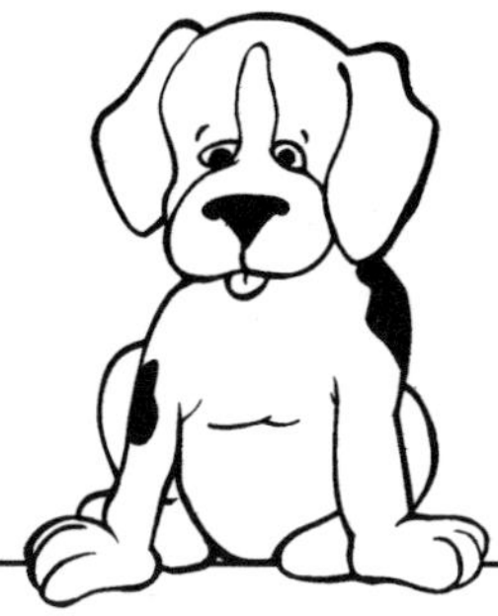

Thank You Very Much for your participation!

Phone Number

Email

Signature

Regular Third Person Singular

Cycle 2, Session 1

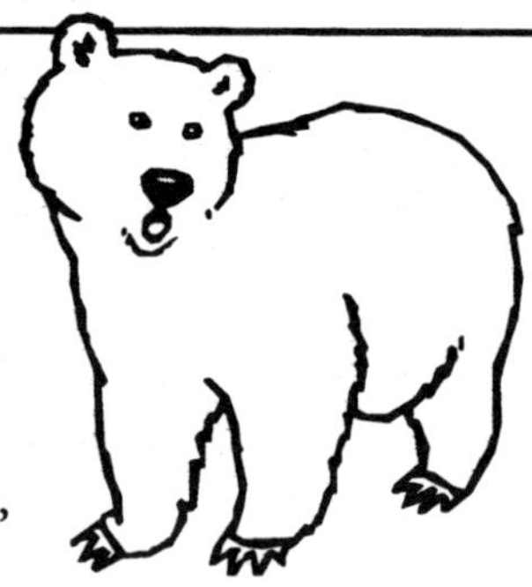

Theme: Animals

Description: Completing activities relating to *Brown Bear, Brown Bear, What Do You See?*

Exemplars: chooses, decorates, feels, gets, glues, likes, looks, makes, puts, sees, shares, uses

Materials:

Brown Bear, Brown Bear, What Do You See? by Bill Martin Jr. and Eric Carle (illustrator)
Felt animal cutouts (see pages 274 and 276–282 for directions and patterns)
Decorations (glitter, google eyes, beads, etc.)
Glue
Felt board

INTRODUCTION TO THEME

EDUCATOR: For the past few weeks, we have been talking about all the fun things we can do with water. Now we are going to talk about something new. We are going to learn about animals! We can find animals in many different places. Does anybody have a pet animal at home? *[Allow children to name the animals they have]* Where else can we find animals? *[Provide cues for places such as the zoo, forest, and farm if necessary]* Today we are going to talk about a bear who **sees** many different animals.

BOOK ACTIVITY

Book: *Brown Bear, Brown Bear, What Do You See?* by Bill Martin Jr. and Eric Carle (illustrator)

Instructions: Read the book with children. Comment on the story using regular third person singular verbs.

Suggested Theme-Related Supplemental Books: *Polar Bear, Polar Bear, What Do You Hear?* by Bill Martin Jr. and Eric Carle (illustrator)
Mouse Creeps by Peter Harris and Reg Cartwright (illustrator)

CYCLE 2

Transition

EDUCATOR: Brown Bear saw many different animals! Now we are going to make some of those animals!

FOCUSED STIMULATION ACTIVITY

Description: Decorating felt animals like those found in the story

Skills Used: Describing and fine motor

Instructions: For sessions with several children, have different children complete different tasks. Comment on what each child is doing or comment on pictures in the book using present tense. For sessions with an individual child, use objects as the subjects of utterances instead of people (e.g., "The glue **feels** sticky," "The hair **looks** shiny," and "The bead **looks** pretty").

Example Script

EDUCATOR: Here are all the things we need to make our animals. *[Present felt pieces, decorations, and glue]* I wonder what kind of animal you would like to make, Maria?

CHILD: I want a dog!

EDUCATOR: Maria **likes** dogs! She **gets** to pick out a felt dog and some decorations to put on it. Let's see what Maria does first.

EDUCATOR: Look, Maria **glues** the eyes on the dog.

EDUCATOR: John, it's your turn to pick out an animal to decorate. It **looks** like John **likes** the sheep. Let's see how John **decorates** his sheep.

EDUCATOR: Now John **makes** the hair shiny. He **uses** glitter to make it shiny.

EDUCATOR: Let's see what Sally **chooses.**

EDUCATOR: Sally **puts** the cap on the glue.

EDUCATOR: Now Sally **makes** a white dog!

EDUCATOR: The dog **feels** soft!

EDUCATOR: Sally **glues** feet on her dog.

EDUCATOR: John **chooses** a blue horse. Maria **likes** John's blue horse!

EDUCATOR: Sally **makes** pretty animals!

EDUCATOR: Maria **shares** her glue. That's so nice!

EDUCATOR: Sally **puts** lots of beads on her animals.

[Continue in a similar manner until numerous third person singular regular verbs have been provided.]

Transition

EDUCATOR: Now that we have made all these beautiful animals, I thought we could act out our story using our animals. Let's look back in our book and see what we should do.

ELICITED PRODUCTION ACTIVITY

Description: Reenacting *Brown Bear, Brown Bear, What Do You See?* using children's felt animals and a felt board

Skills Used: Narrative and sequencing

Goal: 10 productions of regular third person singular verbs per child

Level of Educator Support: Cloze task (____> indicates educator's pause for child to fill in the blank)

Instructions: For sessions with an individual child, use objects as the subjects of utterances instead of people (e.g., "Brown Bear **sees** a bird," "The duck **looks** nice on our board," and "The horse **moves** fast").

Example Script

EDUCATOR: Look at our book. Here Brown Bear **sees** a red bird, and here he ____>

CHILD: **Sees** a yellow duck!

EDUCATOR: Yes, he **sees** a yellow duck. *[Have the child put the yellow duck felt piece on the board]*

EDUCATOR: Hmmm, what does John do with his yellow duck? He ____>

CHILD: **Puts** it on!

EDUCATOR: Yes, he **puts** it on our picture.

EDUCATOR: Now what does Brown Bear do? He ____>

CHILD: **Sees** a blue horse.

EDUCATOR: You're right. He **sees** a blue horse. What does Jake do now? He ____>

CHILD: **Puts** horsey on.

EDUCATOR: Yes, he **puts** the horse on the picture. What does he do, Sally? He ____>

CHILD: **Puts** the horse on.

[Continue in a similar manner until each child has had at least 10 opportunities to use regular third person singular verbs.]

Transition

EDUCATOR: It was fun acting out our story. Now it's time to learn a new song about Brown Bear! Are you ready?

SONG ACTIVITY

Instructions: Sing to the tune of "Mary Had A Little Lamb," emphasizing regular third person singular verbs.

Brown Bear Sees All His Friends

Brown Bear **sees** all his friends,
sees all his friends, **sees** all his friends.
Brown Bear **sees** all his friends.
He **sees** them every day.

Brown Bear **likes** all his friends,
likes all his friends, **likes** all his friends.
Brown Bear **likes** all his friends.
He **likes** them every way!

Regular Third Person Singular

Cycle 2, Session 2

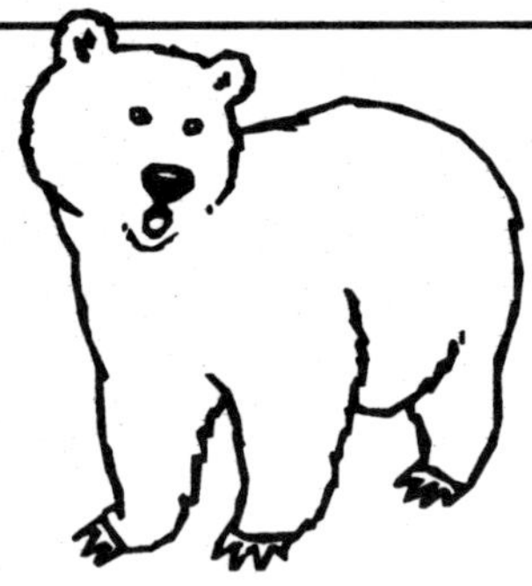

Theme: Animals

Description: Completing activities relating to *Brown Bear, Brown Bear, What Do You See?*

Exemplars: feels, likes, looks, makes, needs, puts, sees, shares, sticks

Materials:

Brown Bear, Brown Bear, What Do You See? by Bill Martin Jr. and Eric Carle (illustrator)
Craft sticks
Brown Bears (see pages 274–275 for directions and a pattern; 1 per child)
Crayons or markers
Decorations (google eyes, brown beads, etc.)
Completed Brown Bear stick puppet (see pages 274–275 for directions and a pattern)
Glue
Pictures of animals (see pages 283–284 for directions and patterns)
Magnifying glass or binoculars (optional)

BOOK ACTIVITY

Book: *Brown Bear, Brown Bear, What Do You See?* by Bill Martin Jr. and Eric Carle (illustrator)

Instructions: Reread the book with children. Comment on the story using regular third person singular verbs.

Suggested Theme-Related Supplemental Books: *Polar Bear, Polar Bear, What Do You Hear?* by Bill Martin Jr and Eric Carle (illustrator)
Mouse Creeps by Peter Harris and Reg Cartwright (illustrator)

Transition

Educator: Brown Bear was an important character in the story. Today we are going to make some Brown Bear puppets!

FOCUSED STIMULATION ACTIVITY

Description: Making Brown Bear stick puppets

Skills Used: Fine motor and direction following

Instructions: Prepare a stick puppet prior to the activity to serve as a model. For sessions with several children, comment on what each child is doing using regular third person singular verbs. For sessions with an individual child, use objects as the subjects of utterances instead of people (e.g., "The bear **looks** scary," "The glue **feels** sticky," and "This eye **moves** a lot").

Example Script

EDUCATOR:	Here are the things we need to make our bear puppets. Let's see what we have. *[Ask a child to hold up the items]*
EDUCATOR:	Jane **sees** some popsicle sticks, some bear faces, and some beads. Each of you will use these things to make a bear puppet that **looks** like this one. *[Present completed model]*
EDUCATOR:	Jane, what do you need?
CHILD:	I need a bear and a stick.
EDUCATOR:	Jane **needs** a bear and a stick.
EDUCATOR:	Start by making his mouth. *[Let the child make a mouth]* That bear **looks** happy.
EDUCATOR:	Jane **sticks** some eyes on her bear and then **puts** the cap on the glue. *[Allow other children to make their bears following the completed model and comment on children's actions or on the bears themselves]*
EDUCATOR:	John **likes** big and scary bears!
EDUCATOR:	Sally **makes** a happy bear.
EDUCATOR:	John's bear **feels** soft.
EDUCATOR:	John **likes** Jane's brown bear!
EDUCATOR:	John **puts** lots of glue on his bear.
EDUCATOR:	Jane **shares** her glue. That's so nice!
EDUCATOR:	Sally **puts** big teeth on her bear.

[Continue in a similar manner until bears have been put together and numerous models of third person singular regular verbs have been provided.]

Transition

EDUCATOR: Remember that in our story, Brown Bear **sees** lots of animals? He **sees** a blue horse who **looks** at him. He **sees** lots and lots of animals, and even some kids! Let's take the bears we just made and have them look around the room. Let's see what they see!

ELICITED PRODUCTION ACTIVITY

Description: Playing a modified game of I Spy (in this case it will be Brown Bear Sees).

Skills Used: Gross motor, searching and finding, and labeling/describing

Goal: 10 productions of regular third person singular verbs per child

Level of Educator Support: Cloze task (____> indicates educator's pause for child to fill in the blank)

Instructions: Prior to the activity, hang up the animal pictures at various eye-level locations around the room or hallway. Have children pretend their Brown Bear puppets are finding the animals. Consider having children use binoculars or a magnifying glass to assist in their search.

Example Script

EDUCATOR: What does your bear see? He ____>

CHILD: **Sees** a yellow duck!

EDUCATOR: Yes, he **sees** a yellow duck.

EDUCATOR: Hmmm, what does your bear see? He ____>

CHILD: **Sees** a blue horse!

EDUCATOR: Yes, he **sees** a blue horse!

EDUCATOR: Now what does the blue horse do? He ____>

CHILD: **Looks** at the bear.

EDUCATOR: You're right. He **looks** at the bear. What does the bear do now? He >

CHILD: **Sees** a white dog.

EDUCATOR: Yes, he **sees** a white dog. And the white dog looks at the bear. What does he do? He ____>

CHILD: **Looks** at the bear!

[Continue in a similar manner until each child has had at least 10 opportunities to use regular third person singular verbs.]

Transition

Educator: We saw lots of interesting animals today. Now it's time to sing our song about those animals!

SONG ACTIVITY

Instructions: Sing to the tune of "Mary Had a Little Lamb," emphasizing regular third person singular verbs.

Brown Bear Sees All His Friends

Brown Bear **sees** all his friends,
sees all his friends, **sees** all his friends.
Brown Bear **sees** all his friends.
He **sees** them every day.

Brown Bear **likes** all his friends,
likes all his friends, **likes** all his friends.
Brown Bear **likes** all his friends.
He **likes** them every way!

Weekly Family Letter

For: ______________________________ **Date:** ______________

Theme

Our theme for language intervention this week is *animals.*

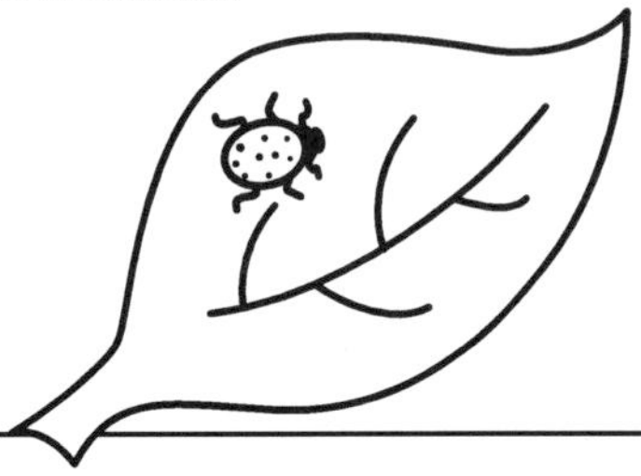

Target

Our target language structures are *irregular past tense verbs.* These verbs indicate past actions, but they do not have the regular *-ed* ending. Examples include:

- She **felt** happy.
- The dog **ran** fast.
- Mom **slept** in the bed.

Book

Our book for the week is *The Grouchy Ladybug* by Eric Carle.

Here are some related books you can read at home: *The Very Quiet Cricket* by Eric Carle, *The Very Lonely Firefly* by Eric Carle, and *Franklin Goes to School* by Paulette Bourgeois and Brenda Clark (illustrator).

Song

Five Little Ladybugs
(Chant: "Five Little Monkeys")

Five little ladybugs jumping on the bed.
One **fell** off and **hurt** his head.

Mama called the doctor and the doctor **said,**
"No more ladybugs jumping on the bed!"

(Repeat for the numbers four, three, two, and one.)

Activities

Our planned activities for the week include:

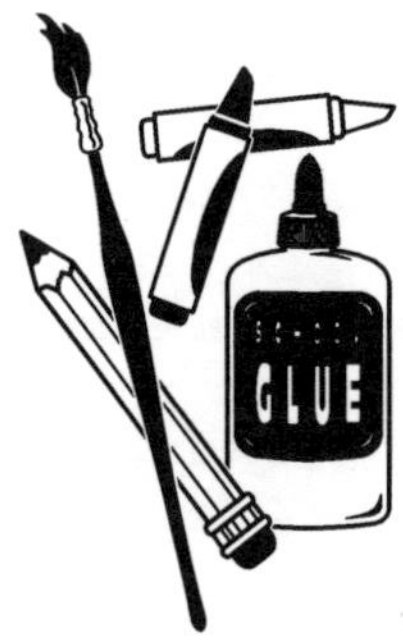

- Making a paper plate ladybug
- Having snacks that look like bugs (raisins)
- Making leaves to stick ladybug stickers on
- Decorating stickers to look like ladybugs

Follow-Up

Suggested follow-up activities for home include:

- Ask your child to tell you the story of the Grouchy Ladybug in his or her own words while using irregular past tense verbs
- Have your child explain how he or she made ladybugs in language intervention, for example:

    I **drew** dots on the bug.

    I **made** a big ladybug.

    I **drew** a smile.

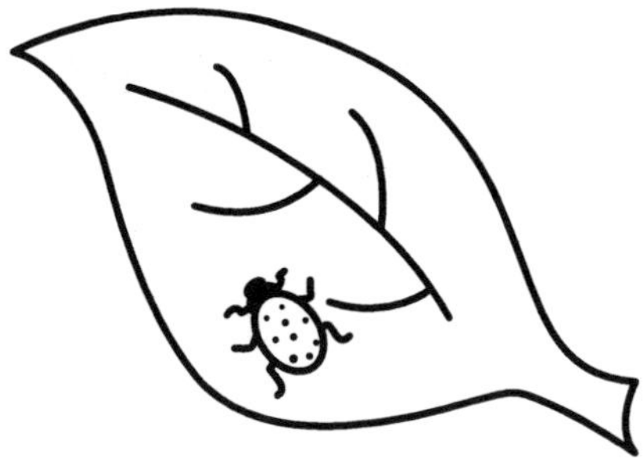

Thank You Very Much
for your participation!

____
Phone Number

____
Email

____
Signature

Irregular Past Tense

Cycle 2, Session 1

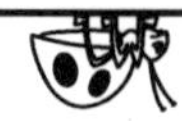

Theme: Animals

Description: Completing activities relating to bugs

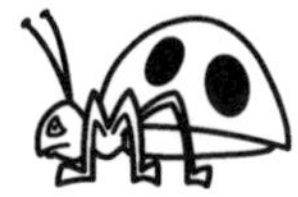

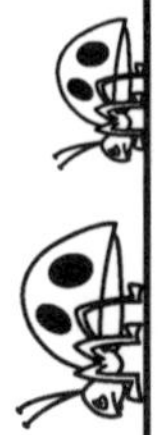

Exemplars: ate, bent, broke, brought, did, drank, fell, felt, found, gave, hurt, made, said

Materials:

The Grouchy Ladybug by Eric Carle
Red paper plates (1 per child)
Pipe cleaners (1 per child)
Black dot stickers
Glue
Scissors
Completed ladybug
(see page 285 for directions)
Raisins
Juice boxes (1 per child)
Bag

INTRODUCTION TO THEME

EDUCATOR: Last week we talked about a bear who **saw** lots of different animals. Bears are really big animals. Today we are going to talk about an animal that is really small. This animal is a bug, and it is red and has black spots. It is a ladybug!

BOOK ACTIVITY

Book: *The Grouchy Ladybug* by Eric Carle

Instructions: Read the book with children, emphasizing irregular past tense verbs.

Suggested Theme-Related Supplemental Books:
The Very Quiet Cricket by Eric Carle
The Very Lonely Firefly by Eric Carle
Franklin Goes to School
by Paulette Bourgeois and Brenda Clark (illustrator)

Transition

Educator: The ladybug in our story was very grouchy until the end of the story. Then she was a happy ladybug! Today we are going to make some happy ladybugs using these plates. *[Hold up plates]*

FOCUSED STIMULATION ACTIVITY

Description: Making ladybugs like those in the story

Skills Used: Fine motor and direction following

Instructions: Prepare a ladybug prior to the activity to serve as a model. After children complete tasks, comment on what they did to obligate irregular past tense verbs.

Example Script

Educator: We will use these things to make our ladybugs. Let's see what I **brought.** I **brought** some red plates, some pipe cleaners, and some spots. I also **brought** some glue and scissors for us to use. Our bugs will look like this when we are done. *[Present model]*

Educator: Let's get started. Look what John **did.**

Educator: John **made** a very spotty ladybug.

Educator: John **broke** his bug's antennae!

Educator: Jake **bent** his bug's antennae!

Educator: Sally **made** very big eyes for her bug.

Educator: That antenna **felt** soft.

Educator: I **brought** lots of spots for our ladybugs.

Educator: Look, I **found** glue in this bag.

Educator: You **gave** Jane the glue. That's so nice!

Educator: You **made** so many nice ladybugs!

[Continue in a similar manner until ladybugs have been made and numerous models of irregular past tense verbs have been provided.]

Transition

EDUCATOR: What great ladybugs you **made! Did** anyone get hungry? I **found** some bugs for snacks! You'll like how they taste!

ELICITED PRODUCTION ACTIVITY

Description: Snacking on "bugs" (raisins) and "bug juice" (juice boxes)

Skills Used: Sharing and turn taking

Goal: 10 productions of irregular past tense verbs per child

Level of Educator Support: Cloze task (____> indicates educator's pause for child to fill in the blank)

Instructions: Hand out raisins and juice boxes, but keep some snacks in the bag.

Example Script

EDUCATOR: We are going to have a snack today. I thought it would be funny if we ate bugs for our snack! Look at these. *[Present raisins]* Are these bugs?

CHILD: No!

EDUCATOR: No, we are just going to pretend that the raisins are bugs.

EDUCATOR: I'm hungry. I think I'm going to eat a bug! *[Eat a raisin]* What **did** I do? I____>

CHILD: **Ate** a bug!

EDUCATOR: Yuck, I **ate** a bug!

EDUCATOR: Hmmm, now it's John's turn. Wow! What **did** he do? He ____>

CHILD: **Ate** another bug!

EDUCATOR: Icky, he **ate** a black bug!

EDUCATOR: John, look in the bag. What **did** you find? You ____>

CHILD: **Found** more bugs.

EDUCATOR: You did? You **found** more bugs!

Continued on next page

Example Script—*Continued*

EDUCATOR:	I'm thirsty. *[Take a drink of juice]* What **did** I do? I ____>
CHILD:	**Drank** some juice.
EDUCATOR:	Yes, I **did** and it was delicious. *[Drop some raisins on the table]*
EDUCATOR:	What happened to our bugs? They ____>
CHILD:	**Fell** down.
EDUCATOR:	I need to pick them up. I can't believe they **fell!**
EDUCATOR:	Wow, Jake is thirsty too. What **did** he do? He ____>
CHILD:	**Drank** juice.

[Continue in a similar manner until each child has had at least 10 opportunities to use irregular past tense verbs.]

Transition

EDUCATOR: That was a delicious snack. It's time to clean up and sing our ladybug song!

SONG ACTIVITY

Instructions: Chant to the rhythm of "Five Little Monkeys" emphasizing irregular past tense verbs. Encourage children to perform motions for the verbs as they are sung.

Five Little Ladybugs

Five little ladybugs jumping on the bed.
One **fell** off and **hurt** his head.

Mama called the doctor and the doctor **said,**
"No more ladybugs jumping on the bed!"

(Repeat for the numbers four, three, two, and one.)

Irregular Past Tense

Cycle 2, Session 2

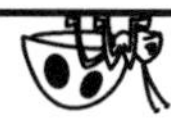

Theme: Animals

Description: Completing activities relating to bugs

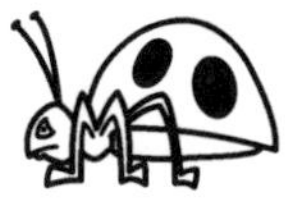

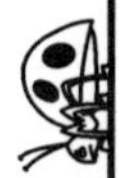

Exemplars: bent, brought, did, drew, fell, felt, found, gave, hung, hurt, made, said, stuck, thought, tore

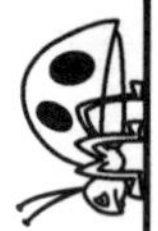

Materials:

- *The Grouchy Ladybug* by Eric Carle
- Photocopies of ladybug leaves (see pages 285–286 for directions and a pattern; 1 per child)
- Child-safe scissors
- Crayons or markers
- Tape
- Bag containing:
  - Red dot stickers
  - Completed ladybug leaves (see pages 285–286 for directions and a pattern)
  - Black markers

BOOK ACTIVITY

Book: *The Grouchy Ladybug* by Eric Carle

Instructions: Reread the book with children, emphasizing irregular past tense verbs.

Suggested Theme-Related Supplemental Books:

The Very Quiet Cricket by Eric Carle
The Very Lonely Firefly by Eric Carle
Franklin Goes to School
by Paulette Bourgeois and Brenda Clark (illustrator)

Transition

EDUCATOR: Remember how the ladybug in our story liked to crawl on leaves? Today we are going to make some leaves and some ladybugs to crawl on them!

FOCUSED STIMULATION ACTIVITY

Description: Coloring and cutting out leaves

Skill Used: Fine motor

Instructions: After children complete tasks, comment on what they did to obligate irregular past tense verbs.

Example Script

EDUCATOR:	Look at this picture. *[Present a picture in the book of ladybugs crawling on leaves]* See how the ladybugs crawled on the leaves? I **thought** that today we could make some leaves for bugs to crawl on. *[Give children leaf templates, scissors, and crayons or markers and instruct them to color and cut out leaves; keep some materials in the bag]*
EDUCATOR:	Look, Sally **made** a leaf!
EDUCATOR:	Uh-oh, Miguel **bent** his leaf!
EDUCATOR:	I **tore** my leaf!
EDUCATOR:	That leaf **felt** rough.
EDUCATOR:	I **brought** lots of leaves for us to make.
EDUCATOR:	Look, I **found** more leaves.
EDUCATOR:	Miguel **gave** Jane a marker. That's so nice!
EDUCATOR:	You **made** so many leaves! Our ladybugs will love to crawl on them!
EDUCATOR:	We need to hang the leaves on the wall.
EDUCATOR:	Sally, see if you can find something we could use to hang our leaves.
EDUCATOR:	Look, Sally **found** some tape.
EDUCATOR:	We can use tape to hang our leaves.
EDUCATOR:	Look, we **hung** up lots of leaves. Now we just need some ladybugs!

[Continue in a similar manner until numerous models of irregular past tense verbs have been provided.]

Transition

EDUCATOR: We made lots of leaves, but we need something to put on them. I thought we could put some ladybugs on them, just like in our story.

ELICITED PRODUCTION ACTIVITY

Description: Making ladybugs to put on leaves

Skills Used: Fine motor and gross motor

Goal: 10 productions of irregular past tense verbs per child

Level of Educator Support: Cloze task (_____> indicates educator's pause for child to fill in the blank)

Example Script

EDUCATOR: Look in this bag. What **did** you find? You _____>

CHILD: **Found** some red stickers!

EDUCATOR: You could use the stickers to make a bug. We need to put something else on these stickers first to make them into bugs. We need to draw some spots on them. *[Present a picture of a ladybug in the book and focus children's attention on the spots; have children draw black dots on the red sticker "bugs"; present a completed model]*

EDUCATOR: Jane, what **did** you do? You _____>

CHILD: **Drew** spots!

EDUCATOR: You **drew** lots of spots!

EDUCATOR: John, look in the bag. What **did** you find? You _____>

CHILD: **Found** more bugs.

EDUCATOR: You **did**? You **found** more bugs! *[After all bugs are made, model sticking them on leaves]*

EDUCATOR: What **did** we do with our bugs after we made them? We _____>

CHILD: **Stuck** them on the leaves.

EDUCATOR: Yes, you **stuck** them on the leaves. Now it's Jane's turn.

CHILD: *[Sticks a bug on a leaf]*

EDUCATOR: What **did** you do? You _____>

CHILD: **Stuck** it.

EDUCATOR: Yes, you **stuck** the bug on the leaf. *[Make a ladybug fall]*

EDUCATOR: Uh-oh, what happened to the bug? He _____>

CHILD: **Fell** down.

[Continue in a similar manner until each child has had at least 10 opportunities to use irregular past tense verbs.]

Transition

Educator: We **made** lots of ladybugs. It's time to clean up and sing our ladybug song!

SONG ACTIVITY

Instructions: Chant to the rhythm of "Five Little Monkeys," emphasizing irregular past tense verbs. Encourage children to perform motions for the verbs as they are sung.

Five Little Ladybugs

Five little ladybugs jumping on the bed.
One **fell** off and **hurt** his head.

Mama called the doctor and the doctor **said,**
"No more ladybugs jumping on the bed!"

(Repeat for the numbers four, three, two, and one.)

Weekly Family Letter

For: ______________________________ **Date:** ____________

Theme

Our theme for language intervention this week is *animals.*

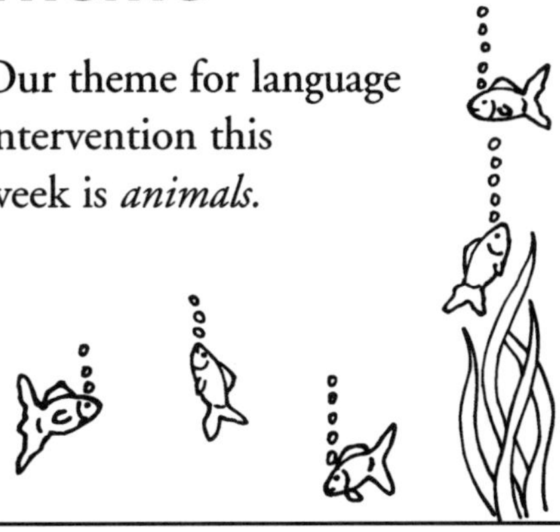

Target

Our target language structures are *regular past tense verbs.* These are verbs that indicate past actions and have regular *-ed* endings. Examples include:

- I **tickled** my baby brother.
- We **played** outside.
- Dad **cleaned** the kitchen.

Book

Our book for the week is *The Rainbow Fish* by Marcus Pfister.

Here are some related books you could read at home: *One Fish, Two Fish, Red Fish, Blue Fish* by Dr. Seuss; *Swimmy* by Leo Lionni; and *Froggy Gets Dressed* by Jonathan London and Frank Remkiewicz (illustrator).

Song

Little Fish, Little Fish
(Tune: "Little Bunny Foo Foo")

Little fish, little fish **moved** in the water.
Little fish, little fish **jumped** in the waves.

Little fish, little fish **moved** in the water.
Little fish, little fish **chased** his friend away.

Little fish, little fish **moved** in the water.
Little fish, little fish **played** all day long!

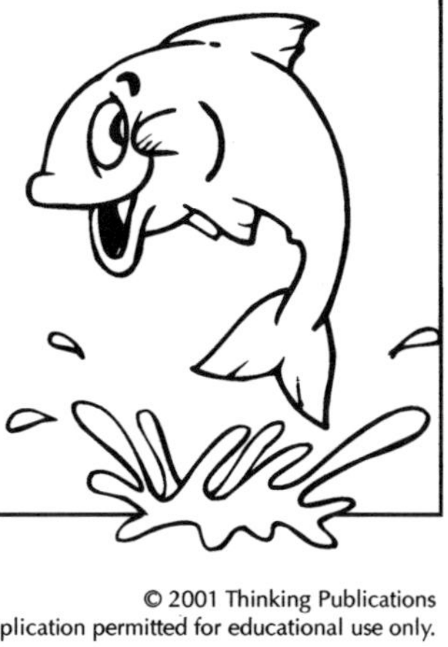

Activities

Our planned activities for the week include:

- Discussing events in the book using regular past tense verbs
- Making a paper plate fish
- Having crackers that look like fish
- Going on a pretend fishing trip

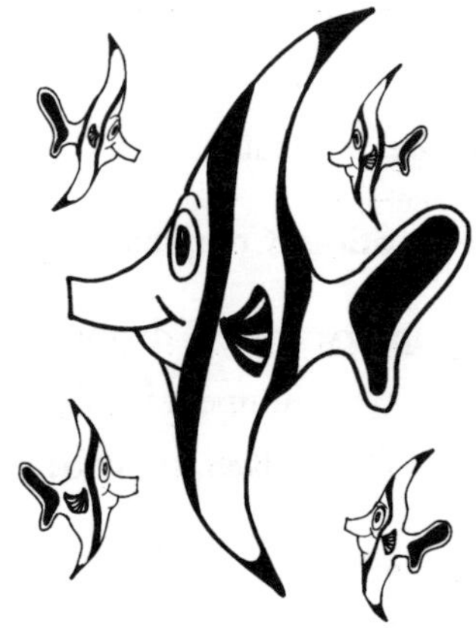

Follow-Up

Suggested follow-up activities for home include:

- Ask your child to retell *The Rainbow Fish* using regular past tense verbs.
- Make a paper plate fish, or have your child tell you how he or she made fish in language intervention using regular past tense verbs, for example:

  I **glued** the beads on the fish.

  I **colored** his mouth.

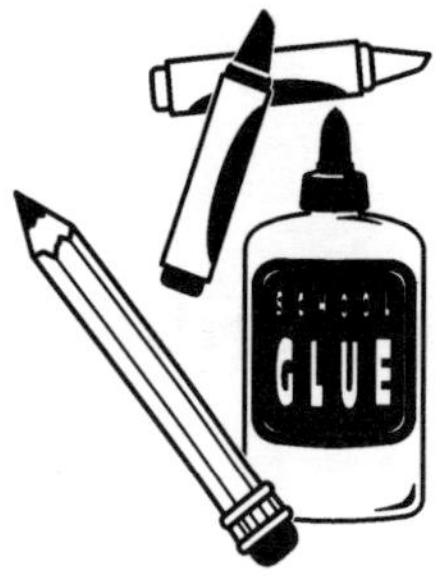

Thank You Very Much for your participation!

____
Phone Number

____
Email

____
Signature

Regular Past Tense

Cycle 2, Session 1

Theme: Animals

Description: Completing activities relating to fish

Exemplars: chased, disappeared, folded, followed, glued, happened, helped, jumped, laughed, liked, lived, looked, moved, played, shared, talked, touched, turned, wanted

Materials:

The Rainbow Fish by Marcus Pfister
Completed Rainbow Fish
(see page 287 for directions)
Rainbow Fish bodies
(see page 287 for directions; 1 per child)
Aluminum foil
Sequins
Glue
Scissors
Google eyes
Puppet

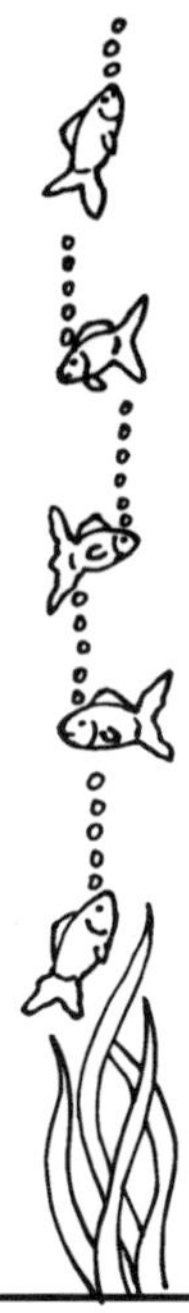

INTRODUCTION TO THEME

Educator: Last week, we **talked** a bit about ladybugs. This week we're going to talk about fish. Let's read our story about fish.

BOOK ACTIVITY

Book: *The Rainbow Fish* by Marcus Pfister

Instructions: Read the book with the children, emphasizing regular past tense verbs.

Suggested Theme-Related Supplemental Books:
One Fish, Two Fish, Red Fish, Blue Fish by Dr. Seuss
Swimmy by Leo Lionni
Froggy Gets Dressed
by Jonathan London and Frank Remkiewicz (illustrator)

Transition

Educator: That was such a nice story. Let's talk a little bit about the Rainbow Fish and look at the pictures in our book.

FOCUSED STIMULATION ACTIVITY

Description: Discussing the story and pictures using regular past tense verbs

Skills Used: Narrative, sequencing, and describing

Example Script

EDUCATOR: The Rainbow Fish **lived** in the sea.

EDUCATOR: Look, the other fish **followed** him wherever he went!

EDUCATOR: Rainbow Fish **liked** the way his scales **looked**.

EDUCATOR: Rainbow Fish didn't share his scales. He **turned** and swam away!

EDUCATOR: The octopus **talked** to the Rainbow Fish.

EDUCATOR: The octopus **helped** Rainbow Fish make friends.

EDUCATOR: Look, the octopus **disappeared!**

EDUCATOR: What **happened** next?

CHILD: The little fish **touched** Rainbow Fish.

CHILD: He **wanted** to be his friend.

EDUCATOR: Rainbow Fish **shared** one of his beautiful scales.

EDUCATOR: Rainbow Fish **shared** all his beautiful scales. He **shared** with all the fish.

EDUCATOR: The fish all **laughed** and **played** together.

EDUCATOR: They became friends because Rainbow Fish **shared** with them.

[Continue in a similar manner until numerous models of regular past tense verbs have been provided.]

Transition

EDUCATOR: What a nice story that was. Today we will make a Rainbow Fish to take home. Look at this pretty Rainbow Fish. *[Present model]* Let's make one just like it.

ELICITED PRODUCTION ACTIVITY

Description: Making paper plate Rainbow Fish

Skills Used: Predicting, fine motor, and sequencing

Goal: 10 productions of regular past tense verbs per child

Level of Educator Support: Cloze task (____> indicates educator's pause for child to fill in the blank)

Instructions: Prepare a Rainbow Fish prior to the activity to serve as a model. Have

Example Script

EDUCATOR: Look at this Rainbow Fish I made. *[Present model]* How do you think I made it? After we figure out how to make it, you are going to make one like it to take home!

EDUCATOR: How did I get these pretty things (sequins) to stay on? *[Point to glue on foil].* I ____>

CHILD: **Glued** them on.

EDUCATOR: Yes I did. I **glued** lots of shiny stuff on the fish.

EDUCATOR: See, I **folded** the shiny stuff on the back like this. *[Demonstrate]*

EDUCATOR: What did I do? I ____>

CHILD: **Folded** it.

EDUCATOR: I **folded** it so that it wouldn't get messed up.

EDUCATOR: Next I **glued** colors on him.

EDUCATOR: What did I do? I ____>

CHILD: **Glued** colors on.

EDUCATOR: Yes, I **glued** the sequins on the fish. *[Have child complete the fish; then present a puppet]*

EDUCATOR: Now let's tell the puppet how we made our fish. First we ____>

CHILD: **Glued** shiny stuff on.

EDUCATOR: Then we ____>

CHILD: **Folded** the shiny stuff.

[Continue in a similar manner until each child has had at least 10 opportunities to use regular past tense verbs.]

Transition

EDUCATOR: Now that we all have a Rainbow Fish to take home, let's sing a song about our fish.

children look at the model Rainbow Fish. Discuss with children what was done to make the fish, targeting regular past tense verbs.

SONG ACTIVITY

Instructions: Sing to the tune of "Little Bunny Foo Foo," emphasizing regular past tense verbs.

Little Fish, Little Fish

Little fish, little fish **moved** in the water.
Little fish, little fish **jumped** in the waves.

Little fish, little fish **moved** in the water.
Little fish, little fish **chased** his friend away.

Little fish, little fish **moved** in the water.
Little fish, little fish **played** all day long!

Regular Past Tense

Cycle 2, Session 2

Theme: Animals

Description: Completing activities relating to fish

Exemplars: chased, chomped, dropped, fixed, handed, helped, jumped, looked, moved, packed, passed, planned, played, poured, pulled, seemed, shared, sipped, tasted, tied

Materials:

- *The Rainbow Fish* by Marcus Pfister
- Bag containing:
  - Fish-shaped crackers
  - Napkins (1 per child)
  - Juice boxes (1 per child)
- Blue blanket or rug
- Fishing pole (see page 288 for directions)
- Fish (see pages 288–289 for directions and patterns)
- Bucket
- Puppet

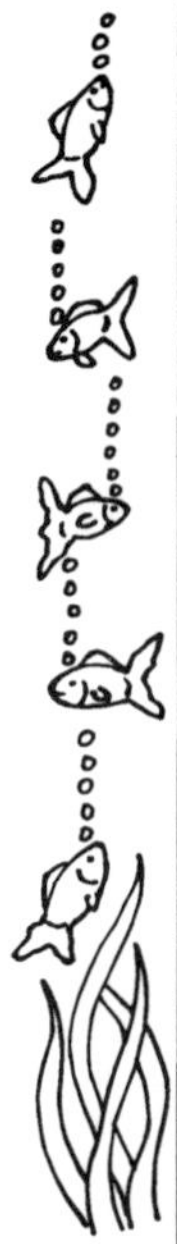

BOOK ACTIVITY

Book: *The Rainbow Fish* by Marcus Pfister

Instructions: Reread the book with children, emphasizing regular past tense verbs.

Suggested Theme-Related Supplemental Books:

One Fish, Two Fish, Red Fish, Blue Fish by Dr. Seuss
Swimmy by Leo Lionni
Froggy Gets Dressed by Jonathan London and Frank Remkiewicz (illustrator)

Transition

Educator: Today we are going to have a snack that reminds me of the story we just read!

FOCUSED STIMULATION ACTIVITY

Description: Having a snack

Skills Used: Sharing and turn taking

Example Script

EDUCATOR: Is anybody hungry? I brought a fish snack for us today. Sally, please look in that bag. Do you see any fish snacks? Please pull them out.

EDUCATOR: See, Sally **looked** in the bag, and she **pulled** out the fish crackers and napkins.

EDUCATOR: John, please pass out these napkins. See, John **passed** out the napkins.

EDUCATOR: Jane, please pour some crackers on Sally's napkin. Jane **poured** the fish out. She **poured** lots of fish.

EDUCATOR: Jake **tasted** his fish. How did it taste, Jake?

EDUCATOR: It looks like it **tasted** good!

EDUCATOR: I'm thirsty. Sally, when you **looked** in the bag, did you see some juice?

EDUCATOR: Sally **handed** me the juice.

EDUCATOR: Please pass out the juice. See, Sally **passed** out the juice.

EDUCATOR: I like to sip my juice through a straw. Watch. See, I **sipped** my juice.

[Continue in a similar manner until numerous models of regular past tense verbs have been provided.]

Transition

EDUCATOR: That was a delicious snack. Let's clean up and get ready to do something new!

ELICITED PRODUCTION ACTIVITY

Description: Going fishing

Skills Used: Gross motor and dramatic play

Goal: 10 productions of regular past tense verbs per child

Level of Educator Support: Cloze task (____> indicates educator's pause for child to fill in the blank)

Instructions: Put the blanket or rug on the floor, and tell children that it is the lake. Complete the fishing activity and then have children tell the puppet what they did using regular past tense verbs.

Example Script

EDUCATOR: Look at what I **planned** for us to do today. I **packed** a fishing pole in my bag. I thought we could go fishing.

EDUCATOR: [*Untie the string from the pole]* Uh-oh, our pole is broken. This broke. *[Show the string]* I need someone to fix it. Can you help me? First you need to tie this string on the stick.

EDUCATOR: What did John do? He ____>

CHILD: **Tied** it.

EDUCATOR: Yes, he **tied** it. Now we can go fishing.

EDUCATOR: I want to look in the lake to see our fish. Does anybody else want to look? What did you do? You ____>

CHILD: **Looked** in the lake.

EDUCATOR: You **looked** in and you saw lots of fish.

EDUCATOR: I need a helper to put these fish on the hook. *[Ask a child to help]*

EDUCATOR: What a good helper! You ____>

CHILD: **Helped.**

EDUCATOR: Chomp, chomp, chomp, the fish likes to chomp on this. *[Show the "hook"]*

EDUCATOR: What did the fish do? He ____>

CHILD: **Chomped** it.

EDUCATOR: He sure **seemed** hungry. I **dropped** him in the bucket.

EDUCATOR: Now it is someone else's turn. Thanks for sharing, John! What did you do? You ____>

CHILD: **Shared** it.

EDUCATOR: That was so nice of you. I am happy you **shared** your pole. *[Continue until each child has had a turn to fish]*

EDUCATOR: It's nice to share. Remember that in our book the fish became friends because Rainbow Fish **shared** with them. *[Present puppet]*

EDUCATOR: Now let's tell the puppet what we did today. First, we ____>

CHILD: **Fixed** our pole.

[Continue in a similar manner until each child has had at least 10 opportunities to use regular past tense verbs.]

Transition

EDUCATOR: I sure like to go fishing! Sometimes when I go fishing I sing songs. Let's sing our song about the little fish!

SONG ACTIVITY

Instructions: Sing to the tune of "Little Bunny Foo Foo," emphasizing regular past tense verbs.

Little Fish, Little Fish

Little fish, little fish **moved** in the water.
Little fish, little fish **jumped** in the waves.

Little fish, little fish **moved** in the water.
Little fish, little fish **chased** his friend away.

Little fish, little fish **moved** in the water.
Little fish, little fish **played** all day long!

Weekly Family Letter

For: ______________________ **Date:** ____________

Theme

Our theme for language intervention this week is *animals.*

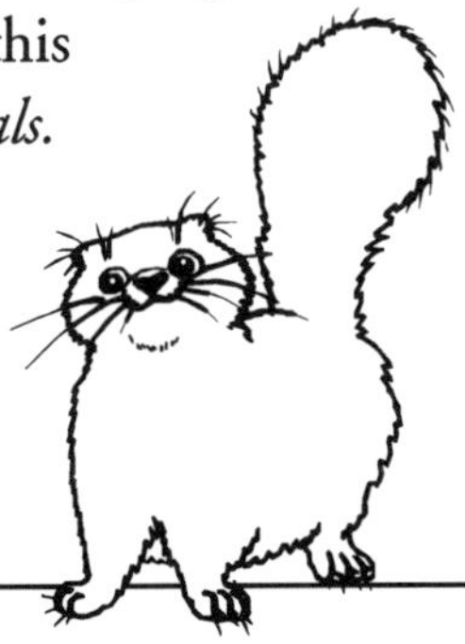

Target

Our target language structures are *copula* be *verbs.* These include the verbs *am ('m), are ('re),* and *is ('s)* when used as the only verb in a sentence. Examples include:

- I **am** happy.
- We'**re** late.
- Daddy **is** tall.

Book

Our book this week is *Have You Seen My Cat?* by Eric Carle.

Here is a related book you could read at home: *The Tale of Tom Kitten* abridged by Marian Hoffman.

Song

Where Is Kitty?
(Tune: "Where Is Thumbkin?")

Where **is** kitty? Where **is** kitty?
Here I **am!** Here I **am!**

I **am** very pretty. I **am** very pretty.
Here I **am!** Here I **am!**

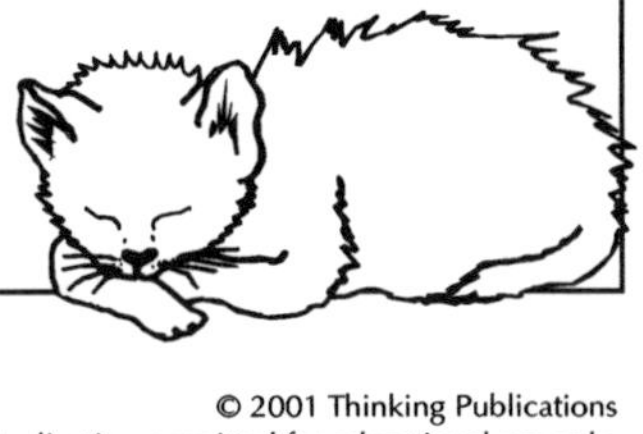

Activities

Our planned activities for the week include:

- Making a cat mask
- Playing show-and-tell using the cat mask
- Going on a "cat hunt" (searching for cat pictures)
- Making a category poster using pictures of cats and other animals

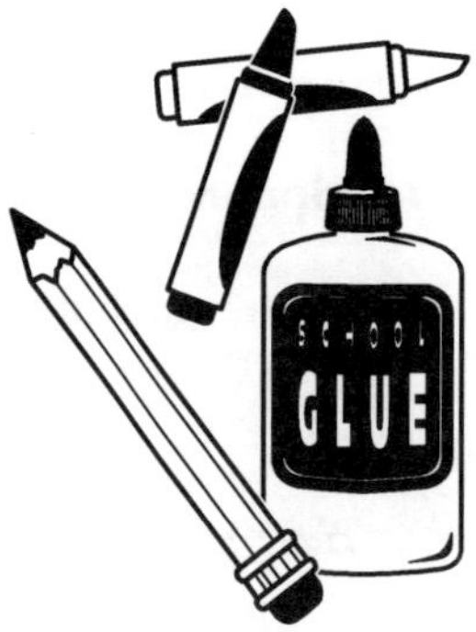

Follow-Up

Suggested follow-up activities for home include:

- Have your child describe features of particular items. Because our theme is cats, you might want to have your child discuss features of a pet cat, if you have one, or cat pictures in a book or magazine, for example:

  This **is** a pretty cat.

  The cat's eyes **are** blue.

  The cat**'s** soft!

- Have your child describe his or her stuffed animals, for example:

  My bear **is** brown.

  My bunnies **are** little.

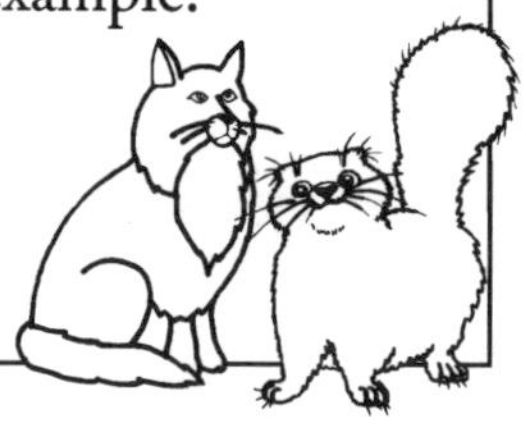

Thank You Very Much for your participation!

____
Phone Number

____
Email

____
Signature

Copula *be*

Cycle 2, Session 1

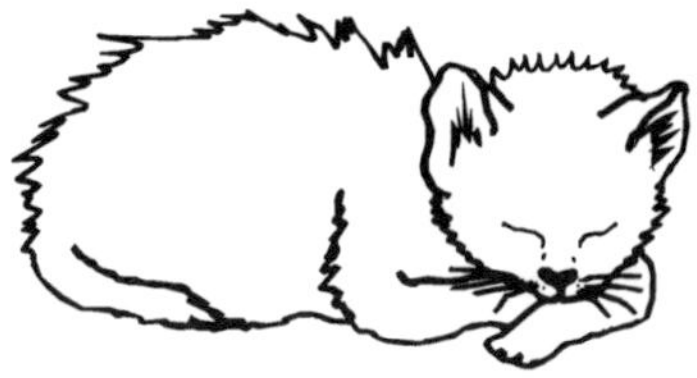

Theme: Animals

Description: Completing activities relating to cats

Exemplars: am ('m), are ('re), is ('s)

Materials:

- *Have You Seen My Cat?* by Eric Carle
- Completed cat ears and nose (see page 290 for directions)
- Paper cups (1 per child)
- Glue
- 3" pipe cleaner pieces (4 per child)
- 12" pieces of yarn (2 per child)
- 24" pieces of yarn (1 per child)
- Ears (see page 290 for directions; 1 pair per child)
- Pompons (1 per child)

INTRODUCTION TO THEME

EDUCATOR: We have been talking a lot about animals. We talked about fish, bugs, and bears. This week we are going to talk about another kind of animal that is a pet. This animal has whiskers, it purrs, and it meows. Can you guess what it is? *[Allow children to guess]* Yes! It**'s** a cat! Let's read our story about cats.

BOOK ACTIVITY

Book: *Have You Seen My Cat?* by Eric Carle

Instructions: Read the book with children, emphasizing copula *be* forms.

Suggested Theme-Related Supplemental Book: *The Tale of Tom Kitten* abridged by Marian Hoffman

Transition

EDUCATOR: Our book was about a cat, and today we are going to do an art project that has to do with cats. Are you ready to get started?

FOCUSED STIMULATION ACTIVITY

Description: Making cat masks (ears and noses)

Skill Used: Fine motor

Instructions: Prepare a mask prior to the activity to serve as a model.

Example Script

EDUCATOR: I thought we could make some masks today. We can wear our masks and pretend to be cats, just like the cat in our book.

EDUCATOR: This **is** a cat mask. *[Present model]*

EDUCATOR: This **is** a pink cat. These **are** his whiskers and these **are** his ears.

EDUCATOR: Let's get our stuff out to make our ears and noses. See, this **is** for the nose *[present nose materials]* and this **is** for the ears *[present ear materials].*

EDUCATOR: This part **is** the string. We tie the ears on our heads with the string.

EDUCATOR: These **are** pipe cleaners. *[Present pipe cleaner]* They **are** for the cat's whiskers.

EDUCATOR: This **is** a soft whisker!

EDUCATOR: These **are** little ears! *[Continue to use copula* be *to discuss attributes of the cat masks as children assemble their cat masks]*

EDUCATOR: This cat **is** so cute!

[Continue in a similar manner until numerous models of copula be *verbs have been provided.]*

Transition

EDUCATOR: You did such nice jobs making your cat masks. Let's show each other what we made!

ELICITED PRODUCTION ACTIVITY

Description: Playing show-and-tell using cat masks

Skills Used: Describing, sharing, and turn taking

Goal: 10 productions of copula *be* verbs per child

Level of Educator Support: Cloze task (____> indicates educator's pause for child to fill in the blank)

Example Script

EDUCATOR:	Let's talk about these neat cat masks. I'll go first. This **is** my cat.
EDUCATOR:	It **is** a girl cat. She **is** a playful cat. She **is** pink. She **is** kind of silly.
EDUCATOR:	Jane, tell us about your cat. Your cat ____>
CHILD:	**Is** little.
EDUCATOR:	Oh, your cat **is** little. **Is** it a boy or a girl? It ____>
CHILD:	**Is** a girl.
EDUCATOR:	Your cat **is** a girl! So **is** mine! They **are** two girl cats.
EDUCATOR:	**Is** your cat nice or mean? She ____>
CHILD:	**Is** mean.
EDUCATOR:	Oh no! Your cat **is** mean! Yikes, watch out everybody. Jane's cat **is** mean!
EDUCATOR:	John, now tell us about your cat. **Is** your cat blue or green? He ____>
CHILD:	**Is** blue.
EDUCATOR:	Your cat **is** blue? So **is** Sally's cat.
EDUCATOR:	**Is** your cat happy or sad? He ____>
CHILD:	**Is** happy.
EDUCATOR:	Great! All these cats ____>
CHILD:	**Are** happy!

[Continue in a similar manner until each child has had at least 10 opportunities to use copula be *verbs.]*

Transition

EDUCATOR: It was fun to talk about our cats. Let's clean up and then sing a song about a kitty!

SONG ACTIVITY

Instructions: Sing to the tune of "Where Is Thumbkin?" emphasizing copula *be* verbs.

Where Is Kitty?

Where **is** kitty? Where **is** kitty?
Here I **am!** Here I **am!**

I **am** very pretty. I **am** very pretty.
Here I **am!** Here I **am!**

Copula *be*

Cycle 2, Session 2

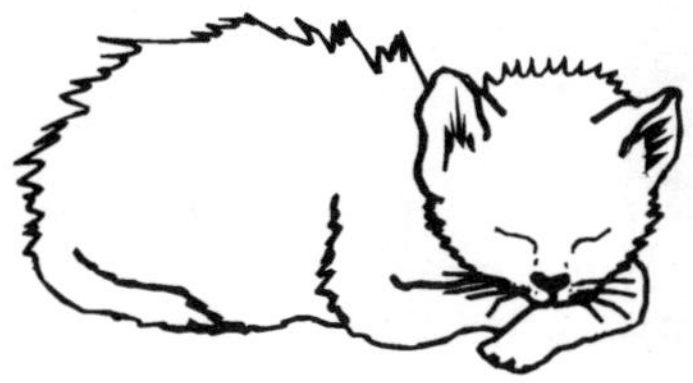

Theme: Animals

Description: Completing activities relating to cats

Exemplars: am ('m), are ('re), is ('s)

Materials:

Have You Seen My Cat? by Eric Carle
10 pictures of various animals (4 pictures that have cats and 4 that do not; see pages 283–284 for directions and patterns)
Poster board

BOOK ACTIVITY

Book: *Have You Seen My Cat?* by Eric Carle

Instructions: Reread the book with the children, emphasizing copula *be* verbs.

Suggested Theme-Related Supplemental Book: *The Tale of Tom Kitten* abridged by Marian Hoffman

Transition

EDUCATOR: I think somebody has been hiding cats in our room. These cats are like the ones we read about in our story! Let's see if we can find them!

FOCUSED STIMULATION ACTIVITY

Description: Going on a cat hunt

Skills Used: Gross motor, searching and finding, and categorization

Instructions: Tape cat pictures back-to-back on other animal pictures. Hide animal pictures prior to the activity.

Example Script

Educator:	Let's go on a cat hunt. We want to know if anyone has seen our cat. Look around the room. When you see a picture, take it off the wall. There **are** pictures of cats and there **are** pictures of other animals too. We want to find the cats! *[Demonstrate walking around the room and selecting a picture]*
Educator:	This **is** not a cat. This **is** a frog!
Educator:	Maria, what **is** that? It **is** a frog! It **is** not a cat!
Educator:	Put it on the table.
Educator:	Where **is** that silly cat? *[Children may comment as they look behind pictures]*
Child:	This **is** not a cat!
Child:	Here**'s** a cat!
Educator:	This **is** not a cat, it **is** a fish!
Educator:	Where **are** all the cats?!
Educator:	**Am** I a cat? No, I **am** not a cat! I **am** a person! Where **is** that cat?
Educator:	Where, oh where, **is** a cat?
Educator:	Cat, where **are** you?
Educator:	This **is** a cat!
Educator:	He **is** so cute!
Educator:	My cat **is** orange.
Educator:	Your cats **are** brown.

[Continue in a similar manner until numerous models of copula be *verbs have been provided.]*

Transition

Educator: We are going to do something with all the pictures we found. Everyone grab your pictures and get ready!

ELICITED PRODUCTION ACTIVITY

Description: Making a "cat" and "not cat" category poster

Skills Used: Fine motor and categorization

Goal: 10 productions of copula *be* verbs per child

Level of Educator Support: Cloze task (___> indicates educator's pause for child to fill in the blank)

Instructions: Draw a vertical line dividing the poster board into two halves: label one side "This **is** a cat" and the other side "This **is** not a cat." Glue the pictures found around the room, and extra copies of other animal pictures if desired, onto the appropriate side of the poster.

Example Script

EDUCATOR: Let's glue the pictures we found on to this poster. Let's put the cats on this side and all the other animals on this side. This side says "This **is** a cat." This side says "This **is** not a cat."

EDUCATOR: **Is** this a cat? *[Present a picture of an animal that is not a cat]* It ___>

CHILD: **Is** not a cat!

EDUCATOR: It**'s** not? Then let's glue it over here.

EDUCATOR: **Is** this a cat? It ___>

CHILD: **Is** an elephant.

EDUCATOR: It **is** an elephant! Then we need to glue it over here.

EDUCATOR: How about this? This ____>

CHILD: **Is** a fish.

EDUCATOR: This **is** a fish. You're right. It **is** not a cat. It **is** over here.

EDUCATOR: Tell me about these. These___>

CHILD: **Are** cats!

[Continue in a similar manner until each child has had at least 10 opportunities to use copula be *verbs.]*

Transition

EDUCATOR: You made a very nice picture with cats and other animals. Now let's clean up and sing our kitty song!

SONG ACTIVITY

Instructions: Sing to the tune of "Where Is Thumbkin?" emphasizing copula *be* verbs.

Where Is Kitty?

Where **is** kitty? Where **is** kitty?
Here I **am!** Here I **am!**

I **am** very pretty. I **am** very pretty.
Here I **am!** Here I **am!**

Weekly Family Letter

For: ______________________________ **Date:** ______________

Theme

Our theme for language intervention this week is *food.*

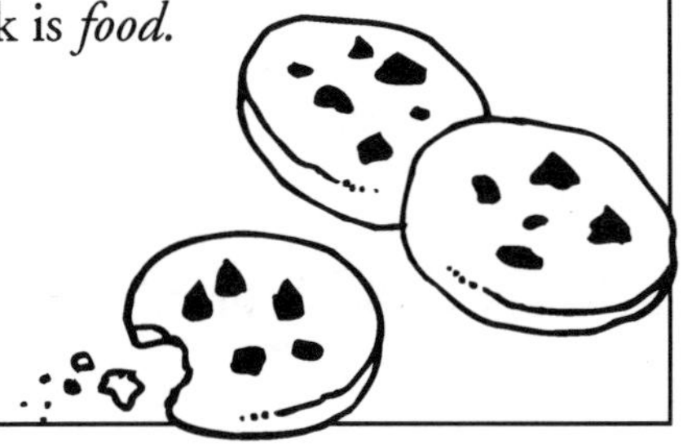

Target

Our target language structures are *regular third person singular verbs.* These verbs indicate actions by a single person or object and have a regular *-s* ending. Examples include:

- She **walks** to school.
- Jenny **eats** dinner every night.
- Dad **works** at a bank.

Book

Our book for the week is *If You Give a Mouse a Cookie* by Laura Joffe Numeroff and Felicia Bond (illustrator).

Here are some related books you could read at home: *If You Give a Pig a Pancake* by Laura Joffe Numeroff and Felicia Bond (illustrator) and *If You Give a Moose a Muffin* by Laura Joffe Numeroff and Felicia Bond (illustrator).

Song

Hungry, Hungry Little Mouse
(Tune: "Twinkle, Twinkle, Little Star")

Hungry, hungry little mouse **eats** all the cookies in the house.

He **eats** them fast. He **eats** them slow.
He **eats** them everywhere he **goes.**

Hungry, hungry little mouse **eats** all the cookies in the house.

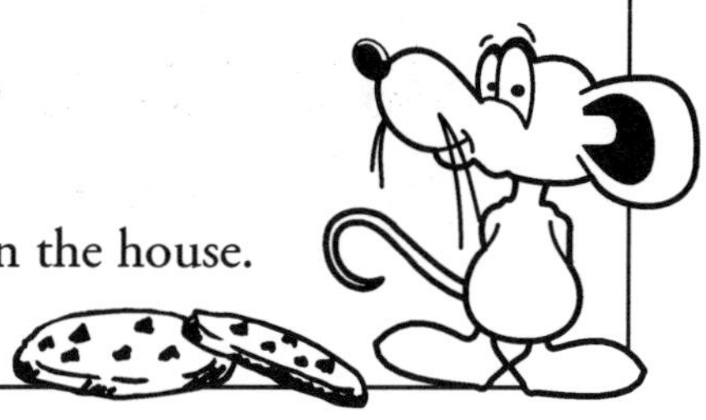

Activities

Our planned activities for the week include:

- Making construction paper cookies and feeding them to a mouse puppet
- Making felt mice to use in a story reenactment
- Reenacting the story *If You Give a Mouse a Cookie*

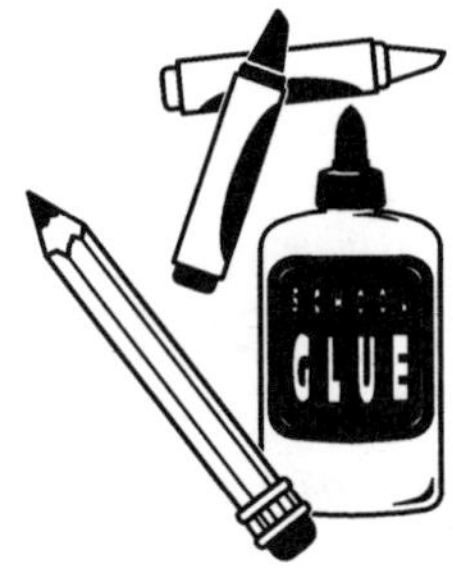

Follow-Up

Suggested follow-up activities for home include:

- Have your child "narrate" actions in a storybook or television show following your model, for example

  The girl **opens** the present.

  The present **looks** like a kitty!

  The girl **hugs** her mom and **tells** her thank you!

- Encourage your child to tell what his or her stuffed animals do, for example:

  Bear **likes** to sleep.

  Monkey **eats** bananas.

Thank You Very Much for your participation!

Phone Number

Email

Signature

Regular Third Person Singular

Cycle 3, Session 1

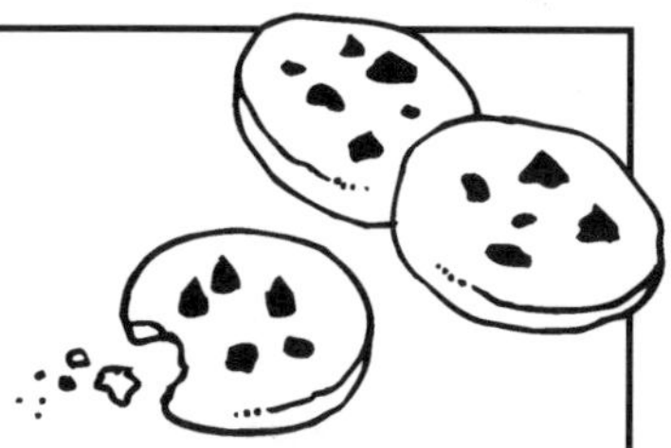

Theme: Food

Description: Completing activities relating to cookies

Exemplars: bites, eats, feeds, feels, finds, gets, gives, goes, grabs, likes, looks, makes, opens, puts, sees, sticks, takes, wants

Materials:

If You Give a Mouse a Cookie by Laura Joffe Numeroff and Felicia Bond (illustrator)
Bag containing:
Glue
Cookies (see page 291 for directions)
Cookie decorations (see page 291 for directions)
Milk carton mouse (see pages 291–292 for directions and a pattern)

INTRODUCTION TO THEME

Educator: For the next few weeks, we are going to be talking about food. What kind of food do you like to eat? *[Allow children to respond]* When do we eat food? *[Allow children to respond]* All people need to eat food. Last time we talked about animals. Animals need to eat food just like people do. A mouse is an animal, and today we are going to talk about a mouse who **likes** to eat a sweet kind of food. Who can guess what kind of food the mouse **likes** to eat? *[Allow children to respond]*

BOOK ACTIVITY

Book: *If You Give a Mouse a Cookie*
by Laura Joffe Numeroff and Felicia Bond (illustrator)

Instructions: Read the book with children. Comment on the story using regular third person singular verbs.

Suggested Theme-Related Supplemental Books: *If You Give a Pig a Pancake* by Laura Joffe Numeroff and Felicia Bond (illustrator)
If You Give a Moose a Muffin by Laura Joffe Numeroff and Felicia Bond (illustrator)

Transition

EDUCATOR: That was a great story! Now let's make some cookies like the mouse ate in our story!

FOCUSED STIMULATION ACTIVITY

Description: Decorating paper cookies

Skill Used: Fine motor

Instructions: Glue construction paper chocolate chips and other decorations (e.g., various colored shapes) on construction paper cookies. For sessions with several children, narrate what children are doing as they do it using names to create natural opportunities to use regular third person singular verbs. For sessions with an individual child, use objects or characters in the story as subjects for utterances instead of people (e.g., "This cookie **tastes** delicious *[Pretend to eat a cookie],"* "This bag **feels** heavy," and "The chocolate chip **sticks** on the cookie").

Example Script

EDUCATOR: I have lots of things we can use to make cookies. Let's see what we have. Let's look in this bag. *[Hold out the bag for children to look in]*

EDUCATOR: Jake **looks** in the bag.

EDUCATOR: He **sees** some scissors.

EDUCATOR: Now Jane **takes** a turn.

EDUCATOR: She **finds** some glue.

EDUCATOR: That **looks** like a chocolate chip.

EDUCATOR: Now John **grabs** his glue.

Continued on next page

Example Script—*Continued*

EDUCATOR:	Look what he does with it!
CHILD:	He **sticks** chips on the cookie.
EDUCATOR:	Next John **puts** glue on his chip.
EDUCATOR:	He **sticks** the chip on the cookie.
EDUCATOR:	Now it's Maria's turn. Maria **likes** the green circles.
EDUCATOR:	She **puts** circles on her cookie.
EDUCATOR:	Maria **makes** very pretty cookies!
EDUCATOR:	Now Jake **sticks** three red squares on the cookie.
EDUCATOR:	Jake's cookie **looks** very yummy!

[Continue in a similar manner until numerous models of regular third person singular verbs have been provided.]

Transition

EDUCATOR: Look at all these yummy cookies we made! Remember the mouse in our story? He liked to eat cookies. Let's feed our cookies to this mouse! *[Present milk carton mouse]*

ELICITED PRODUCTION ACTIVITY

Description: Feeding cookies to the milk carton mouse

Skills Used: Gross motor and dramatic play

Goal: 10 productions of regular third person singular verbs per child

Level of Educator Support: Preparatory set

Instructions: Prepare the milk carton mouse prior to the activity.

Example Script

EDUCATOR:	We have all these cookies. Our mouse **feels** hungry. He **wants** to eat the cookies. Watch. The mouse **opens** his mouth. Jane, tell John what the mouse does.
CHILD:	He **opens** his mouth.
EDUCATOR:	Yes, he **opens** his mouth.
EDUCATOR:	Now Jake **puts** the cookie in the mouse's mouth.
EDUCATOR:	Jane, tell me what the mouse does now.
CHILD:	He **eats** the cookie!
EDUCATOR:	Yes, he **eats** it up.
EDUCATOR:	Now it's Jane's turn to feed the mouse. What does she do?
CHILD:	She **feeds** the mouse.
EDUCATOR:	Yes, Jane **feeds** the mouse and then what happens?
CHILD:	The mouse **eats** the cookie. *[Have the mouse "bite" one of the children's fingers]*
EDUCATOR:	Oh no! What does that mouse do now?
CHILD:	He **bites** me!
EDUCATOR:	Oh, he **gets** in trouble for that!
EDUCATOR:	Look at John. What does he do?
CHILD:	He **gives** the mouse a cookie.

[Continue in a similar manner until each child has had at least 10 opportunities to use regular third person singular verbs.]

Transition

EDUCATOR: Our mouse sure was hungry! Let's sing a song about our hungry little mouse!

SONG ACTIVITY

Instructions: Sing to the tune of "Twinkle, Twinkle, Little Star," emphasizing regular third person singular verbs.

Hungry, Hungry Little Mouse

Hungry, hungry little mouse
eats all the cookies in the house.

He **eats** them fast. He **eats** them slow.
He **eats** them everywhere he **goes.**

Hungry, hungry little mouse
eats all the cookies in the house.

Regular Third Person Singular

Cycle 3, Session 2

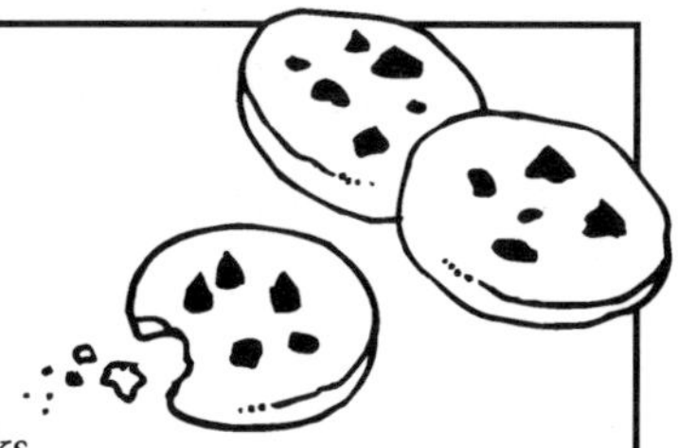

Theme: Food

Description: Completing activities relating to cookies

Exemplars: asks, drinks, eats, gets, glues, goes, happens, likes, looks, makes, needs, picks, puts, takes

Materials:

If You Give a Mouse a Cookie by Laura Joffe Numeroff and Felicia Bond (illustrator)
Completed felt mouse (see pages 293–294 for directions and patterns)
Bag containing:
- Felt mouse cutouts (see pages 293–294 for directions and patterns; 1 set per child)
- Glue

Felt board
Felt mouse story cutouts (see pages 293 and 295–296 for directions and patterns; 1 set)

BOOK ACTIVITY

Book: *If You Give a Mouse a Cookie*
by Laura Joffe Numeroff and Felicia Bond (illustrator)

Instructions: Reread the book to children. Then go back and discuss using regular third person singular verbs.

Suggested Theme-Related Supplemental Books: *If You Give a Pig a Pancake*
by Laura Joffe Numeroff and Felicia Bond (illustrator)
If You Give a Moose a Muffin
by Laura Joffe Numeroff and Felicia Bond (illustrator)

Transition

Educator: Today we are each going to make a mouse like the one in our story.

FOCUSED STIMULATION ACTIVITY

Description: Decorating felt mice

Skill Used: Fine motor

Instructions: Each child will decorate (i.e., put on a face and clothing) a felt mouse. Make a mouse prior to the activity to serve as a model. For sessions with several children, narrate what children are doing as they do it using names to create natural opportunities to use regular third person singular verbs. For sessions with an individual child, use objects or characters in the story as subjects for utterances (e.g., "This bag **feels** heavy," "The shirt **looks** pretty!" and "The mouse **looks** great in his outfit!"

Example Script

EDUCATOR: I have some things in this bag that we can use to make our mouse look more like the one in our story. When we are all done, we can have our mouse eat cookies!

EDUCATOR: John, look in here. See, John **looks** in the bag.

EDUCATOR: Now Sally **gets** the glue.

EDUCATOR: Let's see what she does next. She **picks** some pants.

EDUCATOR: She **glues** the pants on the mouse.

EDUCATOR: Now it's Jane's turn. She **likes** the pink nose.

EDUCATOR: She **puts** the nose on her mouse.

EDUCATOR: Jane **makes** a very cute mouse!

EDUCATOR: Now Jake **puts** some eyes on his mouse.

EDUCATOR: John's mouse **looks** like the mouse in the story.

[Continue in a similar manner until mice have been decorated and numerous models of regular third person singular verbs have been provided.]

Transition

EDUCATOR: Now each person has a mouse that is just like the one in the story. Let's look at our book and make our own story on this. *[Present felt board]* Let's see what **happens** after our mouse eats a cookie.

ELICITED PRODUCTION ACTIVITY

Description: Reenacting the events in *If You Give a Mouse a Cookie*

Skills Used: Narrative, fine motor, and sequencing

Goal: 10 productions of regular third person singular verbs per child

Level of Educator Support: Preparatory set

Instructions: Put one child's felt mouse on the felt board and have children add felt pieces in the order they appeared in the story. For sessions with several children, use the following script. For sessions with an individual child, use objects or characters in the story as subjects for utterances instead of people (e.g., "The mouse **asks** for a cookie," "He **drinks** some milk," and "The mouse **sweeps** the floor").

Example Script

Educator: Let's look at our book. What does the mouse do first?

Child: He **asks** for a cookie.

Educator: Yes, he **asks** for a cookie.

Educator: So look, Jane **puts** a cookie on the felt board.

Educator: Jane, tell us what the mouse does now. *[Consult story]*

Child: He **drinks** milk.

Educator: Yes, he **drinks** milk. Next, the mouse **asks** for a straw.

Educator: What does that silly mouse need now?

Child: He **needs** a straw.

Educator: Look at our story. What does the mouse do now?

Child: He **gets** a napkin.

Educator: Yes he **gets** a napkin, so Jane **puts** a napkin on the felt board.

[Continue in a similar manner until the story has been told and each child has had at least 10 opportunities to use regular third person singular verbs.]

Transition

EDUCATOR: It was fun to retell the story! Now it's time to clean up and sing our mouse song!

SONG ACTIVITY

Instructions: Sing to the tune of "Twinkle, Twinkle, Little Star," emphasizing regular third person singular verbs.

Hungry, Hungry Little Mouse

Hungry, hungry little mouse
eats all the cookies in the house.

He **eats** them fast. He **eats** them slow.
He **eats** them everywhere he **goes.**

Hungry, hungry little mouse
eats all the cookies in the house.

Weekly Family Letter

For: ______________________ **Date:** ____________

Theme

Our theme for language intervention this week is *food.*

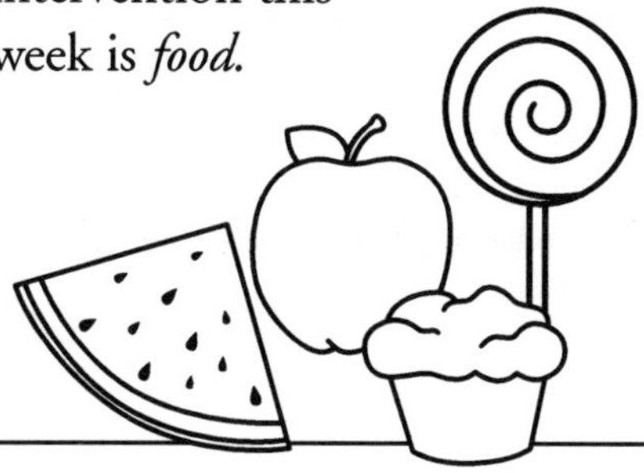

Target

Our target language structures are *irregular past tense verbs.* These verbs indicate past actions, but they do not have the regular *-ed* ending. Examples include:

- The sun **came** out.
- The caterpillar **ate** a plum.
- Mom **broke** the cup.

Book

Our book for the week is *The Very Hungry Caterpillar* by Eric Carle.

Here is a related book you could read at home: *What's for Lunch?* by Eric Carle.

Song

The Hungry Caterpillar
(Tune: "If You're Happy and You Know It")

The hungry caterpillar **ate** his lunch!
The hungry caterpillar **ate** his lunch!

He **ate, ate, ate**
until he cleaned up his plate.

He **ate, ate, ate** all his lunch!

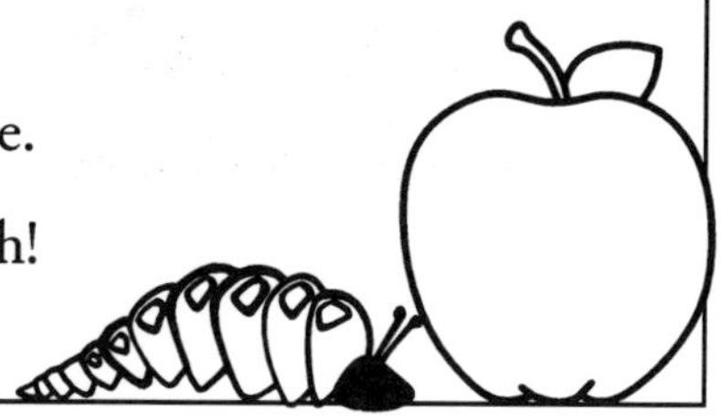

Activities

Our planned activities for the week include:

- Making a hungry caterpillar sock puppet
- Feeding food to the caterpillar puppet
- Cutting out food pictures from magazines
- Making a food collage out of magazine pictures

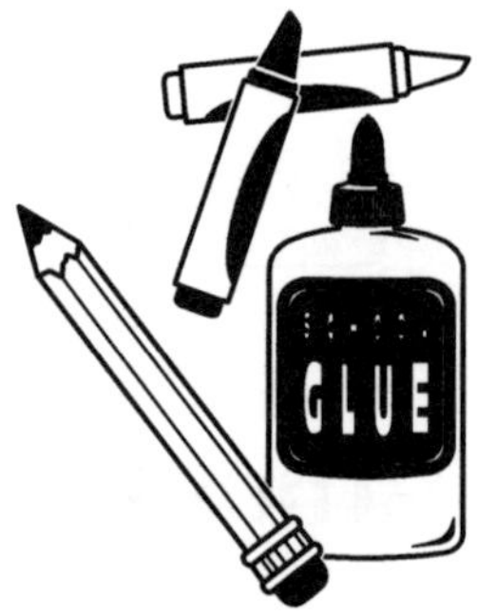

Follow-Up

Suggested follow-up activities for home include:

- Ask your child to tell you the story of *The Very Hungry Caterpillar* using irregular past tense verbs, for example:

  The caterpillar **ate** some cake.

  He **bit** a pear.

  He **had** lots to eat.

- Ask your child to tell you how he or she made the sock puppet, for example:

  We **stuck** eyes on the sock.

  We **made** spots on the caterpillar.

  The caterpillar puppet **ate** his food.

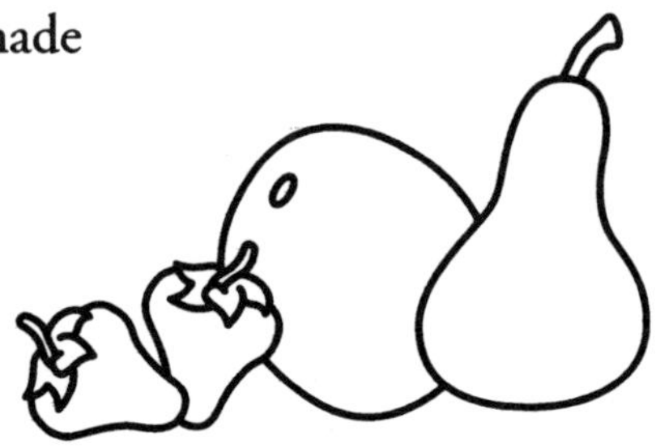

Thank You Very Much for your participation!

Phone Number

Email

Signature

Irregular Past Tense

Cycle 3, Session 1

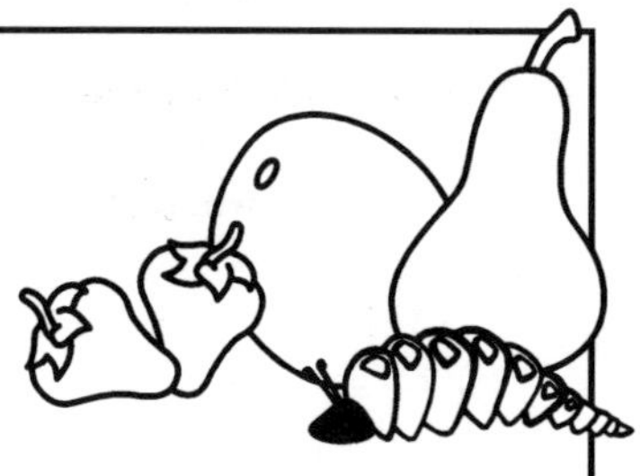

Theme: Food

Description: Completing activities relating to *The Very Hungry Caterpillar*

Exemplars: ate, broke, brought, did, drew, fed, gave, had, made, saw, stuck, thought

Materials:

The Very Hungry Caterpillar by Eric Carle
Completed caterpillar sock puppet (see page 297 for directions)
Light-colored adult socks (1 per child)
Felt mouths (see page 297 for directions; 1 per child)
Decorations (sequins, beads, etc.)
Glue
Pipe cleaner (1 piece per child)
Markers
Felt food (see pages 297–299 for directions and patterns; 1 set per child)
Child-safe scissors

INTRODUCTION TO THEME

EDUCATOR: Last time we talked about a mouse who was hungry. What **did** the mouse eat when he was hungry? *[Allow children to respond].* Yes, he **ate** a cookie. After he **ate** a cookie, he **did** lots of funny things. Today we are going to talk about a caterpillar who was hungry just like the mouse. But this caterpillar was so hungry that he **did**n't eat just one thing, like a cookie. He **ate** lots and lots of food.

BOOK ACTIVITY

Book: *The Very Hungry Caterpillar* by Eric Carle

Instructions: Read the book with children, emphasizing irregular past tense verbs.

Suggested Theme-Related Supplemental Book: *What's for Lunch?* by Eric Carle

Transition

EDUCATOR: Wow, that caterpillar sure was hungry! I **thought** it would be fun to make caterpillars just like the one in the story!

FOCUSED STIMULATION ACTIVITY

Description: Making hungry caterpillar sock puppets

Skills Used: Fine motor and direction following

Instructions: Prepare a caterpillar sock puppet prior to the activity to serve as a model. Narrate children's actions after they complete each task to create natural opportunities to produce irregular past tense verbs.

Example Script

EDUCATOR: You are each going to make a caterpillar puppet today. You will make your puppet with a sock. *[Present sock]* You can use all these things to decorate your puppets. *[Present decorations]* When you are done, your puppet should look something like this. *[Present completed model]* Let's get started and see what our caterpillars will look like.

EDUCATOR: John **made** a big mouth for his caterpillar.

EDUCATOR: You **stuck** two eyes on your caterpillar.

EDUCATOR: I **saw** some strings on Sally's caterpillar.

EDUCATOR: John **drew** eyebrows on his caterpillar.

EDUCATOR: I **broke** my caterpillar's antenna!

EDUCATOR: Jane **had** three spots on her caterpillar.

EDUCATOR: We **made** so many caterpillars!

[Continue in similar manner until all caterpillars have been made and numerous models of irregular past tense verbs have been provided.]

Transition

EDUCATOR: Now we all have caterpillars. Remember what the caterpillar in our story **did?** *[Children respond]* That's right. He **ate** lots of food. What should we do with our caterpillar? *[Children respond]* Good, let's feed him!

ELICITED PRODUCTION ACTIVITY

Description: Feeding caterpillars food (consult the story for order)

Skills Used: Narrative, gross motor, dramatic play, and sequencing

Goal: 10 productions of irregular past tense verbs per child

Level of Educator Support: Preparatory set

Example Script

EDUCATOR: Remember the caterpillar in our story? He was very hungry, so he **ate** lots of food. First he **ate** an apple. Then he **ate** two pears. What did he do next?

CHILD: He **ate** three plums.

EDUCATOR: Yes he **did**! Let's feed our caterpillars this food I **brought**. Who is first? *[Feed the caterpillar something]* What **did** he do?

CHILD: **Ate** an apple!

EDUCATOR: Tell us what the caterpillar did next. *[Look in the book]*

CHILD: He **ate** two pears.

EDUCATOR: Yes, he **ate** two pears.

EDUCATOR: Jane, tell us what the caterpillar **did** next.

CHILD: He **ate** four strawberries.

EDUCATOR: OK, feed him four strawberries, John.

EDUCATOR: Tell me what John **did**.

CHILD: He **fed** the caterpillar.

EDUCATOR: Yes, he **fed** him some strawberries.

EDUCATOR: Then what happened?

CHILD: He **gave** him a plum.

[Continue in a similar manner until all food is eaten and each child has had at least 10 opportunities to use irregular past tense verbs.]

Transition

EDUCATOR: Our caterpillars sure **ate** lots of food! Now it's time to sing a song about a hungry caterpillar who eats lots of food. Do you want to hear it?

SONG ACTIVITY

Instructions: Sing to the tune of "If You're Happy and You Know It," emphasizing irregular past tense verbs. Felt food items may be held up as the children sing about them.

The Hungry Caterpillar

The hungry caterpillar **ate** his lunch!
The hungry caterpillar **ate** his lunch!

He **ate, ate, ate**
until he cleaned up his plate.

He **ate, ate, ate** all his lunch!

Irregular Past Tense

Cycle 3, Session 2

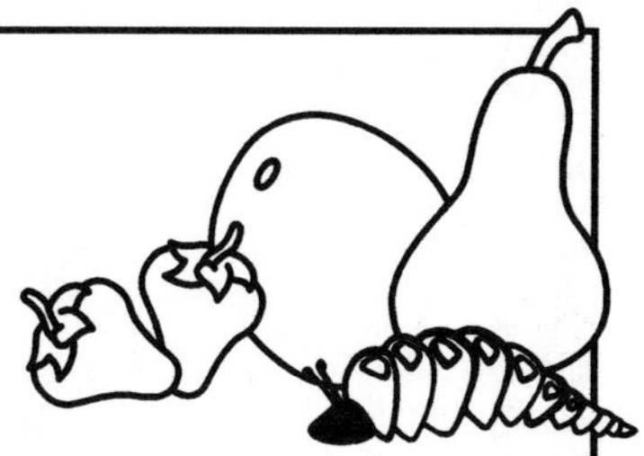

Theme: Food

Description: Completing activities relating to *The Very Hungry Caterpillar*

Exemplars: ate, did, found, gave, had, have, hid, saw, thought, tore

Materials:

The Very Hungry Caterpillar by Eric Carle
Magazines containing food pictures
Child-safe scissors
Glue
Construction paper

BOOK ACTIVITY

Book: *The Very Hungry Caterpillar* by Eric Carle

Instructions: Reread the book with children, emphasizing irregular past tense verbs.

Suggested Theme-Related Supplemental Book: *What's for Lunch?* by Eric Carle.

Transition

Educator: That caterpillar sure **ate** a lot of food! Today we are going to cut out pictures of food in these magazines *[present magazines and child-safe scissors]* and make a project with them. Let's get started.

FOCUSED STIMULATION ACTIVITY

Description: Cutting out food pictures from magazines

Skills Used: Categorization and fine motor

Instructions: Remind children about the food theme, and ask them to cut or tear out food pictures from the magazines.

Example Script

EDUCATOR:	Let's look in these magazines and see if we can find pictures of food in them. Jane, you look in this magazine and see what you can find. *[Wait for the child to find some food pictures]* Jane **found** lots of food pictures.
EDUCATOR:	Jane **found** cookies. *[Look and then put picture out of sight to indicate past tense]*
EDUCATOR:	I **saw** cake!
EDUCATOR:	John **tore** his picture.
EDUCATOR:	Jane **had** five grapes in her picture.
EDUCATOR:	John **found** some more apples.
EDUCATOR:	I **saw** more apples!
EDUCATOR:	Jane **gave** me her picture.
EDUCATOR:	I **found** some fruit.
EDUCATOR:	We **tore** out lots of pictures.

[Continue in a similar manner until numerous models of irregular past tense verbs have been provided.]

Transition

EDUCATOR: We have all these great food pictures. I **thought** we could glue them on this paper and make a really pretty food picture.

ELICITED PRODUCTION ACTIVITY

Description: Making food collages

Skill Used: Fine motor

Goal: 10 productions of irregular past tense verbs per child

Level of Educator Support: Preparatory set

Instructions: Have children glue pictures on construction paper.

Example Script

EDUCATOR:	Look at all the food we found. What **did** Jane do? *[Point to the picture to provide the child with vocabulary and context]*
CHILD:	**Found** grapes.
EDUCATOR:	Yes, she **did.** I **saw** lots of cakes and cookies too.
EDUCATOR:	What **did** Miguel do? *[Point to Miguel's picture to provide vocabulary and context]*
CHILD:	**Saw** cherries.
EDUCATOR:	Let's tell each other what we **found.** I'll go first. I **found** an apple. Now it's your turn.
CHILD:	I **found** a cookie.
EDUCATOR:	Now it's Sally's turn.
CHILD:	I **found** a sandwich.
EDUCATOR:	That sounds good. *[Next, have one child show another child a picture; then have them hide it behind their backs]*
EDUCATOR:	I **saw** a potato. Miguel, tell everyone what you **did.**
CHILD:	I **hid** a cake. *[If this is too difficult, model and recast]*
EDUCATOR:	I **saw** some soup. How about you, Jane?

[Continue in a similar manner until each child has had at least 10 opportunities to use irregular past tense verbs.]

Transition

EDUCATOR: Our caterpillar was very hungry, wasn't he? Our pictures have a lot of food he would like. Let's sing a song about him.

SONG ACTIVITY

Instructions: Sing to the tune of "If You're Happy and You Know It," emphasizing irregular past tense verbs. Felt food items may be held up as children sing about lunch.

The Hungry Caterpillar

The hungry caterpillar **ate** his lunch.
The hungry caterpillar **ate** his lunch.

He **ate, ate, ate**
until he cleaned up his plate.

He **ate, ate, ate** up his lunch!

Weekly Family Letter

For: ______________________________ **Date:** ______________

Theme

Our theme for language intervention this week is *food.*

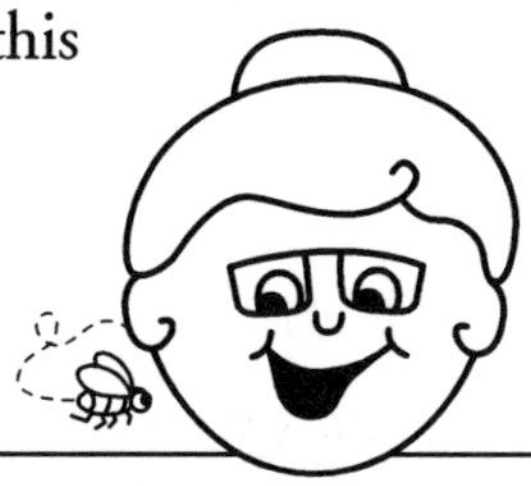

Target

Our target language structures are *regular past tense verbs.* These are verbs that indicate past actions and have regular *-ed* endings. Examples include:

- The lady **swallowed** a fly.
- It **wiggled** and **jiggled** inside her.

Book

Our book for the week is *There Was an Old Lady Who Swallowed a Fly* by Pam Adams (illustrator).

Here is a related book you could read at home: *Golly Gump Swallowed a Fly* by Joanna Cole and Bari Weissman (illustrator).

Song

There Was an Old Lady Who Swallowed a Fly
(Chant)

There was an old lady who **swallowed** a fly.
I don't know why she **swallowed** the fly.

I don't know why!

There was an old lady who **swallowed** a spider.
It **wiggled** and **wiggled** and **jiggled** inside her.

She **swallowed** the spider to catch the fly.
But I don't know why she **swallowed** the fly.

I don't know why!

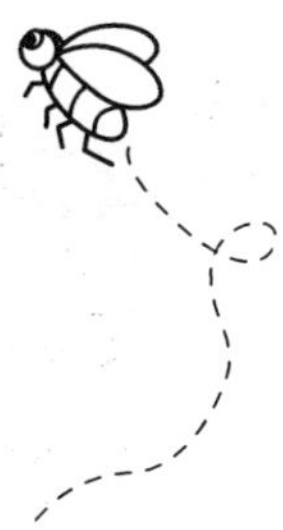

(Continue with the verses for the bird, cat, dog, cow, and horse.)

Activities

Our planned activities for the week include:

- Making "food" for an old lady puppet to eat
- Feeding food to the Old Lady
- Making a paper plate Old Lady

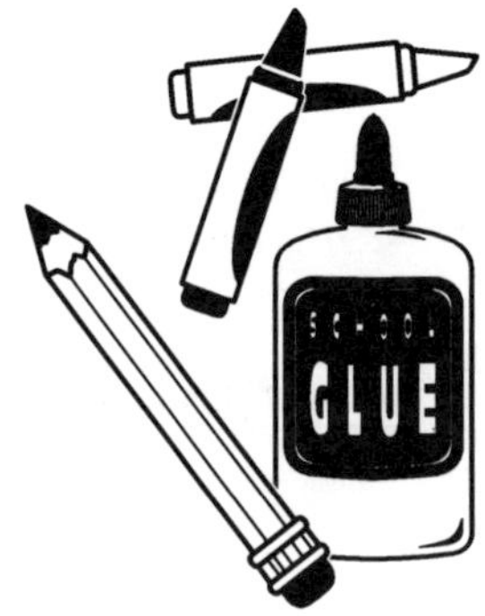

Follow-Up

Suggested follow-up activities for home include:

- Ask your child to sing the "There Was an Old Lady Who Swallowed a Fly" song with you (lyrics are on the previous page). Or read the story with your child, emphasizing the many regular past tense verbs.
- Have your child help you prepare some simple food (e.g., peanut butter and jelly sandwiches). Talk about what you did using regular past tense verbs, for example:

  We **opened** the bread bag.

  We **counted** two pieces of bread.

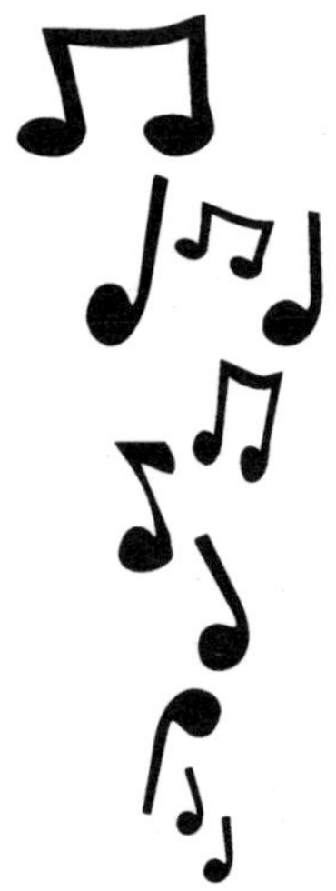

Thank You Very Much for your participation!

Phone Number

Email

Signature

Regular Past Tense

Cycle 3, Session 1

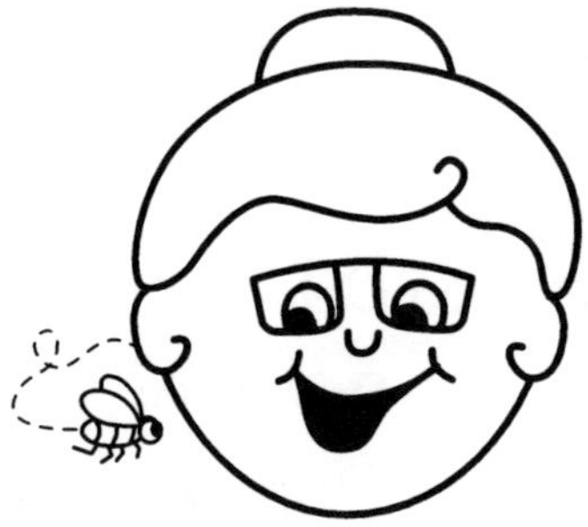

Theme: Food

Description: Completing activities relating to *There Was an Old Lady Who Swallowed a Fly*

Exemplars: colored, crawled, gobbled, happened, jiggled, nibbled, swallowed, talked, wiggled

Materials:

There Was an Old Lady Who Swallowed a Fly by Pam Adams (illustrator)
Old Lady food (see pages 300 and 302 for directions and patterns; 1 set)
Crayons or markers
Old Lady jar (see pages 300–301 for directions and a pattern)

INTRODUCTION TO THEME

Educator: Last week we **talked** about a caterpillar who was very hungry. When he was hungry, what did he do? *[Allow children to respond]* That's right, he ate food! Today we are going to talk about an old lady who was hungry like our caterpillar. She was so hungry that she **swallowed** a fly and lots of other silly things!

BOOK ACTIVITY

Book: *There Was an Old Lady Who Swallowed a Fly* by Pam Adams (illustrator)

Instructions: Read the book with children, emphasizing regular past tense verbs.

Suggested Theme-Related Supplemental Book: *Golly Gump Swallowed a Fly* by Joanna Cole and Bari Weissman (illustrator)

Transition

Educator: Today we are going to make some food for our Old Lady to eat! *[Present Old Lady jar]* We need to look in our story to see what kinds of food we need to make.

FOCUSED STIMULATION ACTIVITY

Description: Coloring "food" (animals) for the Old Lady to eat

Skill Used: Fine motor

Instructions: Have each child color 2–3 animals. Provide numerous regular past tense verb models in a naturalistic way during this activity.

Example Script

Educator: First, the old lady swallowed a fly. Let's color a fly. *[Narrate children's/educator's actions after they occur]*

Educator: Jane **colored** lots of wings on her fly.

Educator: Next, the Old Lady **swallowed** a spider. So let's color a spider.

Educator: John **colored** lots of legs on his spider.

Educator: Next, the Old Lady **swallowed** a bird.

Educator: Jane **colored** a blue bird.

Educator: Now the Old Lady **gobbled** up a cat!

Educator: Jake **colored** a big smile on his cat.

Educator: Now the Old Lady **swallowed** a dog!

[Continue in similar manner until all animals have been colored and numerous models of regular past tense verbs have been provided.]

Transition

Educator: We have all this food for the Old Lady. Now she wants to eat it!

ELICITED PRODUCTION ACTIVITY

Description: Feeding the Old Lady

Skills Used: Fine motor and dramatic play

Goal: 10 productions of regular past tense verbs per child

Level of Educator Support: Preparatory set

Instructions: Prepare the Old Lady prior to the activity. Have children feed the Old Lady jar.

Example Script

EDUCATOR: The old lady in our story **swallowed** lots of things. I need your help to tell me what the Old Lady **swallowed.** We will take turns. After you tell me what she **swallowed,** you can feed her. We will be able to see all the things that the Old Lady **swallowed** when we are done! I'll start *[model]:* I know an old lady who **swallowed** a fly. Now it's your turn, Jane.

CHILD: She **swallowed** a spider.

EDUCATOR: Yes, and I bet it **jiggled** and **crawled** insider her! What **happened** next, John?

CHILD: The lady **swallowed** a bird!

EDUCATOR: How absurd! What **happened** next?

CHILD: She **swallowed** a cat.

EDUCATOR: Look, the lady **gobbled** up a cat!

EDUCATOR: Then what **happened?**

CHILD: She **gobbled** a dog.

EDUCATOR: Then she **nibbled** on a cow!

EDUCATOR: I bet it **wiggled** inside her!

[Continue in a similar manner until all items have been eaten and each child has had at least 10 opportunities to use regular past tense verbs.]

Transition

Educator: The Old Lady ate all the food. Let's clean up and sing our song about the Old Lady who **swallowed** a fly.

SONG ACTIVITY

Instructions: Chant while emphasizing regular past tense forms. Pictures of food items can be held up as children sing about them.

There Was an Old Lady Who Swallowed a Fly

There was an old lady who **swallowed** a fly.
I don't know why she **swallowed** the fly.

I don't know why!

There was an old lady who **swallowed** a spider.
It **wiggled** and **wiggled** and **jiggled** insider her.

She **swallowed** the spider to catch the fly.
But I don't know why she **swallowed** the fly.

I don't know why!

(Continue with the verses for the bird, cat, dog, cow, and horse.)

Regular Past Tense

Cycle 3, Session 2

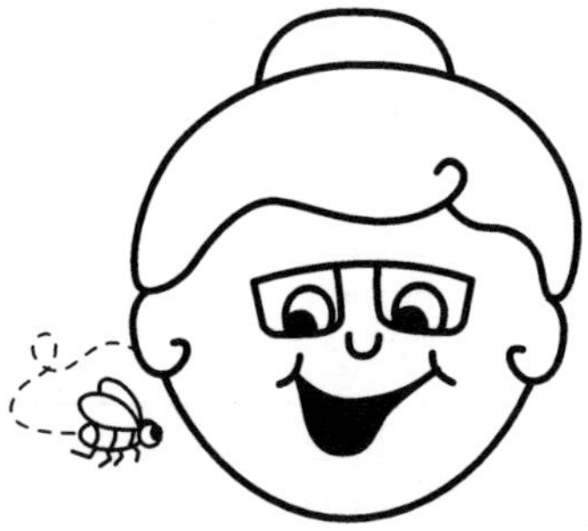

Theme: Food

Description: Completing activities relating to *There Was an Old Lady Who Swallowed a Fly*

Exemplars: colored, glued, jiggled, swallowed, wiggled

Materials:

There Was an Old Lady Who Swallowed a Fly by Pam Adams (illustrator)
Old Lady animals (see pages 303 and 305–308 for directions and patterns; 1 set per child)
Crayons and markers
Completed Old Lady plate (see pages 303–308 for directions and patterns)
Old Lady plates (see pages 303–304 for directions and patterns; 1 per child)
Glue

BOOK ACTIVITY

Book: *There Was an Old Lady Who Swallowed a Fly* by Pam Adams

Instructions: Reread the book with children, emphasizing regular past tense verbs.

Suggested Theme-Related Supplemental Book: *Golly Gump Swallowed a Fly* by Joanna Cole and Bari Weissman (illustrator)

Transition

EDUCATOR: The Old Lady is still hungry, so we need to make more food for her! We need to look in our story to see what kinds of food we need to make.

FOCUSED STIMULATION ACTIVITY

Description: Coloring "food" (animals) for the Old Lady to eat

Skills Used: Fine motor and sequencing

Instructions: Have each child color every animal in his or her set.

Example Script

EDUCATOR: First, the old lady **swallowed** a fly. Let's color our flies.

EDUCATOR: Jane **colored** lots of wings on her fly.

EDUCATOR: Now the old lady **swallowed** a spider.

EDUCATOR: John **colored** lots of legs on his spider.

EDUCATOR: Now the old lady **swallowed** a bird.

EDUCATOR: John **colored** his bird blue.

EDUCATOR: Now the old lady **swallowed** a cat!

EDUCATOR: Jake **colored** eyes on his cat.

EDUCATOR: Now the old lady **swallowed** a dog!

EDUCATOR: Sally **colored** her dog yellow.

EDUCATOR: It looks like John **colored** his dog green.

EDUCATOR: Look at Jane's goat. She **colored** it purple!

[Continue in similar manner until all animals have been colored and numerous models of regular past tense verbs have been provided.]

Transition

EDUCATOR: Our food pictures look so nice. Now we are going to put all these pictures in the Old Lady's tummy so that we can see all the things she ate!

ELICITED PRODUCTION ACTIVITY

Description: Gluing the animals (from largest to smallest) on paper plates

Skills Used: Fine motor and sequencing

Goal: 10 productions of regular past tense verbs per child

Level of Educator Support: Preparatory set

Instructions: Prepare an Old Lady plate prior to the activity to serve as a model.

Example Script

EDUCATOR: Our Old Lady **swallowed** lots of things. Now we are going to glue all the things she **swallowed** on this plate like this. *[Present completed model]* Before we glue each thing on, I want you to tell me what the Old Lady **swallowed.** I'll go first. I know an Old Lady who **swallowed** a horse. Now it's your turn, John. We are going to glue on the biggest animals first.

CHILD: She **swallowed** a cow.

EDUCATOR: Yes she did. I like how John **glued** his cow on the horse.

EDUCATOR: Jane, tell us what John did.

CHILD: He **glued** the cow.

EDUCATOR: Yes. What do you think the Old Lady did next?

CHILD: She **swallowed** a dog!

EDUCATOR: Yes, she **swallowed** a whole dog! Tell us what Sally did to the dog.

CHILD: She **glued** it on the lady's tummy!

EDUCATOR: Yes, she **glued** it!

[Continue in a similar manner until all items have been glued on and each child has had at least 10 opportunities to use regular past tense verbs.]

Transition

EDUCATOR: Let's sing our song about the Old Lady who **swallowed** all those animals!

SONG ACTIVITY

Instructions: Chant while emphasizing regular past tense forms. Pictures of food items can be held up as the children sing about them.

There Was an Old Lady Who Swallowed a Fly

There was an old lady who **swallowed** a fly.
I don't know why she **swallowed** the fly.

I don't know why!

There was an old lady who **swallowed** a spider.
It **wiggled** and **wiggled** and **jiggled** insider her.

She **swallowed** the spider to catch the fly.
But I don't know why she **swallowed** the fly.

I don't know why!

(Continue with the verses for the bird, cat, dog, cow, and horse.)

Weekly Family Letter

For: ______________________________ **Date:** ______________

Theme

Our theme for language intervention this week is *food.*

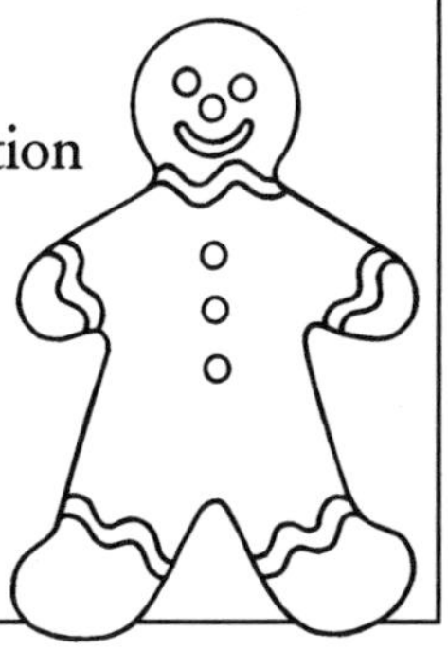

Target

Our target language structures are *copula* be *verbs.* These include *am ('m), are ('re),* and *is ('s)* when used as the only verb in a sentence. Examples include:

- I **am** sleepy.
- It**'s** hot out today.
- We**'re** angry.

Book

Our book for the week is *The Gingerbread Man* by Karen Schmidt (illustrator).

Here are some related books you could read at home: *Whiff, Sniff, Nibble, and Chew: The Gingerbread Boy Retold* by Charlotte Pomerantz and Monica Incisa (illustrator) and *The Runaway Pancake* by P.C. Asbjorsen, Jorgen Moe, and Otto Svend (illustrator).

Song

Where Is Gingerbread Man?
(Tune: "Where Is Thumbkin?")

Where **is** gingerbread man (or woman)?
Where **is** gingerbread man?

Here I **am!** Here I **am!**

I**'m** so fast. I**'m** so fast.

Yes I **am!** Yes I **am!**

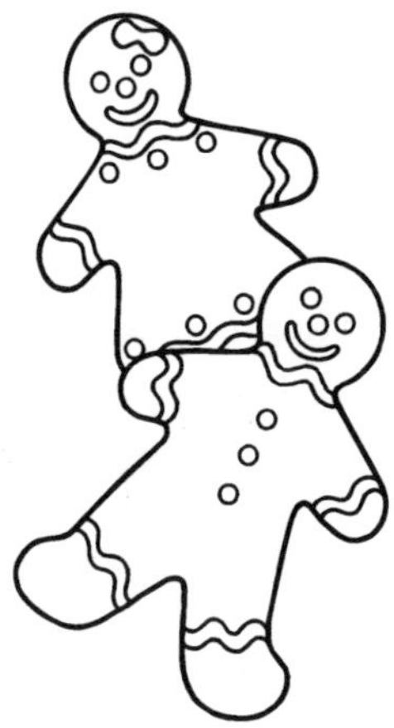

Activities

Our planned activities for the week include:

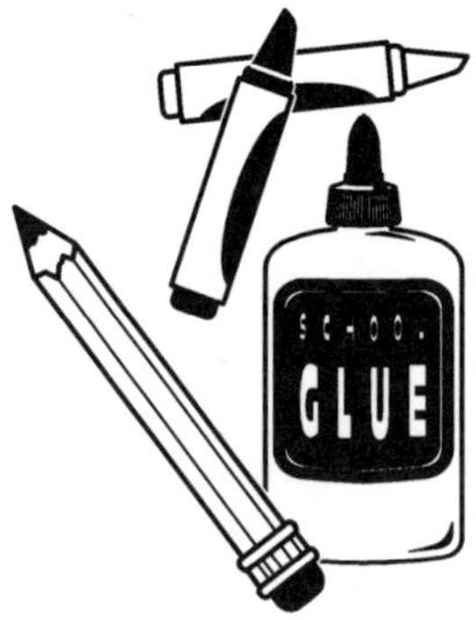

- Making a gingerbread person stick puppet
- Playing show-and-tell with the stick puppet
- Having a race with the stick puppet
- Decorating and eating gingerbread people cookies

Follow-Up

Suggested follow-up activities for home include:

- Have your child discuss the features of a particular item. Because our theme is food, with a focus on gingerbread people, it might be fun to bake and decorate gingerbread people cookies and have your child describe them, for example:

  Her coat **is** brown.

  These **are** his eyes.

- Look through a cookbook with pictures or a food magazine with your child. Talk about what you see, for example:

  These **are** muffins.

  This soup **is** white.

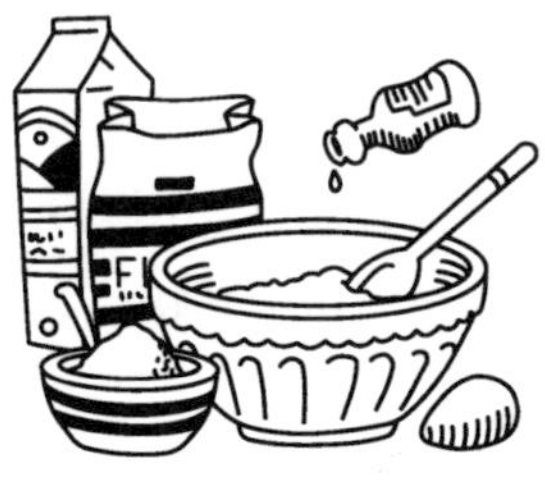

Thank You Very Much for your participation!

Phone Number

Email

Signature

Copula *be*

Cycle 3, Session 1

Theme: Food

Description: Completing activities relating to gingerbread people

Exemplars: am ('m), are ('re), is ('s)

Materials:

The Gingerbread Man by Karen Schmidt (illustrator)
Completed gingerbread person stick puppet
(see pages 309–310 for directions and patterns)
Brass fasteners (2 per child)
Gingerbread people cutouts
(see pages 309–310 for directions and patterns; 1 set per child)
Glue
Single hole punch
Craft sticks (1 per child)
Puppet (for individual sessions only)

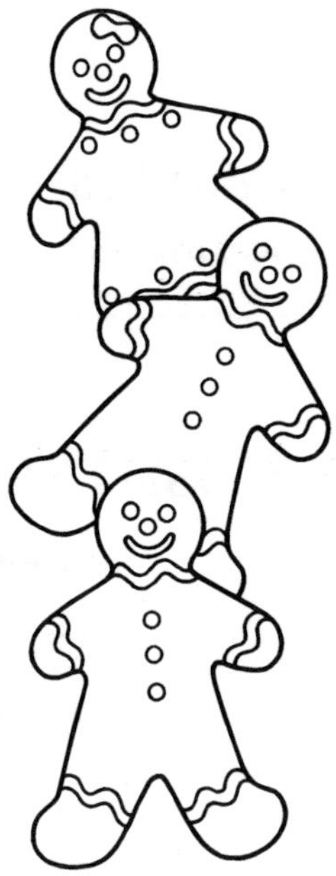

INTRODUCTION TO THEME

Educator: For the past few weeks, we have been talking about food. We learned about a mouse who liked to eat cookies. We talked about a caterpillar who ate all kinds of food. Last week we sang songs and read a story about an old lady who ate lots of different things, like a spider and a horse. This week, we are going to talk about some food that turns into a little person. We are going to talk about a gingerbread person. Has anyone ever eaten a gingerbread person cookie? *[Allow children to respond]* Well, the gingerbread man in our story does not want to get eaten so he runs away.

BOOK ACTIVITY

Book: *The Gingerbread Man* by Karen Schmidt (illustrator)

Instructions: Read the book with children, emphasizing copula *be* verbs. This story is quite lengthy, so it may be necessary to shorten the story, depending on the educator's time constraints and children's attention spans.

Suggested Theme-Related Supplemental Books: *Whiff, Sniff, Nibble, and Chew: The Gingerbread Boy Retold* by Charlotte Pomerantz and Monica Incisa (illustrator)
The Runaway Pancake by P.C. Asbjorsen, Jorgen Moe, and Otto Svend (illustrator)

Transition

EDUCATOR: Today we are going to make gingerbread people like the one in the story.

FOCUSED STIMULATION ACTIVITY

Description: Making gingerbread people stick puppets

Skill Used: Fine motor

Instructions: Show children the example gingerbread person, and explain that they are going to make one.

Example Script

EDUCATOR: Remember that the gingerbread man was a runner, so we need to be sure that our gingerbread people's legs move. That is why we need these. *[Present fasteners]* These **are** movers.

EDUCATOR: These *[present legs]* **are** the gingerbread person's legs.

EDUCATOR: These *[present arms]* **are** the gingerbread person's arms.

EDUCATOR: These *[present eyes]* **are** the eyes.

EDUCATOR: This *[present nose]* **is** the nose.

EDUCATOR: This *[present head]* **is** the head

EDUCATOR: This *[present mouth]* **is** the body.

EDUCATOR: This stick **is** for the gingerbread person. *[Glue a craft stick on the back of the puppet]*

[Continue in similar manner until each child has assembled a gingerbread person and numerous models of copula be *verbs have been provided.]*

Transition

Educator: We made some really nice gingerbread people today. Now I thought we could tell each other about what we made. Then we can have a race with our gingerbread people.

ELICITED PRODUCTION ACTIVITY

Description: Playing show-and-tell with gingerbread people and having a race with gingerbread people

Skills Used: Describing, sharing, and gross motor

Goal: 10 productions of copula *be* verbs per child

Level of Educator Support: Preparatory set

Instructions: For sessions with an individual child, have a puppet "participate" in the race.

Example Script

Educator: We all have very nice gingerbread people. Let's talk about them and then we are going to have a race. Remember how the gingerbread man in the story ran so fast? Well, that's what our gingerbread people are going to do.

Educator: I'll tell you about my gingerbread man first. He **is** a man. He **is** very little and he **is** fast. Now it**'s** your turn, John. Tell us about your gingerbread man.

Child: This **is** my gingerbread man. He **is** funny.

Educator: Good. Maria, tell us about yours.

Child: She **is** happy.

Educator: Tell me, who **is** fast?

Child: She **is.**

Educator: Who **is** slow?

Child: He **is.**

Continued on next page

Example Script—*Continued*

EDUCATOR:	Let's have a race now. *[Children should have a mini race in pairs. Then discuss the race using copula* be *verbs. Designate a staring and finishing point for the race, and have children hold their gingerbread people and run or walk]* Sally's man **is** in the lead. Now Sally's man **is** behind.
EDUCATOR:	It looks like Sally's man **is** slow. Tell me about her man.
CHILD:	He **is** slow.
EDUCATOR:	Now tell me about this woman. *[Point to the "fast" gingerbread person]*
CHILD:	She **is** fast! You **are** the winner!

[Continue in a similar manner until each child has had at least 10 opportunities to use copula be *verbs.]*

Transition

EDUCATOR: Our gingerbread people were very fast! Let's sing our gingerbread man song now.

SONG ACTIVITY

Instructions: Sing to the tune of "Where Is Thumbkin?" emphasizing copula *be* verbs. Use gingerbread people puppets as visual aids.

Where Is Gingerbread Man?

Where **is** the gingerbread man (or woman)?
Where **is** the gingerbread man?

Here I **am!**
Here I **am!**

I'**m** so fast.
I'**m** so fast.

Yes I **am!**
Yes I **am!**

Copula *be*

Cycle 3, Session 2

Theme: Food

Description: Completing activities relating to gingerbread people

Exemplars: am ('m), are ('re), is ('s)

Materials:

The Gingerbread Man by Karen Schmidt (illustrator)
Gingerbread people cookies
Decorations (sprinkles, candy, etc.)
Frosting
Napkins (1 per child)
Juice boxes (1 per child)

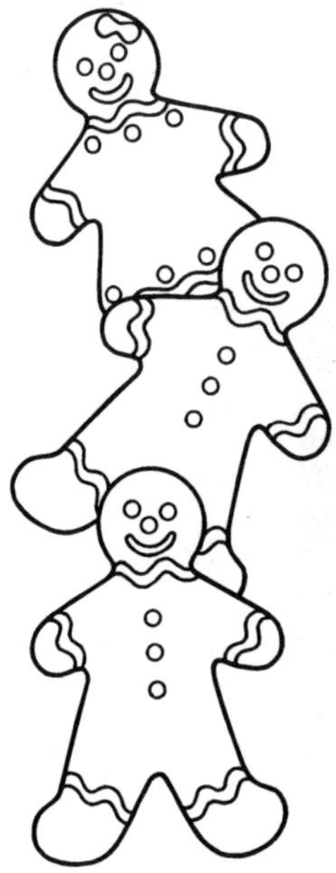

BOOK ACTIVITY

Book: *The Gingerbread Man* by Karen Schmidt (illustrator)

Instructions: Reread the book with children, emphasizing copula *be* verbs.

Suggested Theme-Related Supplemental Books: *Whiff, Sniff, Nibble, and Chew: The Gingerbread Boy Retold* by Charlotte Pomerantz and Monica Incisa (illustrator)
The Runaway Pancake by P.C. Asbjorsen, Jorgen Moe, and Otto Svend (illustrator)

Transition

EDUCATOR: Remember in our story how the farmer and his wife wanted to eat the gingerbread man? Well, today I thought it would be fun if we made gingerbread people to eat!

FOCUSED STIMULATION ACTIVITY

Description: Decorating gingerbread people cookies

Skills Used: Describing and fine motor

Instructions: Bake or purchase gingerbread people cookies prior to the activity. Show children an example decorated gingerbread person cookie and explain that they are going to decorate their own.

Example Script

EDUCATOR: Today we are going to make gingerbread people cookies to eat. See, here's mine. He **is** little and he **is** yummy! He **is** a cookie! There are lots of things we can use to make our gingerbread people look good.

EDUCATOR: These *[present sprinkles]* **are** sprinkles.

EDUCATOR: These *[present candies]* **are** pieces of candy. They **are** round. They **are** buttons for the gingerbread person's shirt.

EDUCATOR: These *[present round candy]* **are** the eyes.

EDUCATOR: This *[present frosting]* is frosting. It **is** sticky. This **is** for us to stick the candy on the cookie.

EDUCATOR: This **is** messy. We need napkins. **Is** this a napkin? No, but this **is**!

[Continue in similar manner until gingerbread people have been decorated and numerous models of copula be *verbs have been provided.]*

Transition

EDUCATOR: These gingerbread people cookies look really good. They look good enough to eat! **Are** you hungry? I **am!** Let's eat our gingerbread people.

ELICITED PRODUCTION ACTIVITY

Description: Eating gingerbread people cookies and drinking juice

Skills Used: Sharing, turn taking, and describing

Goal: 10 productions of copula *be* verbs per child

Level of Educator Support: Preparatory set

Example Script

EDUCATOR:	We all have very nice gingerbread people. I would like us to talk about our cookies, and then we are going to eat them up.
EDUCATOR:	I'll tell you about my gingerbread man first. He **is** a man. He **is** very little and he **is** cute. Now it**'s** your turn, Jane. Tell us about your gingerbread woman.
CHILD:	This **is** my cookie. It **is** yummy.
EDUCATOR:	Good. Sally, tell us about yours.
CHILD:	He **is** a man. *[Continue for all children]*
EDUCATOR:	Who **is** hungry?
CHILD:	I **am.**
EDUCATOR:	Who **is** thirsty?
CHILD:	I **am.**
EDUCATOR:	Let's drink our juice and eat our cookies. *[Pass out juice boxes]*
EDUCATOR:	Sally, ask Jane if her cookie **is** good.
CHILD:	**Is** it good?
EDUCATOR:	John, ask Jane which one **is** a woman cookie.
CHILD:	Which **is** a woman?
CHILD:	This **is!**

[Continue in a similar manner until each child has had at least 10 opportunities to use copula be *verbs.]*

Transition

EDUCATOR: That snack sure was good! Now it's time to clean up and sing our gingerbread man song.

SONG ACTIVITY

Instructions: Sing to the tune of "Where Is Thumbkin?" emphasizing copula *be* verbs. Use gingerbread people stick puppets as visual aids.

Where Is Gingerbread Man?

Where **is** gingerbread man (or woman)?
Where **is** gingerbread man?

Here I **am!**
Here I **am!**

I'**m** so fast.
I'**m** so fast.

Yes I **am!**
Yes I **am!**

Part II: Supplementary Morphemes

Weekly Family Letter

For: ______________________________ **Date:** ____________

Theme

Our theme for language intervention this week is *water.*

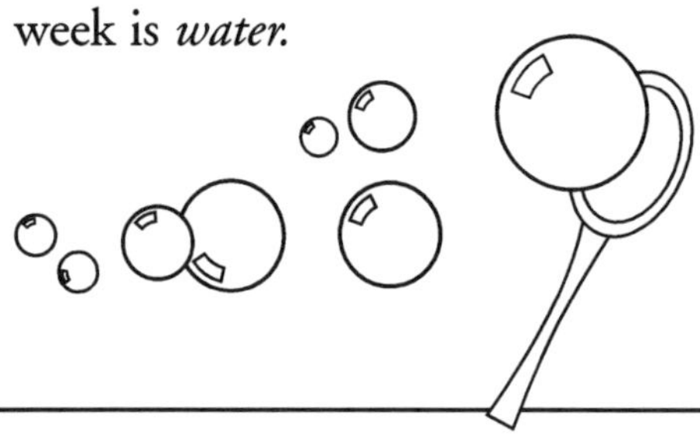

Target

Our target language structures are *regular plurals.* These are words ending in *-s* that indicate more than one of something. Examples include:

- I have two **dogs**.
- Matt ate lots of **chips**.
- Mom gave me **kisses**.

Book

Our book for the week is *Bubble Trouble* by Mary Packard and Elena Kucharik (illustrator).

Here are some related books you could read at home: *Bubble Bubble* by Mercer Mayer and *Clifford Counts Bubbles* by Norman Bridwell.

Song

This Is the Way We Blow Our Bubbles
(Tune: "This Is the Way We…")

This is the way we blow our **bubbles,**
blow our **bubbles,** blow our **bubbles.**

This is the way we blow our **bubbles**
early in the morning!

(Repeat using the words *stomp, pop,* and *poke.)*

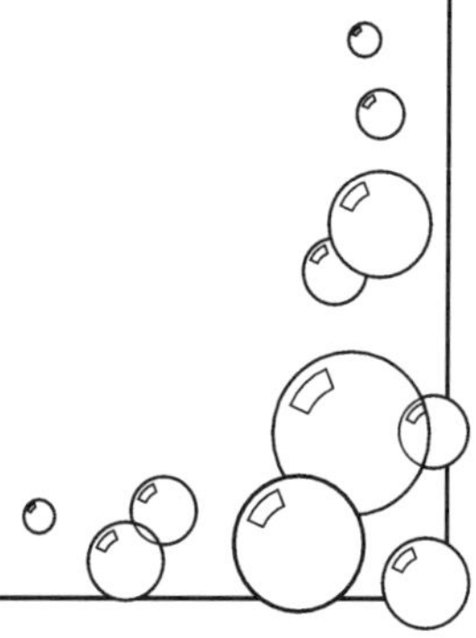

Activities

Our planned activities for the week include:

- Making bubble blowers out of milk cartons and pipe cleaners
- Making colored bubbles in a jar
- Creating a picture using colored bubble soap

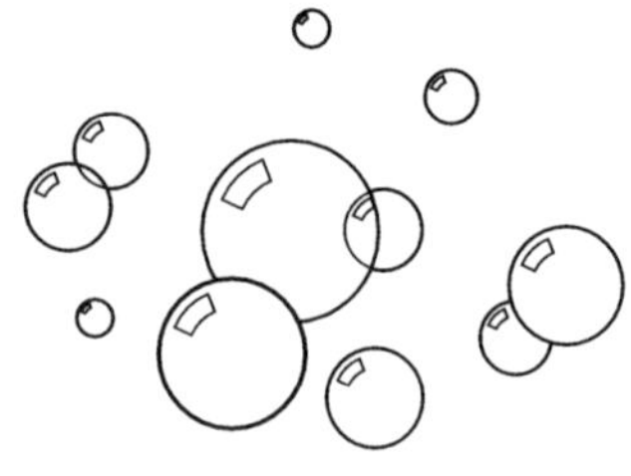

Follow-Up

Suggested follow-up activities for home include:

- Talk about items used during bath time. While your child takes a bath, discuss items using regular plurals, for example:

  Look at all the **bubbles!**

  Wash your **toes.**

- Round up all your child's stuffed animals and pretend to give them baths. Talk about what you are doing using regular plurals, for example:

  The **bears** look really dirty.

  The **bunnies** need to wash their **ears.**

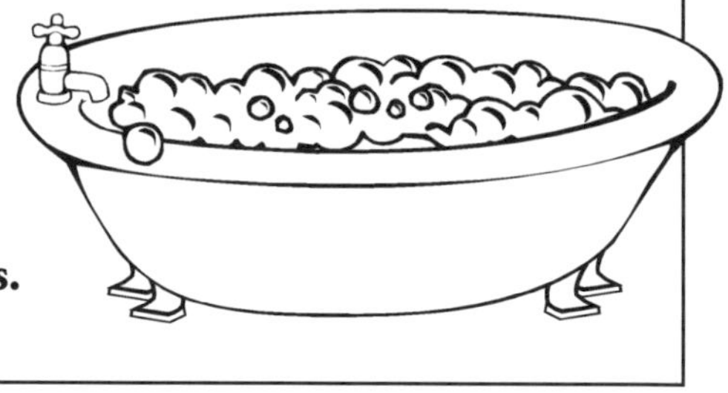

Thank You Very Much
for your participation!

Phone Number

Email

Signature

Regular Plurals

Cycle 1, Session 1

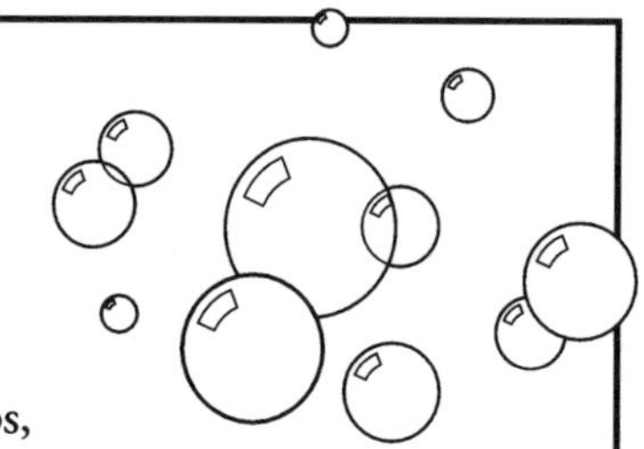

Theme: Water

Description: Creating bubbles

Exemplars: animals, blowers, bubbles, cartons, circles, cups, drops, forks, hands, holes, lots, pencils, plates, rocks, shapes, spoons, squares, sticks, straws, things, tops

Materials:

Bubble Trouble by Mary Packard
Half-pint milk cartons (1 per child)
Pencils
Bubble soap materials (see page 271 for recipe and directions)
Straws (2 per child)
Pipe cleaners (1 per child)
2 Styrofoam cups

INTRODUCTION TO THEME

Educator: We are going to talk about water today. We use water every day. We use water when we take a bath, and we drink water when we are thirsty. There are lots of different **things** we can do with water. One thing people do with water is make **bubbles. Bubbles** are made of water. Who likes to play with **bubbles?** *[Allow children to respond]* You do? Me too! Well, today we are going to read a book about **bubbles** and we are going to do a special activity with **bubbles.** Are you ready? *[Allow children to respond]* Let's read our bubble book.

BOOK ACTIVITY

Book: *Bubble Trouble* by Mary Packard and Elena Kucharik (illustrator)

Instructions: Read the book with children, emphasizing regular plurals.

Suggested Theme-Related Supplemental Books: *Bubble Bubble* by Mercer Mayer
Clifford Counts Bubbles by Norman Bridwell

Transition

Educator: The **animals** in our story made lots of **bubbles** in their bathtub! Now we are going to make **lots** of **bubbles** too!

FOCUSED STIMULATION ACTIVITY

Description: Making bubble blowers using half-pint milk cartons

Skills Used: Fine motor, direction following, and sequencing

Instructions: Poke a hole in the top of each child's straw using a safety pin so he or she will not be able to drink the bubble soap.

Example Script

Educator: Today we are going to make a special kind of bubble blower. We will use milk **cartons** for our bubble **blowers.**

Educator: First, we need to put **holes** in the top so that the **bubbles** can come out.

Educator: Let's use these **pencils** to poke **holes** in the tops of the **cartons.** *[Poke one hole on each side of the tops of the milk cartons]*

Educator: Then, we need to put water in the **cartons.** We'll pour the water in the **holes.** *[Pour 1/2 cup of water in each carton]*

Educator: Now we need to measure our soap. This is a spoon. Let's pour three **spoons** of soap in the **holes.**

Educator: We need to put two **spoons** of sugar in our soap and water. Sugar makes our **bubbles** stronger.

Educator: Now let's put **straws** in the **holes** and shake up the soap, water, and sugar.

Educator: We'll shake it up with our **hands.** Try not to spill **bubbles** on the table!

Educator: Now that we have shaken our bubble soap, let's blow through one of these **straws.** *[Demonstrate]*

Educator: Look what happened! **Bubbles** came out of the other straw.

Educator: Look at all these **bubbles!** There are **bubbles** everywhere!

Educator: I like bubble **blowers** like these!

[Continue in a similar manner until numerous models of regular plurals have been provided.]

Transition

EDUCATOR: Now we're going to make some different bubble **blowers.** Then we'll blow more **bubbles!**

ELICITED PRODUCTION ACTIVITY

Description: Making bubble blowers using pipe cleaners

Skills Used: Direction following and fine motor

Goal: 10 productions of regular plurals per child

Level of Educator Support: Forced choice

Example Script

EDUCATOR: We are going to make more bubble **blowers.** This time, we are going to use these **things** to make our **bubbles.** What are these? *[Present pipe cleaners]* Are they **sticks** or **rocks?**

CHILD: **Sticks.**

EDUCATOR: We will make bubble **blowers** with these **sticks.**

EDUCATOR: We need to make **shapes** with our **sticks.** *[Demonstrate how to make an enclosed shape, such as a circle or square, at the top of the pipe cleaner]*

EDUCATOR: I made **circles** on the **tops** of my **sticks.**

EDUCATOR: What **shapes** do you want to make today? **Circles** or **squares?**

CHILD: **Squares!**

EDUCATOR: OK, let's make some **squares.** I'll help you.

EDUCATOR: Now that we have our **blowers** made, we need something else. What will we dip our bubble **blowers** in to get them wet?

CHILD: Soap!

EDUCATOR: You're right! Let's make some bubble soap!

EDUCATOR: Remember, we need soap, sugar and water to make our bubble soap.

EDUCATOR: Jane, let's use this first. *[Present water]* What should we pour our water into? **Cups** or **plates?**

Continued on next page

Example Script—*Continued*

CHILD: **Cups.**

EDUCATOR: Yes, let's pour it into some **cups**. *[Have children pour 1/2 cup of water into each cup]*

EDUCATOR: This is what we need next. *[Present soap]* Do we want three **spoons** or three **drops** of soap?

CHILD: Three **spoons!**

EDUCATOR: Yes, please put three **spoons** of soap into each cup.

EDUCATOR: This is kind of funny, but we need to put this white stuff in our bubble soap. It is sugar. Sugar helps make our **bubbles** stronger. How many **spoons** of sugar should we put in our bubble soap? Two **spoons** or three **spoons**? *[Either response is acceptable]*

CHILD: Two **spoons**!

EDUCATOR: Sounds good! Go ahead and pour two **spoons** of sugar in each cup of our bubble soap.

EDUCATOR: Now we need to mix up our bubble soap. Should we use **spoons** or **forks**?

CHILD: **Spoons!**

EDUCATOR: Great idea! Go ahead and use the **spoons** to mix up our soap.

EDUCATOR: Now we are ready to use our bubble **sticks** to blow **bubbles.**

EDUCATOR: What **shapes** are our **sticks**? **Squares** or **circles**?

CHILD: **Squares!**

EDUCATOR: Yes, our **sticks** have **squares** on the end.

EDUCATOR: Let's dip our **sticks** in the soap and blow some **bubbles**!

EDUCATOR: Wow! What did we make? **Bubbles** or **squares**?

CHILD: **Bubbles!**

[Continue in a similar manner until each child has had at least 10 opportunities to use regular plurals.]

Transition

EDUCATOR: Wow, **bubbles** are fun! Let's clean up and get ready to sing our song about **bubbles.**

SONG ACTIVITY

Instructions: Sing to the tune of "This Is The Way We…," emphasizing regular plurals. Use a different child's name for each verse. (When using the song with an individual child, use his or her name.) Encourage children to take turns performing gestures that match the lyrics. For example, as Jane sings, Jake can perform the gestures.

This Is the Way We Blow Our Bubbles

This is the way we blow our **bubbles,**
blow our **bubbles,** blow our **bubbles.**

This is the way we blow our **bubbles**
early in the morning!

(Repeat for the words *stomp, pop,* and *poke.)*

Regular Plurals

Cycle 1, Session 2

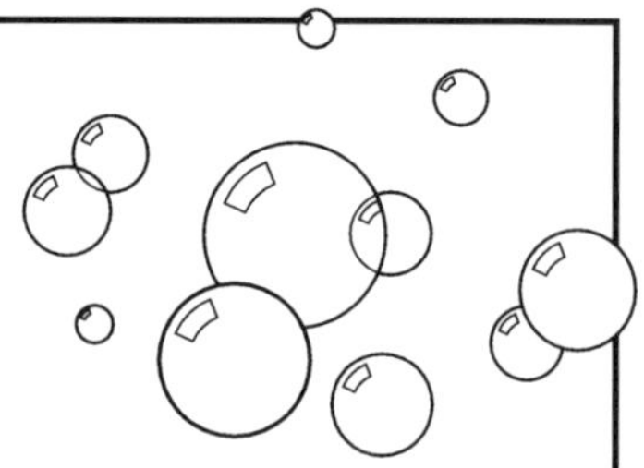

Theme: Water

Description: Creating bubbles

Exemplars: blocks, blowers, bubbles, colors, cups, drops, forks, hands, jars, lids, lots, papers, pictures, smears, spoons, tables, things, wands

Materials:

Bubble Trouble by Mary Packard and Elena Kucharik (illustrator)

Bag containing:

- Baby food jars with lids (1 or more per color)
- Bubble soap materials (see page 271 for recipe and instructions)
- Food coloring (3–4 colors)
- Bubble wands
- White construction paper

BOOK ACTIVITY

Book: *Bubble Trouble* by Mary Packard and Elena Kucharik (illustrator)

Instructions: Reread the book with children, emphasizing regular plurals.

Suggested Theme-Related Supplemental Books: *Bubble Bubble* by Mercer Mayer
Clifford Counts Bubbles by Norman Bridwell

Transition

EDUCATOR: There were **lots** of **bubbles** in our story. Remember last time you were here when we made **bubbles?** Well, that was so much fun that we are going to make even more **bubbles** today!

FOCUSED STIMULATION ACTIVITY

Description: Making and shaking colored bubbles

Skills Used: Fine motor, gross motor, direction following, sharing, and sequencing

Example Script

EDUCATOR:	We have been playing with **bubbles**. Last time we made bubble **blowers**. Today we are going to make **lots** of little **bubbles** in **jars**.
EDUCATOR:	Look at these **things** I brought for us. *[Pull items out of the bag and discuss]*
EDUCATOR:	First, we need these **jars**.
EDUCATOR:	These **things** on the top are called **lids**.
EDUCATOR:	We need to open the **lids** and put water in our **jars**. Let's fill them up this high. *[Point to the half full point on a jar]*
EDUCATOR:	Let's use **cups** to pour the water in. *[Pour water in]*
EDUCATOR:	We also need soap in our **jars**. We need to put three **spoons** of soap and two **spoons** of sugar in our **jars**.
EDUCATOR:	Pour them in.
EDUCATOR:	Now we have soap and water. We can make **bubbles** now. I thought we could make different **colors**. Do you want green **bubbles** or red **bubbles**?
CHILD:	Green **bubbles**!
EDUCATOR:	Let's put our food coloring in the **jars**. Let's put two **drops** of green in our **jars**.
EDUCATOR:	Now we need to close our **lids**. Now let's shake our **jars** with our **hands**.
EDUCATOR:	Wow! Look what we made!
CHILD:	**Bubbles**!
EDUCATOR:	We made **lots** and **lots** of **bubbles**.
EDUCATOR:	Do you want to make our **bubbles** be different **colors**? Let's put different **colors** in our **jars**. *[Repeat the same procedure for different colors]*
EDUCATOR:	Let's see what happens when we shake it up. Do it.
EDUCATOR:	Wow! That was fun.

Transition

EDUCATOR: That sure was fun. Now we are going to use the **bubbles** in our **jars.** We are going to make **pictures.**

ELICITED PRODUCTION ACTIVITY

Description: Making pictures using bubble soap

Skills Used: Fine motor, direction following, and oral motor

Goal: 10 productions of regular plurals per child

Level of Educator Support: Forced choice

Example Script

EDUCATOR: You did such a good job making all those **colors** in your **jars.** I thought we could make **pictures** with your **bubbles.** We need our bubble soap.

EDUCATOR: I wonder what **things** we could use to blow our **bubbles. Wands** or **blocks**?

CHILD: **Wands**!

EDUCATOR: Good idea! We could use **wands.**

EDUCATOR: If we want to make a picture, what should we blow our **bubbles** on? **Papers** or **tables**?

CHILD: **Papers**!

EDUCATOR: If we blow **bubbles** on **papers,** we can make pretty **pictures.**

EDUCATOR: What will happen when the **bubbles** pop? Will they make **pictures** or **smears**?

CHILD: **Pictures**!

EDUCATOR: When the **bubbles** pop, they will make our **papers** lots of different **colors.**

EDUCATOR: I want to make a green picture. I wonder what color **bubbles** I should blow.

Continued on next page

Example Script—*Continued*

EDUCATOR:	Green **bubbles** or red **bubbles?**
CHILD:	Green **bubbles.**
EDUCATOR:	Good idea. I'm going to blow green **bubbles.** Now I want some red on my picture. What should I do? Blow red **bubbles** or blue **bubbles?**
CHILD:	Blow red **bubbles!**
EDUCATOR:	What are we using to blow our **bubbles**? **Wands** or **forks?**
CHILD:	**Wands.**

[Continue in a similar manner until each children has had at least 10 opportunities to use regular plurals.]

Transition

EDUCATOR: I had fun shaking up the **bubbles** and making bubble **pictures!** Now it's time to clean up and sing our bubble song!

SONG ACTIVITY

Instructions: Sing to the tune of "This Is the Way We…," emphasizing regular plurals. Use a different child's name for each verse. (When using the song with an individual child, use his or her name.) Encourage children to take turns performing gestures that match the lyrics. For example, as Jane sings, Jake can perform the gestures.

This Is the Way We Blow Our Bubbles

This is the way we blow our **bubbles,**
blow our **bubbles,** blow our **bubbles.**

This is the way we blow our **bubbles**
early in the morning!

(Repeat using the words *stomp, pop,* and *poke.)*

Weekly Family Letter

For: ______________________________ **Date:** ______________

Theme

Our theme for language intervention this week is *water.*

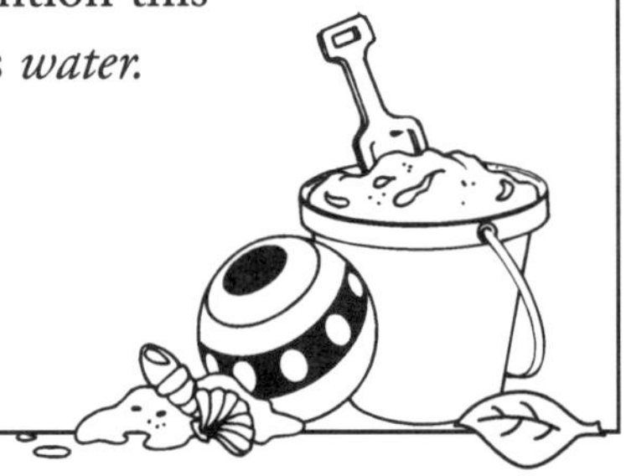

Target

Our target language structures are *possessives.* Possessives indicate ownership and usually have an *'s* ending. Examples include:

- **Jenny's** mom is nice.
- I like my **brother's** teacher.
- It's **daddy's** turn.

Book

Our book for the week is *At the Beach* by Anne Rockwell and Harlow Rockwell.

Here are some related books you could read at home: *Curious George Goes to the Beach* by Margaret Rey and H.A. Rey and *For Sand Castles or Seashells* by Gail Hartman and Ellen Weiss (illustrator).

Song

Down by the Seashore
(Tune: "Little Bunny Foo Foo")

Down by the seashore early in the morning, I saw the **baby's** toy lying on the beach.
I saw **[child's name]'s** family having so much fun!

Down by the seashore early in the morning, I saw **mommy's** boat floating in the water.
I saw **[child's name]'s** family having so much fun!

Down by the seashore early in the morning,
I saw the **baby's** seashell shining like the sun.
I saw **[child's name]'s** family having so much fun!

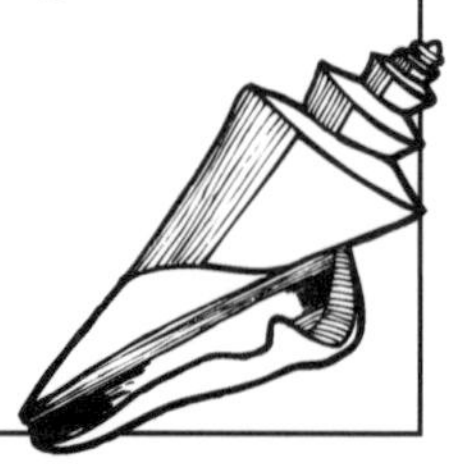

Activities

Our planned activities for the week include:

- Discussing events in the book using possessives
- Sinking and floating objects in water
- Having a boat race with index card boats
- Making a milk carton sailboat

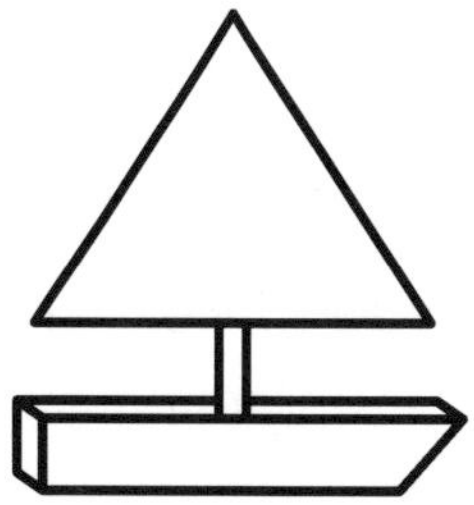

Follow-Up

Suggested follow-up activities for home include:

- Discuss features of items that belong to different people. For example, your child and you or a brother, sister, or friend might each draw a picture related to the beach. Afterward you can discuss similarities and differences of each picture, focusing on possessive forms, for example:

  Sally's picture has lots of waves.

  Tom's boat is blue and **Sally's** boat is red.

- Gather your child's dolls and/or stuffed animals and take turns telling each other what to touch, for example:

  Touch the **doll's** nose.

  Touch the **bear's** tummy.

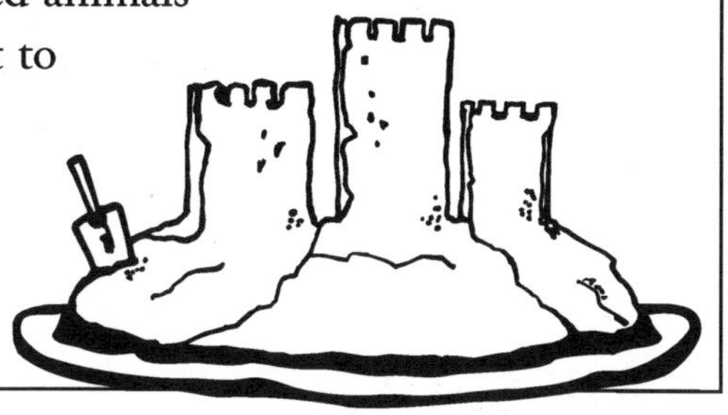

Thank You Very Much for your participation!

Phone Number

Email

Signature

Possessives

Cycle 1, Session 1

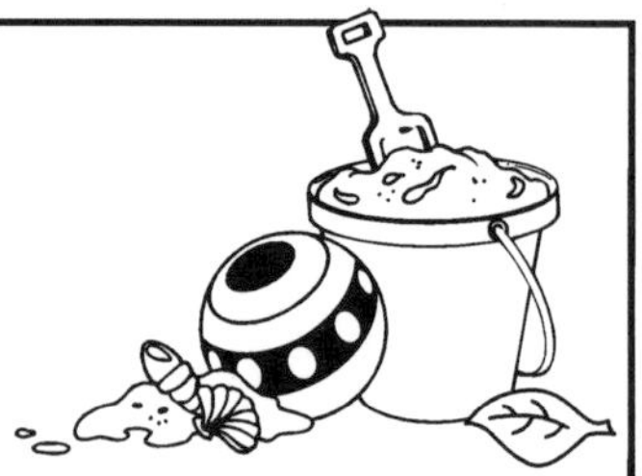

Theme: Water

Description: Sinking and floating objects in water

Exemplars: baby's, boy's, [child's name]'s, girl's, lifeguard's, man's, mom's, sandpiper's, shell's, someone's

Materials:

At the Beach by Anne Rockwell and Harlow Rockwell
Stuffed animal or puppet (for individual sessions only)
Bag filled with objects that sink (e.g., rocks and seashells) and objects that float (e.g., sponges and feathers)
Container filled with water

INTRODUCTION TO THEME

EDUCATOR: Remember how we made bubbles with water last week? Well, this week we are going to talk about something else we can do with water. We are going to talk about things to do with water at the beach. *[Ask children if they have been to the beach and discuss what they have done there]* There are lots of fun things we can do in the water when we go to the beach.

BOOK ACTIVITY

Book: *At the Beach* by Anne Rockwell and Harlow Rockwell

Instructions: Read the book with children, emphasizing possessives. When possessives do not occur naturally in the book, comment on the story using them (e.g., "That is the **girl's** shell" and "She grabbed the **shovel's** handle").

Suggested Theme-Related Supplemental Books:
Curious George Goes to the Beach by Margaret Rey and H.A. Rey
For Sand Castles or Seashells by Gail Hartman and Ellen Weiss (illustrator)

Transition

EDUCATOR: The girl in our book went to the beach and played in the water. Let's look at our story again and talk about the things she saw.

FOCUSED STIMULATION ACTIVITY

Description: Discussing the story using possessives

Skills Used: Narrative, labeling, and describing

Instructions: Start at the beginning of the book and discuss items.

Example Script

EDUCATOR: This is the **girl's** shovel.

EDUCATOR: The **mom's** umbrella is pretty.

EDUCATOR: The little **girl's** cup has a flower on it.

EDUCATOR: The **sandpiper's** feet make prints in the sand.

EDUCATOR: This **shell's** colors are beautiful!

EDUCATOR: The boy shares the **girl's** shovel.

EDUCATOR: The **boy's** boat is sailing in the water. *[Consider having children name the boy and the girl and use the names instead of "boy's" and "girl's"]*

EDUCATOR: The **man's** tummy is covered in sand!

EDUCATOR: The **girl's** toe is getting pinched by a crab!

EDUCATOR: The **lifeguard's** station is on the beach.

EDUCATOR: The **mom's** hands are holding the girl.

EDUCATOR: The **girl's** hair is wet from playing in the water.

EDUCATOR: The **girl's** lunch looks yummy!

[Continue in a similar manner until the story is completed and numerous models of possessives have been provided.]

Transition

Educator: I liked the part of the story when the girl played in the water. Today we are going to do something fun with water! Let's get started!

ELICITED PRODUCTION ACTIVITY

Description: Sinking and floating items

Skills Used: Fine motor and direction following

Goal: 10 productions of possessives per child

Level of Educator Support: Forced choice

Instructions: The following script works best for sessions with several children. If using this script for sessions with an individual child, have a stuffed animal or puppet "participate" in the activity and give it a name to create natural opportunities to use possessives.

Example Script

Educator: We can do lots of things with water. The girl in the book played by the water. We made bubbles with water last time. We drink water and we swim in water. Some things float in water and some things sink. Remember how the **boy's** boat floated in the water in our story? Today we are going to put some things in water and see if they sink or float.

Educator: Let's each look in this bag and choose something. *[Each child reaches in the bag and gets something]* Now let's see what each of us has.

Educator: Jake found a penny. Whose penny is it? Is it **Jake's** or **Sally's**?

Child: It's **Jake's**.

Educator: Whose shell is this? **Sally's** or **John's**?

Child: **Sally's**.

Educator: I wonder whose eraser this is. Is it **Sally's** or **Maria's**?

Example Script—*Continued*

CHILD:	**Maria's**. *[Continue using this format for all items/children]*
EDUCATOR:	Now let's drop our objects in the water. *[Present container filled with water]*
EDUCATOR:	Look, **someone's** penny sank in the water! Whose was it? **Jake's** or **Sally's**?
CHILD:	**Jake's.**
EDUCATOR:	**Someone's** sponge floated. Whose was it? **John's** or **Maria's**?
CHILD:	**John's.**
EDUCATOR:	I wonder whose turn it is now to sink and float. Is it **Sally's** or **Maria's** turn?
CHILD:	**Sally's.**

[Continue in a similar manner until each child has had at least 10 opportunities to use possessives.]

Transition

EDUCATOR: I really had fun sinking and floating things in water. Now it's time to clean up and sing our beach song.

SONG ACTIVITY

Instructions: Sing to the tune of "Little Bunny Foo Foo," emphasizing possessives.

Down by the Seashore

Down by the seashore early in the morning,
I saw the **baby's** toy lying on the beach.
I saw **[child's name]'s** family having so much fun!

Down by the seashore early in the morning,
I saw **mommy's** boat floating in the water.
I saw **[child's name]'s** family having so much fun!

Down by the seashore early in the morning,
I saw the **baby's** seashell shining like the sun.
I saw **[child's name]'s** family having so much fun!

Possessives

Cycle 1, Session 2

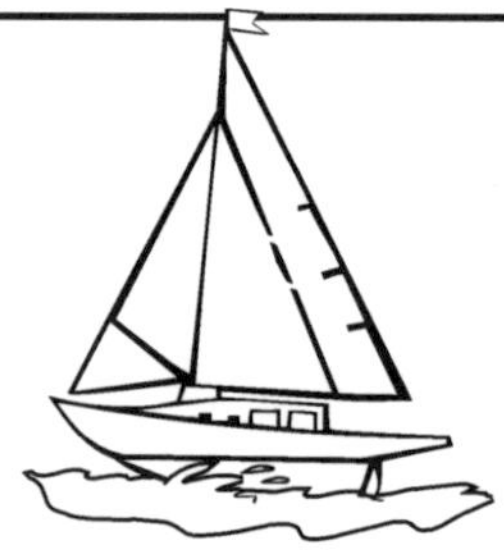

Theme: Water

Description: Completing activities relating to boats

Exemplars: baby's, boat's, [child's name]'s, girl's, mommy's

Materials:

- *At the Beach* by Anne Rockwell and Harlow Rockwell
- Completed sailboat (see page 272 for directions)
- Puppet (for individual sessions only)
- Milk cartons (cut in half lengthwise; 1 half per child)
- Tape
- Styrofoam (cut in 1 square inch pieces; 1 piece per child)
- Craft sticks
- Boat sails (see page 272 for directions; 2 per child)
- Glue
- Stickers (optional)
- Index cards (1 per child)
- Pen
- Container filled with water

BOOK ACTIVITY

Book: *At the Beach* by Anne Rockwell and Harlow Rockwell

Instructions: Reread the book with children, emphasizing possessives. When possessives do not occur naturally in the book, comment on the book using possessives (e.g., "That is the **girl's** shell" and "She grabbed the **shovel's** handle").

Suggested Theme-Related Supplemental Books: *Curious George Goes to the Beach* by Margaret Rey and H.A. Rey
For Sand Castles or Seashells by Gail Hartman and Ellen Weiss (illustrator)

Transition

EDUCATOR: The girl in our book played with a boat when she went to the beach. Today we are going to make some boats too!

FOCUSED STIMULATION ACTIVITY

Description: Making milk carton sailboats

Skills Used: Fine motor and direction following

Special Instructions: Prepare a sailboat prior to the activity to serve as a model. The following script is most appropriate for sessions with several children. If using this script for sessions with an individual child, have a puppet make a sailboat while the child does and give it a name to create natural opportunities to produce possessives.

Example Script

EDUCATOR: Let's see what we've got. *[Distribute materials]* Look at **Jane's** milk carton. I wonder what we'll do with **Jane's** milk carton.

EDUCATOR: Look at **John's** tape, Styrofoam, sticks, and sails.

EDUCATOR: **Sally's** paper is blue. **John's** paper is red.

EDUCATOR: **Jane's** milk carton is blue and white.

EDUCATOR: **John's** Styrofoam is very crumbly!

EDUCATOR: **Sally's** stick is in the Styrofoam.

EDUCATOR: **Jane's** stick is big.

EDUCATOR: **Jane's** boat needs a sail. So does **John's** boat.

EDUCATOR: **Sally's** boat will have a blue sail. **Jake's** boat will have a red sail.

EDUCATOR: Let's put our boats together. First, use **Jake's** glue to glue the foam in the **boat's** bottom *[i.e., the milk carton cut in half]*.

EDUCATOR: Now **Sally's** stick gets stuck in the foam.

EDUCATOR: Let's glue **Jake's** sail on the stick.

EDUCATOR: **John's** stickers will make his sail pretty.

[Continue in a similar manner until the sailboats have been completed and numerous models of possessives have been provided.]

Transition

EDUCATOR: The girl in our story liked to do things in the water. She went to the beach and made sandcastles. The **girl's** mom played too. Another fun thing to do in water is ride on boats. Today we are going to make more boats and have a race in water to see whose boat is the fastest!

ELICITED PRODUCTION ACTIVITY

Description: Having a boat race

Skills Used: Fine motor, turn taking, and oral motor

Goal: 10 productions of possessives per child

Level of Educator Support: Forced choice

Special Instructions: Cut a boat shape out of each child's index card. Children's names should be written on their boats. Then laminate the boats. Using the container, have children, two at a time, race their boats by blowing on them. For sessions with an individual child, have a hand puppet a "participate" in the race to create natural opportunities to use possessives.

Example Script

EDUCATOR: We are going to use these for our boats. *[Present index cards]*

EDUCATOR: I wrote your names on them.

EDUCATOR: Whose boat is this? **Jane's** or **Jake's?**

CHILD: **Jane's.**

EDUCATOR: Whose name is this? **John's** or **Sally's?**

CHILD: **Sally's.** *[Continue in similar manner for each child]*

EDUCATOR: Now that you all have your boats, we are going to have a race.

EDUCATOR: Let's have our race here in this water. *[Present container filled with water]*

Example Script—*Continued*

EDUCATOR: Here is **Jane's** boat and here is **Jake's.** Put your boats in the water. We are going to start on this end. If you want your boats to move, you have to blow on them like this. *[Demonstrate]* Are you ready? *[Allow children to respond]* Go!

EDUCATOR: Whose boat is this? **Jake's** or **Sally's?**

CHILD: **Sally's.**

EDUCATOR: Whose boat won? **Sally's** or **Jake's?**

CHILD: **Jake's.** *[Repeat elicitations for each pair of children, and discuss features of different children's boats]*

[Continue in a similar manner until each child has had at least 10 opportunities to use possessives.]

Transition

EDUCATOR: It was fun sailing our boats! Let's finish up by singing our beach song.

SONG ACTIVITY

Instructions: Sing to the tune of "Little Bunny Foo Foo," emphasizing possessives.

Down by the Seashore

Down by the seashore early in the morning,
I saw the **baby's** toy lying on the beach.
I saw **[child's name]'s** family having so much fun!

Down by the seashore early in the morning,
I saw **mommy's** boat floating in the water.
I saw **[child's name]'s** family having so much fun!

Down by the seashore early in the morning,
I saw the **baby's** seashell shining like the sun.
I saw **[child's name]'s** family having so much fun!

Weekly Family Letter

For: ______________________________ **Date:** ______________

Theme

Our theme for language intervention this week is *water.*

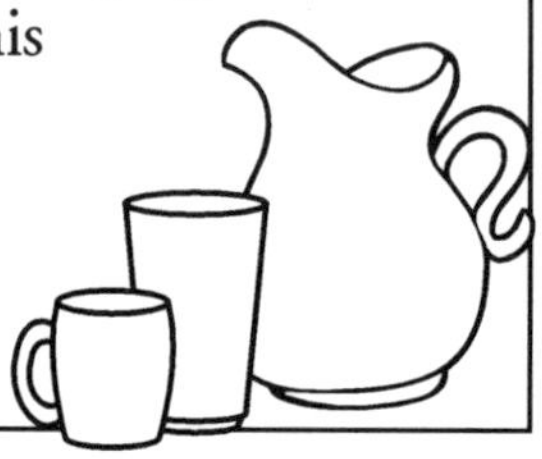

Target

Our target language structures are *pronouns.* Pronouns take the place of proper names. Examples include:

- **She** frosted the cake.
- The dog barked at **him.**
- **Her** bike is pink.

Book

Our book for the week is *Miss Spider's Tea Party* by David Kirk.

Here is a related book you could read at home: *Let's Have a Tea Party* by Emilie Barnes and Michal Sparks and Sue Junker (illustrators).

Song

Our Tea Party
(Tune: "She'll Be Coming Around the Mountain")

She was pouring, pouring, pouring **her** tea!
She was pouring, pouring, pouring **her** tea!
She was happy as **she** could be because **she** was pouring **her** tea!
She was happy, happy, happy as could be!

He was putting some sugar in **his** tea!
He was putting some sugar in **his** tea!
He was stirring, stirring, stirring and **he** was in a big hurry.
He was stirring, stirring, stirring up **his** tea!

They were all having a tea party!
They were all having a tea party!
They had such fun at **their** little tea party
because **they** were sipping, sipping, sipping up **their** tea!

Activities

Our planned activities for the week include:

- Making a drink with sugar, water, and drink mix
- Drawing a sequence picture of making a drink
- Having a pretend tea party
- Smelling tea bags

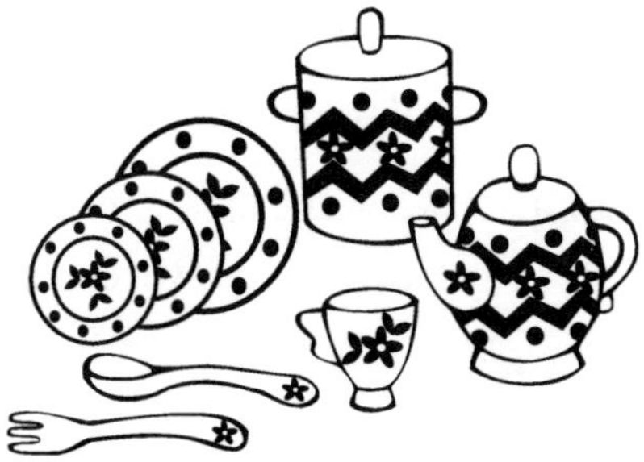

Follow-Up

Suggested follow-up activities for home include:

- Have a tea party with your child and talk about what you are doing using pronouns, for example:

  We poured water in **our** cups.

  We stirred up **our** drink.

- Play a game where your child identifies correct pronoun usage. For example, say "**Her** drank the tea or **she** drank the tea?" and have your child pick an answer.

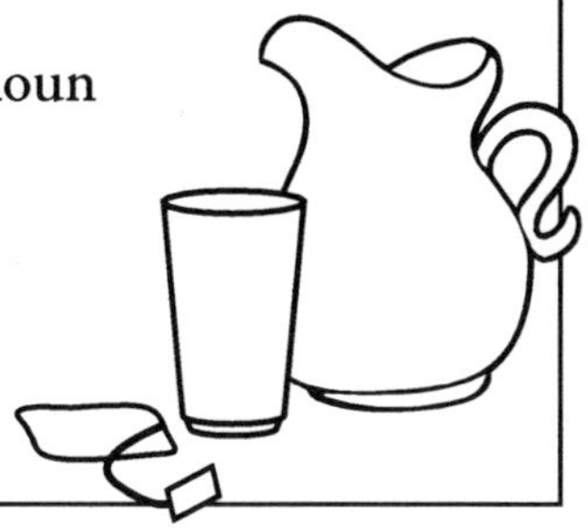

Thank You Very Much for your participation!

____
Phone Number

____
Email

____
Signature

Pronouns

Cycle 1, Session 1

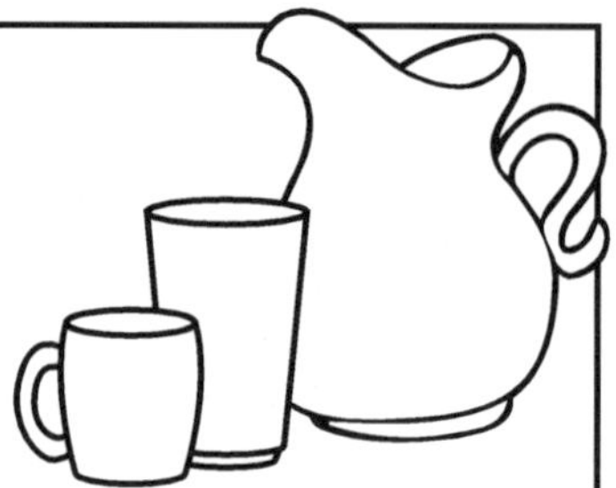

Theme: Water

Description: Making beverages with water

Exemplars: he, her, hers, him, his, I, me, my, our, she, their, they, us, we, our, you, it, your

Materials:

Miss Spider's Tea Party by David Kirk
Wet paper towels
Stuffed animal or puppet (for individual sessions only)
Cups (1 per child; 1 for educator)
Bottle of water
Drink mix (sweetened or unsweetened)
Tablespoons and teaspoons (1 each per child; 1 each for educator)
Sugar (if using unsweetened drink mix)
Paper
Markers or crayons

INTRODUCTION TO THEME

EDUCATOR: **We** have been doing lots of interesting things with water. **We** made bubbles with water. **We** talked about places where **we** can find water, like the beach. **We** sank and floated things in water. There are other things **we** can do with water too. Can anyone tell **me** something else **we** can do with water? *[If children do not generate the response "drink it," provide a gestural or other type of cue]* That's right! **We** can drink water. Sometimes **we** drink water all by itself and sometimes **we** put things in water to make yummy drinks. Let**'s** read **our** story and find out what Miss Spider likes to drink.

BOOK ACTIVITY

Book: *Miss Spider's Tea Party* by David Kirk

Instructions: Read the book with children, emphasizing pronouns.

Suggested theme-related supplemental book: *Let's Have a Tea Party* by Emilie Barnes and Michal Sparks and Sue Junker (illustrators)

Transition

EDUCATOR: Miss Spider had a nice tea party. Today **we** are going to have a tea party like **hers.**

FOCUSED STIMULATION ACTIVITY

Description: Making drinks

Skills Used: Sharing, direction following, and turn taking

Instructions: For the following script, use the product name in place of "drink mix." For sessions with an individual child, have a stuffed animal or puppet "participate" in the tea party to create natural opportunities to use the pronouns *he/his/him* or *she/hers/her.* Or focus on the pronouns *me/my/mine, we/our/ours,* and *you/your/yours* instead.

Example Script

EDUCATOR: **You** can sit at the table, and **I** will show you how to make **our** tea. *[Wash or wipe hands]*

EDUCATOR: **I** washed **my** hands. *[Take out a cup, some water, the drink mix, and a spoon]*

EDUCATOR: **I** looked for **my** spoon. **I** looked for the drink mix, and **I** poured some water in **my** cup. *[Scoop out the drink mix and dump it in the cup]*

EDUCATOR: **I** scooped out some drink mix and poured **it** in **my** cup. *[Scoop sugar into drink mix if necessary; then stir and take a sip]*

EDUCATOR: **I** stirred and stirred. Then **I** sipped **my** drink.

EDUCATOR: OK, now it's **your** turn to make a drink. *[Pass out spoons and cups to each child]*

EDUCATOR: Oh, John grabbed **his** spoon and Jane grabbed **her** spoon. Here is **her** water and here is **his** water. Here is some water for Jake. I will give **it** to **him.**

EDUCATOR: **He** poured drink mix in **his** cup.

EDUCATOR: Oops, **she** spilled drink mix on the table.

EDUCATOR: Look, **she** got some drink mix.

EDUCATOR: Do **you** remember what **I** did next?

Continued on next page

Example Script—*Continued*

CHILD:	**<u>You</u>** stirred it.
EDUCATOR:	That's right, **<u>I</u>** stirred the drink mix into **<u>my</u>** water.
EDUCATOR:	After **<u>I</u>** stirred the drink mix, what did **<u>I</u>** get to do?
CHILD:	**<u>You</u>** tasted **<u>it</u>**.
EDUCATOR:	That's right, **<u>I</u>** tasted it! Now **<u>John</u>** can taste **<u>his</u>** drink mix. **<u>We</u>** made good drinks today!

[Continue in a similar manner until numerous models of pronouns have been provided.]

Transition

EDUCATOR: Our drinks were delicious! Now **we** are going to draw pictures to show what **we** did today. Then **we** can take them home to show **our** families.

ELICITED PRODUCTION ACTIVITY

Description: Drawing sequence pictures of making drinks

Skills Used: Sequencing and fine motor

Goal: 10 productions of pronouns per child

Level of Educator Support: Forced choice

Instructions: For the following script, use the product name in place of "drink mix." If children are unable or not interested in drawing all pictures of the sequence, they can draw a picture of one aspect of the project or, as a group, discuss the steps and the educator can draw a picture.

Example Script

EDUCATOR:	**<u>We</u>** are going to draw a picture of what **<u>we</u>** did today.
EDUCATOR:	Jane, who made a drink? **<u>We</u>** did or **<u>I</u>** did?
CHILD:	**<u>We</u>** did.
EDUCATOR:	First, someone poured in water.
EDUCATOR:	John, then someone scooped in the drink mix. Who did that? **<u>I</u>** did or **<u>you</u>** did?
CHILD:	**<u>I</u>** did.
EDUCATOR:	That's right, **<u>you</u>** scooped up some drink mix.

Example Script—*Continued*

EDUCATOR: Let'**s** draw a picture of that.

EDUCATOR: Then Sally did something. Sally stirred the drink mix. Who stirred it? **She** did or **he** did?

CHILD: **She** did.

EDUCATOR: Yes, **she** stirred the drink. Let'**s** draw a picture of that.

EDUCATOR: Then what happened? **He** tasted it or **I** tasted it?

CHILD: **He** tasted it.

EDUCATOR: Yes, **he** did! Who did let taste the drink mix? I let **him** or **her?**

CHILD: **Him.**

[Continue in a similar manner until each child has had at least 10 opportunities to use pronouns.]

Transition

EDUCATOR: I had such a good time at **our** tea party! **Our** drinks were great! **Our** pictures look nice too. Now let'**s** clean up and sing the tea party song.

SONG ACTIVITY

Instructions: Sing to the tune of "She'll Be Coming Around the Mountain," emphasizing pronouns.

Our Tea Party

She was pouring, pouring, pouring **her** tea!
She was pouring, pouring, pouring **her** tea!
She was happy as **she** could be because **she** was pouring **her** tea!
She was happy, happy, happy as could be!

He was putting some sugar in **his** tea!
He was putting some sugar in **his** tea!
He was stirring, stirring, stirring and **he** was in a big hurry.
He was stirring, stirring, stirring up **his** tea!

They were all having a tea party!
They were all having a tea party!
They had such fun at **their** little tea party
because **they** were sipping, sipping, sipping up **their** tea!

Pronouns

Cycle 1, Session 2

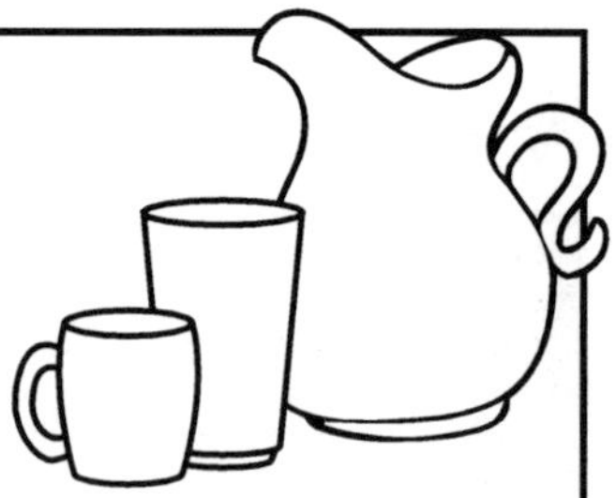

Theme: Water

Description: Making beverages with water

Exemplars: he, her, him, his, I, it, me, my, our, she, theirs, they, us, we, you

Materials:

- *Miss Spider's Tea Party* by David Kirk
- Stuffed animal or puppet (for individual sessions only)
- Bag containing:
  - Cups, spoons, and small paper plates OR child's tea set
  - Tea bags in a variety of flavors
  - Hot water (in insulated container)
  - Sugar
  - Cookies

BOOK ACTIVITY

Book: *Miss Spider's Tea Party* by David Kirk

Instructions: Reread the book with children, emphasizing pronouns.

Suggested theme-related supplemental book: *Let's Have a Tea Party* by Emilie Barnes and Michal Sparks and Sue Junker (illustrators)

Transition

EDUCATOR: Miss Spider had a good time at **her** tea party, so **I** thought **we** could have a tea party too!

FOCUSED STIMULATION ACTIVITY

Description: Having a tea party

Skill Used: Dramatic play

Instructions: For sessions with an individual child, have a stuffed animal or puppet "participate" in the tea party to create natural opportunities to use *he/his/him* or *she/hers/her.* Or focus on the pronouns *you/your/yours, we/our/ours,* or *me/mine/my* instead.

Example Script

EDUCATOR:	Let'**s** have a tea party like Miss Spider.
EDUCATOR:	**I** have everything **we** need to set **our** table. **You** can take the stuff out of this bag.
CHILD:	*[Removes items from bag]*
EDUCATOR:	**You** pulled out a cup.
EDUCATOR:	Now **you** found a spoon.
EDUCATOR:	**I** wonder what **she** will pull out next.
EDUCATOR:	**She** pulled out another spoon.
EDUCATOR:	Remember **our** story? What did Miss Spider do after **she** set **her** table? *[Consult pictures in the story if necessary]*
CHILD:	**She** poured tea.
EDUCATOR:	**You** think **she** poured some tea. **I** think **she** poured tea too.
EDUCATOR:	**You** and **I** can make some tea. **We** need some hot water and some tea bags.
EDUCATOR:	**I** pulled out some water and some tea bags. *[Unwrap a tea packet]*
EDUCATOR:	**I** opened the tea and **I** poured **it** in **my** cup.
CHILD:	*[Pours water in cup]*
EDUCATOR:	Then **she** poured some hot water in **it.**
CHILD:	*[Stirs the tea]*
EDUCATOR:	**He** stirred **his** tea.
CHILD:	*[Scoops up sugar and pours it into tea]*
EDUCATOR:	**She** scooped up some sugar and put **it** in **her** tea.
EDUCATOR:	Now Sally will find **our** snack.
CHILD:	*[Passes out cookies]*
EDUCATOR:	She gave cookies to **him.** **She** gave cookies to **her.**
EDUCATOR:	**We** tasted **her** cookies.

[Continue in a similar manner until numerous models of pronouns have been provided.]

Transition

EDUCATOR: I had fun at **our** tea party. **I** noticed something when **we** opened up the tea bags. **I** noticed that some of the tea bags smelled really good! Today **we** are going to do something special with these tea bags.

ELICITED PRODUCTION ACTIVITY

Description: Smelling tea bags

Skills Used: Sensory exploration and describing

Goal: 10 productions of pronouns per child

Level of Educator Support: Forced choice

Instructions: For sessions with an individual child, focus on the pronouns *you/your/yours, we/our/ours,* or *me/my/mine* as opposed to *he/his/him* and *she/hers/her.* Or have a puppet "participate" to create natural opportunities to use *he/his/him* and *she/hers/her.*

Example Script

EDUCATOR:	Look, **I** have some tea bags in here. **I**'ll take one out. Maria, smell this.
EDUCATOR:	Who smelled **it**? **He** did or **she** did?
CHILD:	**She** did.
EDUCATOR:	Now whose turn is **it**? **His** turn or **her** turn?
CHILD:	**Her** turn.
EDUCATOR:	Who smelled **it**? **You** did or **she** did?
CHILD:	**She** did.
EDUCATOR:	*[Rip open a tea packet]*
EDUCATOR:	Who ripped open the packet? **I** did or **he** did?
CHILD:	**You** did!
EDUCATOR:	Right, **I** ripped open the packet.
EDUCATOR:	Here's a bag for **you.** Who did I give the bag to, **him** or **her**?
CHILD:	**Her**.
EDUCATOR:	Who does this bag belong to? **Him** or **me**?

Example Script—*Continued*

CHILD: **Him.**

EDUCATOR: Who ripped open this packet? **He** did or **she** did?

CHILD: **She** did.

EDUCATOR: *[Have a different child rip open a tea packet]*

EDUCATOR: Look who ripped this bag open. **She** did or **he** did?

CHILD: **He** ripped it. *[Educator and children clean up]*

EDUCATOR: Who cleaned up? **We** did or **he** did?

CHILD: **We** cleaned up!

[Continue in a similar manner until each child has had at least 10 opportunities to use pronouns.]

Transition

EDUCATOR: **We** had a busy day. First **we** had a tea party like Miss Spider's, and then **we** smelled some delicious tea. Before **we** go, let**'s** sing the tea party song.

SONG ACTIVITY

Instructions: Sing to the tune of "She'll Be Coming Around the Mountain," emphasizing pronouns.

Our Tea Party

She was pouring, pouring, pouring **her** tea!
She was pouring, pouring, pouring **her** tea!
She was happy as **she** could be because **she** was pouring **her** tea!
She was happy, happy, happy as could be!

He was putting some sugar in **his** tea!
He was putting some sugar in **his** tea!
He was stirring, stirring, stirring and **he** was in a big hurry.
He was stirring, stirring, stirring up **his** tea!

They were all having a tea party!
They were all having a tea party!
They had such fun at **their** little tea party
because **they** were sipping, sipping, sipping up **their** tea!

Weekly Family Letter

For: ______________________________ **Date:** ______________

Theme

Our theme for language intervention this week is *water.*

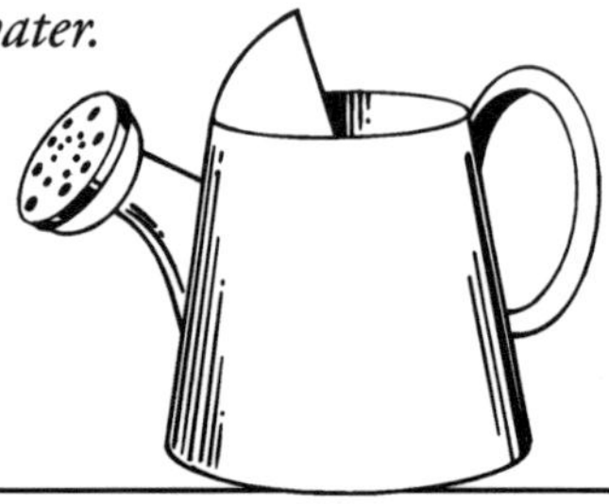

Target

Our target language structures are *auxiliary* be *verbs.* These are the verbs *am ('m), are ('re),* and *is ('s)* when used as "helping" verbs in a sentence. Generally, these verbs are used in front of verbs with *-ing* endings. Examples include:

- **I'm** going home.
- My sister **is** taking a ballet class.
- The dogs **are** barking loudly.

Book

Our book for the week is *This Is Your Garden* by Maggie Smith.

Here is a related book you could read at home: *The Tiny Seed* by Eric Carle.

Song

Little Seed
(Tune: "Mary Had a Little Lamb")

Jane **is** growing a little seed, little seed, little seed.
Jane **is** growing a little seed. Soon it will grow.

John **is** watering his little seed, little seed, little seed.
John **is** watering his little seed. Soon it will grow.

Maria **is** watching her little seed, little seed, little seed.
Maria **is** watching her little seed. Now it's all grown!

(Repeat using your child's name and other names.)

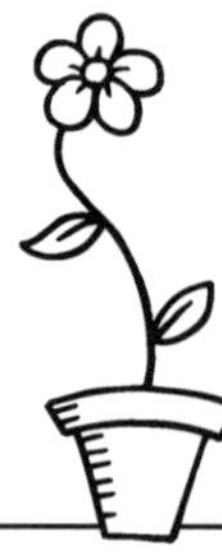

Activities

Our planned activities for the week include:

- Decorating a flower pot
- Planting seeds
- Drawing a sequence picture of planting seeds

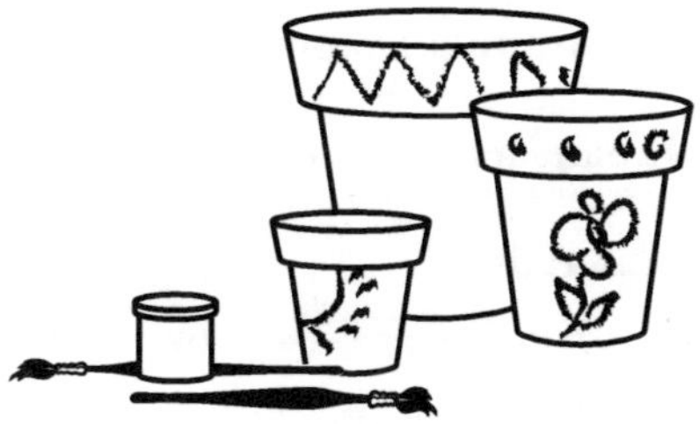

Follow-Up

Suggested follow-up activities for home include:

- Discuss ongoing actions, perhaps during a television show or story, using auxiliary *be* verbs, for example:

  They **are** driving a big car.

  He **is** hugging a friend.

- Plant seeds (either inside in a pot or outside in the ground). As you complete the activity, you can "narrate" actions, emphasizing auxiliary *be* verbs.

  We **are** digging a hole for our seeds.

  I **am** using a shovel to dig in the dirt.

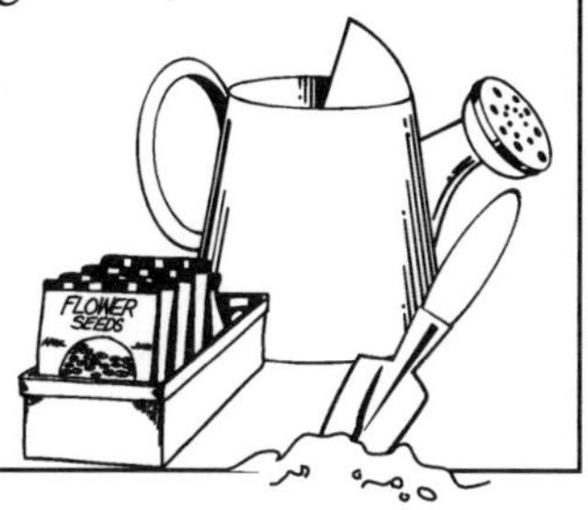

Thank You Very Much for your participation!

Phone Number

Email

Signature

Auxiliary *be*

Cycle 1, Session 1

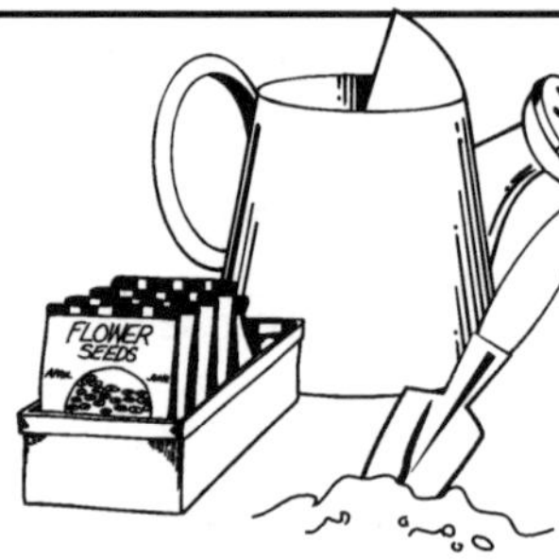

Theme: Water

Description: Decorating a flower pot

Exemplars: am ('m), are ('re), is ('s)

Materials:

This Is Your Garden by Maggie Smith
Styrofoam cups (1 per child)
Completed flower pot (see page 273 for directions and patterns)
Photocopies of facial features (see page 273 for directions and patterns; 1 per child)
Child-safe scissors
Crayons or markers
Glue

INTRODUCTION TO THEME

EDUCATOR: We have been talking about many different things we can do with water. Who remembers what we used water for last week? *[Allow children to guess/respond]* That's right! We used water to make yummy things for us to drink. People like to drink water. There is something that needs water to grow. I will give you some hints about what it might be. The thing I **am** thinking about needs sunlight. It grows in the ground and it is very pretty. Can you guess what it is? *[Children may choose to guess what it is]* That's right! **I'm** talking about flowers and plants.

BOOK ACTIVITY

Book: *This Is Your Garden* by Maggie Smith

Instructions: Read the book with children, emphasizing auxiliary *be* verbs. When these forms do not occur naturally in the story, comment on the story using them (e.g., "The water **is** moving" and "They **are** walking").

Suggested Theme-Related Supplemental Book: *The Tiny Seed* by Eric Carle

Transition

EDUCATOR: The girl in our story planted a whole garden. We can plant seeds and give them water too. If we want to plant seeds, we'll need something to put them in. Look at this. *[Present cup]* It is a white cup. We **are** going to put these things on it. *[Present photocopies of facial features]*

FOCUSED STIMULATION ACTIVITY

Description: Preparing items for flower pots, which will be made in the elicited production activity.

Skill Used: Fine motor

Instructions: Complete a flower pot prior to the activity to serve as a model. Discuss actions as they are being completed to create natural opportunities to use auxiliary *be* verbs.

Example Script

EDUCATOR We can plant seeds and give them water so they will grow. If we want to plant seeds, we'll need something to put them in. Look at this. *[Present a cup]* It's a white cup. We **are** going to put a face on it like this. *[Present model]*

EDUCATOR: Look at these mouths. This mouth **is** smiling but this mouth **is** frowning.

EDUCATOR: Let's cut out some eyes for the cup. Jane **is** cutting out two eyes.

EDUCATOR: It looks like Miguel **is** cutting out a nose for his cup.

EDUCATOR: Sally and Jane **are** cutting out ears.

EDUCATOR: I **am** making a nose for my cup.

EDUCATOR: Our cups **are** going to look so good!

EDUCATOR: I **am** coloring my mouth red.

EDUCATOR: Sally **is** making her eyes green.

EDUCATOR: Miguel **is** using some glue.

EDUCATOR: Jane **is** borrowing the yellow crayon from Sally.

EDUCATOR: We **are** coloring lots of things to put on our cups!

EDUCATOR: Our cups **are** going to look like faces when we are done!

[Continue in a similar manner until the cups have been decorated and numerous models of auxiliary be *verbs have been provided.]*

Transition

EDUCATOR: We **are** going to have very pretty cups to grow our seeds in! Let's get started!

ELICITED PRODUCTION ACTIVITY

Description: Decorating flower pots

Skill Used: Fine motor

Goal: 10 productions of auxiliary *be* verbs per child

Level of Educator Support: Forced choice

Instructions: Remember that contracted (e.g., He**'s** walking) and uncontracted (e.g., It **is** raining) auxiliary *be* verbs are acceptable.

Example Script

EDUCATOR: Now we need to put our mouths, noses, and eyes on our cups, like this one. *[Present model]*

EDUCATOR: Who **is** gluing? Jane **is** gluing or John **is** gluing?

CHILD: John **is** gluing.

EDUCATOR: Who **is** taping on eyes? Sally **is** taping or Jake **is** taping?

CHILD: Sally **is** taping.

EDUCATOR: Tell me about John. He**'s** coloring or he**'s** gluing?

CHILD: He**'s** coloring.

EDUCATOR: Now tell me about Sally. She**'s** cutting or she**'s** gluing?

CHILD: She**'s** gluing.

EDUCATOR: Who **is** gluing on a pink mouth? John **is** gluing or Jane **is** gluing?

CHILD: Jane **is** gluing.

EDUCATOR: Who **is** working faster? We **are** working faster or they **are** working faster?

CHILD: They **are** working faster.

EDUCATOR: Tell me about the face on this cup. It**'s** smiling or it**'s** crying?

CHILD: It**'s** smiling.

EDUCATOR: Who **is** putting on ears? I **am** putting them on or you **are** putting them on?

CHILD: I **am** putting them on.

[Continue in a similar manner until each child has had at least 10 opportunities to use auxiliary be *verbs.]*

Transition

EDUCATOR: Our flower pots look great! Let's clean up and sing our song about the little seed.

SONG ACTIVITY

Instructions: Sing to the tune of "Mary Had a Little Lamb," emphasizing auxiliary *be* verbs. Use a different child's name for each verse. (When using the song with an individual child, use his or her name.)

Little Seed

Jane **is** growing a little seed, little seed, little seed.
Jane **is** growing a little seed. Soon it will grow.

John **is** watering his little seed, little seed, little seed.
John **is** watering his little seed. Soon it will grow.

Maria **is** watching her little seed, little seed, little seed.
Maria **is** watching her little seed. Now it's all grown!

(Repeat, if necessary, using other names.)

Auxiliary *be*

Cycle 1, Session 2

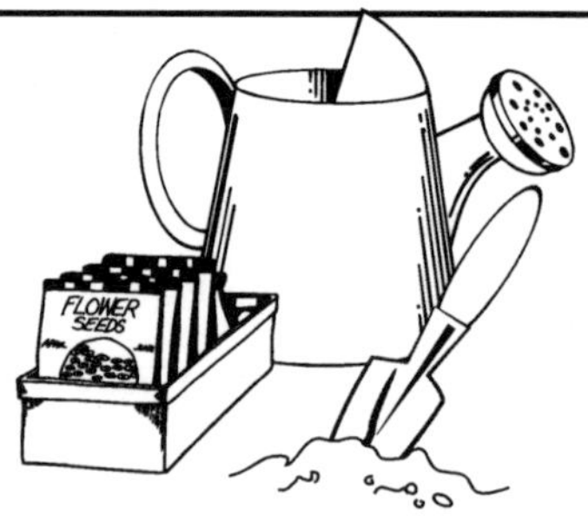

Theme: Water

Description: Using water to grow plants

Exemplars: am ('m), are ('re), is ('s)

Materials:

This Is Your Garden by Maggie Smith
Cups (decorated in previous session)
Potting soil
Spoons
Seeds (grass or wheat seeds work best)
Water
Paper
Crayons or markers

BOOK ACTIVITY

Book: *This Is Your Garden* by Maggie Smith

Instructions: Reread the book with children, emphasizing auxiliary *be* verbs. When these forms do not occur naturally in the story, comment on the story using them (e.g., "The water **is** moving" and "They **are** walking").

Suggested theme-related supplemental book: *The Tiny Seed* by Eric Carle

Transition

EDUCATOR: Remember how we made our face cups last time? Well, today we **are** going to use our cups. We **are** going to do something like the girl in the story. We **are** going to put dirt, seeds, and water in our cups and grow grass!

FOCUSED STIMULATION ACTIVITY

Description: Planting seeds

Skills Used: Fine motor and gross motor

Instructions: Narrate actions as they are occurring to create natural opportunities for auxiliary *be* verbs.

Example Script

EDUCATOR:	Here are the cups we made last time. *[Present cups]* Today, we **are** going to plant seeds in our cups. The seeds **are** going to grow into grass. After the seeds grow, it **is** going to look like the faces on our cups have hair!
EDUCATOR:	Let's get started. I **am** putting dirt in my cup. Now it is Sally's turn.
EDUCATOR:	Sally **is** putting dirt in her cup. She **is** using a spoon to put her dirt in the cup.
EDUCATOR:	Jake **is** filling up his cup too.
EDUCATOR:	Oh no! John's dirt **is** spilling on the floor, so Jake **is** helping him clean up.
EDUCATOR:	Our cups have dirt so let's see what's next.
EDUCATOR:	We need some seeds! Sally**'s** finding the seeds for us.
EDUCATOR:	What should we do now? It looks like John and Jake **are** digging a little hole to put their seeds in.
EDUCATOR:	We all **are** planting our seeds.
EDUCATOR:	Now we **are** covering our seeds with dirt.
EDUCATOR:	I think we need one last thing to help our seeds grow.
CHILD:	Water!
EDUCATOR:	Yes! Sally **is** going to find some water for us.
EDUCATOR:	I wonder what we should do with the water.
CHILD:	Pour it on the seeds!
EDUCATOR:	Yes, I **am** pouring the water on my seeds.
EDUCATOR:	I**'m** pouring too much water! Our seeds only need a little water.
EDUCATOR:	I wonder where we should put our seed cups.
CHILD:	In the sun!
EDUCATOR:	What a good idea! You **are** all looking hard to find a sunny place for our seeds.
EDUCATOR:	It looks like Jane **is** finding lots of sunny places. Let's put our seeds over here.
EDUCATOR:	When our seeds **are** growing, we will be able to watch them!

[Continue in a similar manner until numerous models of auxiliary be *verbs have been provided.]*

Transition

EDUCATOR: It was fun planting our seeds. If we give them water and sunshine, they will grow in a few days. Then our cups will have hair! Let's draw pictures of what we did with our seeds.

ELICITED PRODUCTION ACTIVITY

Description: Drawing sequence pictures of planting seeds

Skills Used: Sequencing and fine motor

Goal: 10 productions of auxiliary *be* verbs per child

Level of Educator Support: Forced choice

Instructions: If children are unable or not interested in drawing all pictures of the sequence, they can draw a picture of one aspect of the project or, as a group, discuss the steps and the educator can draw a picture.

Example Script

EDUCATOR: Now we **are** going to draw pictures of what we did with our seeds.

EDUCATOR: We **are** going to take our pictures home and show our families what we did.

EDUCATOR: Look what I **am** doing. I **am** drawing or I **am** running?

CHILD: You **are** drawing.

EDUCATOR: Let's draw a picture of what we did first. First, we filled our cups with dirt. Let's draw that. *[Allow children time to draw this]*

EDUCATOR: Look at Jane's picture. What **is** she doing in that picture? She**'s** filling her cup or she**'s** dumping out her cup?

CHILD: She**'s** filling her cup.

EDUCATOR: Let's draw a picture of what we did after we filled our cups with dirt.

EDUCATOR: Look at John's picture. Tell me about it. He**'s** digging a hole or he**'s** spilling his dirt?

CHILD: He **is** digging a hole.

Example Script—*Continued*

EDUCATOR: I think he**'s** digging a hole to put his seeds in.

EDUCATOR: Let's draw what we did next.

EDUCATOR: Look at my picture and tell me what **I'm** doing to the seeds. **I'm** covering them or **I'm** eating them?

CHILD: You**'re** covering them.

EDUCATOR: Let's draw a picture of what we did last. Look at Jane's picture. What **is** Jane doing in this picture? She **is** pouring water or she **is** drinking water?

CHILD: She **is** pouring water.

[Continue in a similar manner until each child has had at least 10 opportunities to use auxiliary be *verbs.]*

Transition

EDUCATOR: We all planted seeds and soon they will grow into plants. Then we drew pictures of planting seeds. That reminds me of our little seed song. Let's sing it now!

SONG ACTIVITY

Instructions: Sing to the tune of "Mary Had a Little Lamb," emphasizing auxiliary *be* verbs. Use a different child's name for each verse. (When using the song with an individual child, use his or her name.)

Little Seed

Jane **is** growing a little seed, little seed, little seed.
Jane **is** growing a little seed. Soon it will grow.

John **is** watering his little seed, little seed, little seed.
John **is** watering his little seed. Soon it will grow.

Maria **is** watching her little seed, little seed, little seed.
Maria **is** watching her little seed. Now it's all grown!

(Repeat, if necessary, using other names.)

Weekly Family Letter

For: ______________________________ **Date:** ____________

Theme

Our theme for language intervention this week is *animals.*

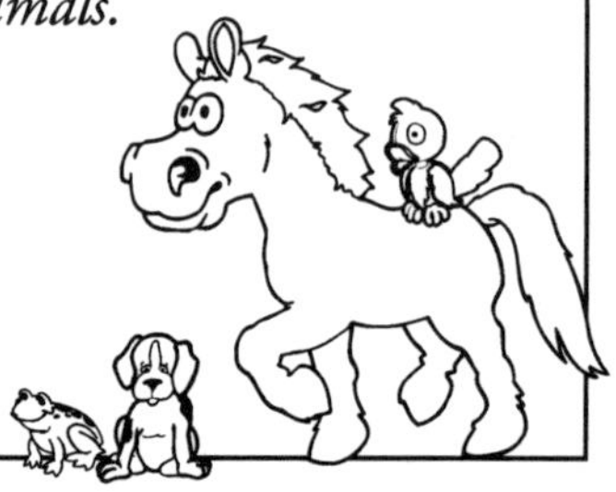

Target

Our target language structures are *regular plurals.* These are words ending in *-s* that indicate more than one of something. Examples include:

- I have two **brothers.**
- My **dogs** play all day long.
- I can't find my **shoes.**

Book

Our book for the week is *Brown Bear, Brown Bear, What Do You See?* by Bill Martin Jr. and Eric Carle (illustrator).

Here are some related books you could read at home: *Polar Bear, Polar Bear, What Do You Hear?* by Bill Martin Jr. and Eric Carle (illustrator) and *Mouse Creeps* by Peter Harris and Reg Cartwright (illustrator).

Song

Brown Bear Sees All His Friends
(Tune: "Mary Had a Little Lamb")

Brown Bear sees all his **friends,** all his **friends,** all his **friends.**
Brown Bear sees all his **friends.** He sees them every day.
Brown Bear likes all his **friends,**
all his **friends,** all his **friends.**
Brown Bear likes his **friends.**
He likes them every way!

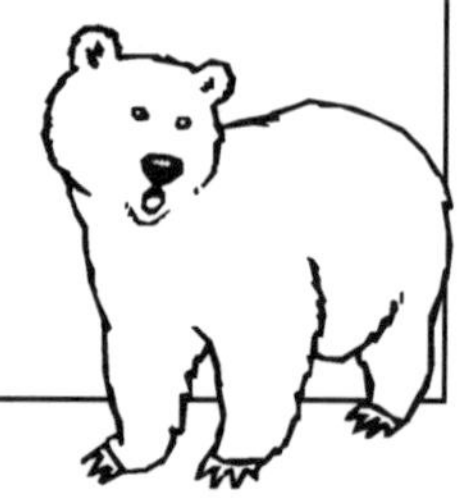

Activities

Our planned activities for the week include:

- Decorating felt animals
- Reenacting the story *Brown Bear, Brown Bear, What Do You See?*
- Making a Brown Bear stick puppet
- Playing I Spy using various animals hidden around the room

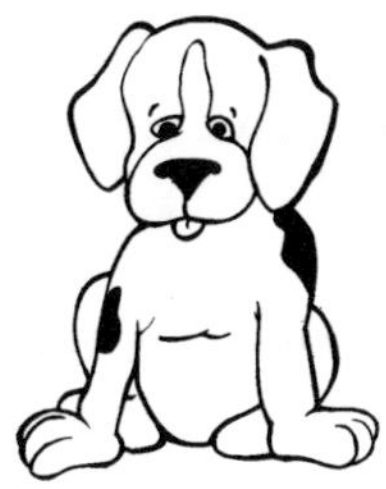

Follow-Up

Suggested follow-up activities for home include:

- Look through a book about animals and discuss it focusing on regular plurals, for example:

  Look at all those **cats!**

  I see a lot of **dogs** on this page!

- Play a fun "What if…" game, and encourage your child to think of possibilities, for example:

  What if we put two **ants** in your bed?

  What if we put ten **elephants** in our bathtub?

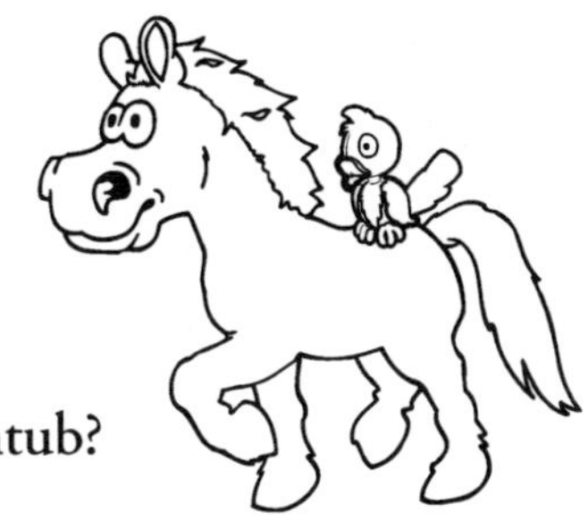

Thank You Very Much for your participation!

Phone Number

Email

Signature

Regular Plurals

Cycle 2, Session 1

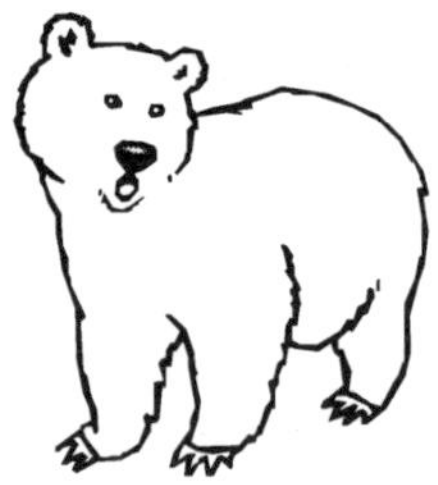

Theme: Animals

Description: Completing activities relating to
Brown Bear, Brown Bear, What Do You See?

Exemplars: animals, beads, cats, dogs, eyes, friends, horses, kids, legs, pets, places, sparkles, spots, things, weeks

Materials:

Brown Bear, Brown Bear, What Do You See? by Bill Martin Jr. and Eric Carle (illustrator)
Felt animal cutouts (see pages 274 and 276–282 for directions and patterns; 1 set)
Glue
Decorations (glitter, google eyes, beads, yarn, etc.)
Felt board

INTRODUCTION TO THEME

EDUCATOR: For the past few **weeks,** we have been talking about all the fun **things** we can do with water. Now we are going to talk about something new. We are going to learn about **animals!** We can find **animals** in many different **places.** Does anybody have a pet animal at home? *[Allow children to name the animals they have]* Where else can we find **animals?** *[Provide cues for places such as the zoo, forest, and farm if necessary]* Today we are going to talk about a bear who sees many different **animals.**

BOOK ACTIVITY

Book: *Brown Bear, Brown Bear, What Do You See?*
by Bill Martin Jr. and Eric Carle (illustrator)

Instructions: Read the book with children. Comment on the story using regular plurals.

Suggested Theme-Related Supplemental Books: *Polar Bear, Polar Bear, What Do You Hear?*
by Bill Martin Jr. and Eric Carle (illustrator)
Mouse Creeps by Peter Harris and Reg Cartwright (illustrator)

Transition

EDUCATOR: Brown Bear saw many different **animals!** Now we are going to make some of those **animals.**

FOCUSED STIMULATION ACTIVITY

Description: Decorating felt animals

Skills Used: Describing and fine motor

Instructions: Have each child make 2–3 animals. Consulting the pictures in the story is encouraged.

Example Script

EDUCATOR: This horse needs **eyes**. Here are some **eyes** for you to use.

EDUCATOR: I wonder what other **things** he needs?

CHILD: **Legs**!

EDUCATOR: Yes, he needs **legs**. He needs four **legs**.

EDUCATOR: This duck needs **eyes** too.

EDUCATOR: Feel this horse and this dog. Our **animals** are so soft!

EDUCATOR: We have lots of **animals**!

EDUCATOR: John has three **animals**!

EDUCATOR: Jane makes good **animals**!

EDUCATOR: Sally likes to use the googly **eyes** for her **animals**!

EDUCATOR: Jane puts lots of **beads** on her **animals**.

EDUCATOR: The **beads** look like **spots**.

EDUCATOR: I like to use these **sparkles** *[glitter]* on my **animals**.

EDUCATOR: **Sparkles** make the **animals** look shiny and pretty.

[Continue in a similar manner until the animals have been decorated and numerous models of regular plurals have been provided.]

Transition

Educator: Now that we have all these beautiful **animals,** I thought we could act out our story using our **animals.** Let's look back in our book and see what we should do.

ELICITED PRODUCTION ACTIVITY

Description: Reenacting *Brown Bear, Brown Bear, What Do You See?* using children's felt animals and a felt board

Skills Used: Narrative and sequencing

Goal: 10 productions of regular plurals per child

Level: Cloze task (____> indicates educator's pause for child to fill in the blank)

Instructions: Place animals on the felt board as they are discussed in the story.

Example Script

Educator: Look at our book. Brown Bear sees lots of ____>

Child: **Pets.**

Educator: Yes, he sees lots of **pets.**

Educator: I like **dogs.** How about you? You like ____>

Child: **Cats.**

Educator: Let's put our **animals** on our board. We have lots of ____>

Child: **Things** on our board.

Educator: We sure do have lots of **things.**

Educator: He sees some **kids** too.

Educator: Let's put these on our board. *[Hold up horses]* They are ____>

Child: **Horses.**

Educator: Now it's time to put these on. They are ____>

Child: **Cats.**

Educator: It looks like we need these now. They are ____>

Child: **Dogs.**

[Continue in a similar manner until all felt animals have been placed on the felt board and each child has had at least 10 opportunities to use regular plurals.]

Transition

Educator: It was fun acting out our story. Now it's time to learn a new song about Brown Bear! Are you ready?

SONG ACTIVITY

Instructions: Sing to the tune of "Mary Had A Little Lamb," emphasizing regular plurals.

Brown Bear Sees All His Friends

Brown Bear sees all his **friends,**
all his **friends,** all his **friends.**

Brown Bear sees all his **friends.**
He sees them every day.

Brown Bear likes all his **friends,**
all his **friends,** all his **friends.**

Brown Bear likes his **friends.**
He likes them every way!

Regular Plurals

Cycle 2, Session 2

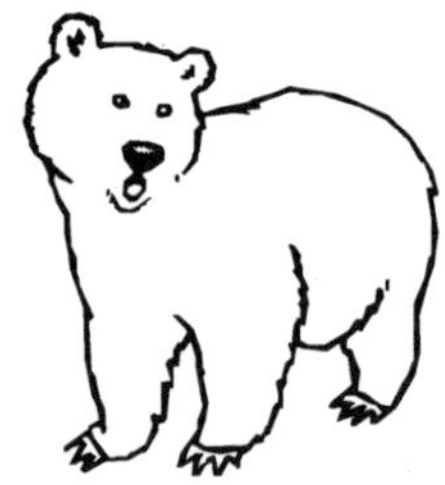

Theme: Animals

Description: Completing activities relating to *Brown Bear, Brown Bear, What Do You See?*

Exemplars: beads, bears, bottles, cats, ears, eyes, horses, friends, kids, lots, markers, pigs, puppets, sticks, stripes, things

Materials:

Brown Bear, Brown Bear, What Do You See? by Bill Martin Jr. and Eric Carle (illustrator)
Completed Brown Bear stick puppet (see pages 274–275 for directions and a pattern)
Brown Bears (see pages 274–275 for directions and a pattern; 1 per child)
Bag containing:
- Glue
- Decorations (google eyes, beads, etc.)
- Craft sticks
- Markers

Pictures of animals (see pages 283–284 for directions and patterns)
Magnifying glass or binoculars (optional)

BOOK ACTIVITY

Book: *Brown Bear, Brown Bear, What Do You See?* by Bill Martin Jr. and Eric Carle (illustrator)

Instructions: Reread the book with children. Comment on the story using regular plurals.

Suggested Theme-Related Supplemental Books: *Polar Bear, Polar Bear, What Do You Hear?* by Bill Martin Jr. and Eric Carle (illustrator)
Mouse Creeps by Peter Harris and Reg Cartwright (illustrator)

Transition

EDUCATOR: Brown Bear was an important character in the story. Today we are going to make some Brown Bear **puppets.**

FOCUSED STIMULATION ACTIVITY

Description: Making Brown Bear stick puppets

Skills Used: Fine motor and direction following

Instructions: Prepare a Brown Bear stick puppet prior to the activity to serve as a model. Give each child a Brown Bear.

Example Script

EDUCATOR: Let's make some bear **puppets** today. Here's a bag that has all the **things** we need inside it. *[Present bag]*

EDUCATOR: Jane finds some **bottles** of glue.

EDUCATOR: John sees some **beads.** We can use **beads** to decorate our bear **puppets.**

EDUCATOR: Sally gets the google **eyes.** Google **eyes** are funny!

EDUCATOR: Here are some **markers** so we can draw on our **bears.**

EDUCATOR: Miguel draws lots of **stripes** on his bear.

EDUCATOR: Jane likes the **beads.** She puts lots of **beads** on her bear.

EDUCATOR: Maria uses **beads** for the bear's **ears.**

EDUCATOR: Don't forget to put **eyes** on your bear!

EDUCATOR: I see some **sticks** *[craft sticks].* We can put our **bears** on **sticks** so that we can hold them like **puppets.**

[Continue in a similar manner until the bears have been decorated and numerous models of regular plurals have been provided.]

Transition

EDUCATOR: Remember that in our story Brown Bear sees **lots** of **animals?** He sees a blue horse who looks at him. He sees **lots** and **lots** of **animals,** and even some **kids!** Let's take the **bears** we just made and have them look around the room. Let's find out what they see!

ELICITED PRODUCTION ACTIVITY

Description: Playing a modified game of I Spy (in this case it will be Brown Bear Sees)

Skills Used: Gross motor, searching and finding, and labeling/describing

Goal: 10 productions of regular plurals per child

Level of Educator Support: Cloze task (____> indicates educator's pause for child to fill in the blank)

Instructions: Prior to activity, hang up the animal pictures at various eye-level locations around the room or hallway. Have children pretend their Brown Bear puppets are finding the animals. Consider having children use binoculars or a magnifying glass to assist in their search. Hang up multiple pictures of the same animals to obligate plurals.

Example Script

EDUCATOR: What does your bear see? He sees ____>

CHILD: **Animals.**

EDUCATOR: Hmmm, what does your bear see? He sees ____>

CHILD: **Pigs!**

EDUCATOR: My bear is looking at some funny **animals** over there. They are ____>

CHILD: **Cats!**

EDUCATOR: You're right. Now he sees some other **things.** They are ____>

CHILD: **Bears.**

EDUCATOR: Yes, they are. Now our **bears** see those **animals** over here. They are ____>

CHILD: **Horses!**

[Continue in a similar manner until each child has had at least 10 opportunities to use regular plurals.]

Transition

EDUCATOR: We saw **lots** of interesting **animals** today! Now it's time to sing our song about those **animals!**

SONG ACTIVITY

Instructions: Sing to the tune of "Mary Had A Little Lamb," emphasizing plurals.

Brown Bear Sees All His Friends

Brown Bear sees all his **friends,**
all his **friends,** all his **friends.**

Brown Bear sees all his **friends.**
He sees them every day.

Brown Bear likes all his **friends,**
all his **friends,** all his **friends.**

Brown Bear likes his **friends.**
He likes them every way!

Weekly Family Letter

For: ______________________________ **Date:** ______________

Theme

Our theme for language intervention this week is *animals.*

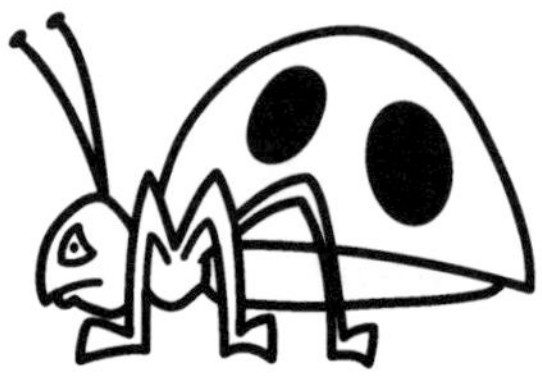

Target

Our target language structures are *possessives.* Possessives indicate ownership and usually have an *'s* ending. Examples include:

- **Jessie's** dog is cute.
- I like to eat **Mom's** apple pie.
- It's **Mike's** turn to play on the swings.

Book

Our book for the week is *The Grouchy Ladybug* by Eric Carle.

Here are some related books you could read at home: *The Very Quiet Cricket* by Eric Carle, *The Very Lonely Firefly* by Eric Carle, and *Franklin Goes to School* by Paulette Bourgeois and Brenda Clark (illustrator).

Song

Ladybug's Leaf
(Tune: "Mary Had a Little Lamb")

This is the **ladybug's** leaf, **ladybug's** leaf, **ladybug's** leaf.
This is the **ladybug's** leaf. See how it grows.

This is the **ladybug's** leaf, **ladybug's** leaf, **ladybug's** leaf.
This is the **ladybug's** leaf. See how it blows.

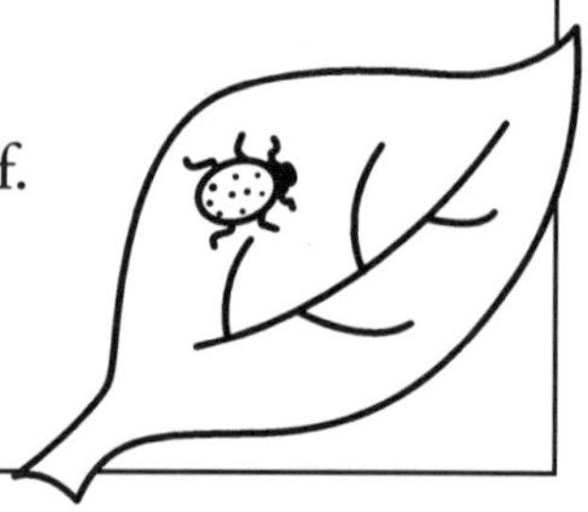

Activities

Our planned activities for the week include:

- Making a paper plate ladybug
- Having snacks that look like bugs (raisins)
- Making leaves to stick ladybug stickers on
- Decorating stickers to look like ladybugs

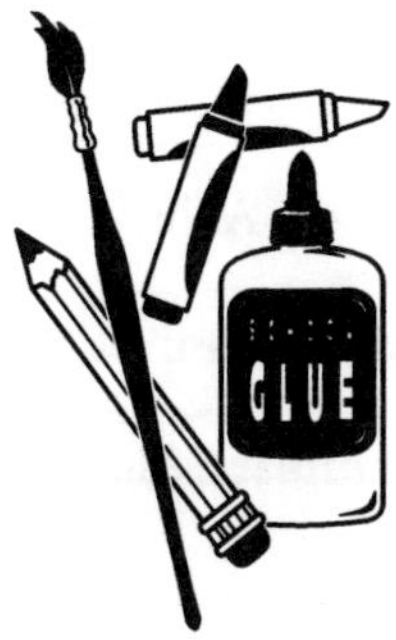

Follow-Up

Suggested follow-up activities for home include:

- Draw pictures of bugs with your child. After the drawings are completed, take turns discussing features of each person's picture, emphasizing possessive forms, for example:

  Jane's ladybug has lots of spots,
  but **Sally's** only has a few.

  Jane's bug is green and
  Sally's is yellow.

- Collect personal items from around the house. Then label and sort them, for example:

  This is **Josh's** shoe.

  This is **daddy's** sock.

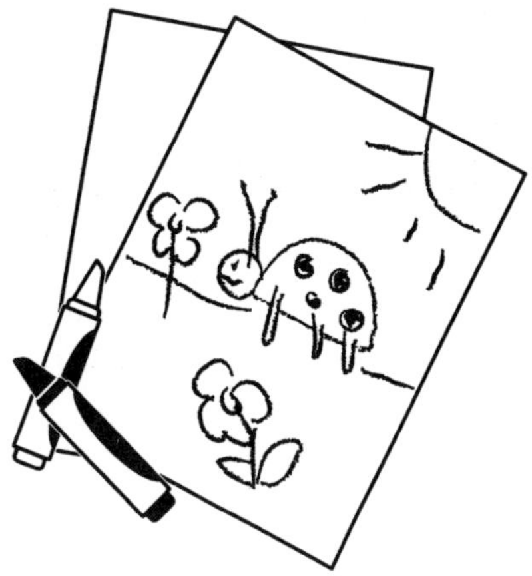

Thank You Very Much
for your participation!

Phone Number

Email

Signature

Possessives

Cycle 2, Session 1

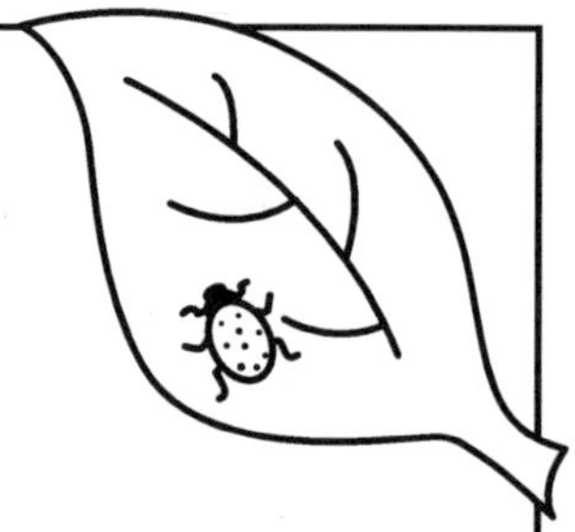

Theme: Animals

Description: Completing activities relating to bugs

Exemplars: bug's, [child's name]'s, ladybug's

Materials:

- *The Grouchy Ladybug* by Eric Carle
- Completed ladybug (see page 285 for directions)
- Red paper plates (1 per child)
- Black dot stickers
- Pipe cleaners (1 per child)
- Google eyes (2 per child)
- Glue
- Stuffed animal or hand puppet (for individual sessions only)
- Raisins
- Juice boxes (1 per child)

INTRODUCTION TO THEME

EDUCATOR: Last week we talked about a bear who saw lots of different animals. Bears are really big animals. Today we are going to talk about an animal that is really small. This animal is a bug, and it is red and has black spots. It is a ladybug!

BOOK ACTIVITY

Book: *The Grouchy Ladybug* by Eric Carle

Instructions: Read the book with the children, emphasizing possessives. When possessive forms do not naturally occur in the book, discuss the story emphasizing them (e.g., "That is the **ladybug's** leaf").

Suggested Theme-Related Supplemental Books:

The Very Quiet Cricket by Eric Carle
The Very Lonely Firefly by Eric Carle
Froggy Goes to School by Paulette Bourgeois and Brenda Clark (illustrator)

Transition

EDUCATOR: The ladybug in our story was very grouchy until the end of the story. Then she was a happy ladybug! Today we are going to make some happy ladybugs using these plates. *[Hold up plates]*

FOCUSED STIMULATION ACTIVITY

Description: Making ladybugs out of paper plates

Skills Used: Fine motor and direction following

Instructions: Prepare a ladybug prior to the activity to serve as a model. For sessions with an individual child, use possessives with the bugs or other objects as the subject as opposed to children. Examples of using *bug's* as the possessive model are in the script below.

Example Script

EDUCATOR: This is the kind of ladybug you are going to make today. *[Present completed ladybug project to serve as a model]* These are the **bug's** eyes.

EDUCATOR: These are the **bug's** spots. *[Have children make ladybugs]*

EDUCATOR: Look at **Jane's** bug!

EDUCATOR: **Miguel's** bug has three eyes!

EDUCATOR: **Sally's** bug is big.

EDUCATOR: The **bug's** antennae are long and skinny.

EDUCATOR: Look at **Jake's** smile.

EDUCATOR: **Miguel's** bug is red and **Jake's** bug is red too!

[Continue in a similar manner until children have constructed their ladybugs and numerous models of possessives have been provided.]

Transition

EDUCATOR: What great ladybugs you made! Did anyone get hungry? I found some bugs for snacks! You'll like how they taste!

ELICITED PRODUCTION ACTIVITY

Description: Snacking on "bugs" (raisins) and "bug juice" (juice boxes)

Skills Used: Sharing and turn taking

Goal: 10 productions of possessives per child

Level of Educator Support: Cloze task (______> indicates educator's pause for child to fill in the blank)

Instructions: For sessions with an individual child, have a stuffed animal or hand puppet "participate" and give it a name to create natural opportunities for possessives affixed onto a proper name.

Example Script

EDUCATOR: I'm hungry. I think I'm going to eat a bug! *[Eat a raisin]* Now it's your turn, Sally. Whose bug is this? It's ____>

CHILD: **Sally's** bug!

EDUCATOR: Yes, it's **Sally's** bug!

EDUCATOR: Hmmm, now whose turn is it? It's ______>

CHILD: **John's** turn!

EDUCATOR: Yes, it's **John's** turn.

EDUCATOR: Jane, look in the bag. What did you find? Whose is it? It's ______>

CHILD: **Jane's.**

EDUCATOR: Whose juice box is this? It's ____>

CHILD: **Jake's.**

[Continue in a similar manner until each child has had at least 10 opportunities to use possessives.]

Transition

EDUCATOR: That was a delicious snack! It's time to clean up and sing our ladybug song!

SONG ACTIVITY

Instructions: Sing to the tune of "Mary Had a Little Lamb," emphasizing possessives. Consider using a leaf (real or silk) as a visual aid for the song.

Ladybug's Leaf

This is the **ladybug's** leaf, **ladybug's** leaf, **ladybug's** leaf.
This is the **ladybug's** leaf. See how it grows.

This is the **ladybug's** leaf, **ladybug's** leaf, **ladybug's** leaf.
This is the **ladybug's** leaf. See how it blows.

Possessives

Cycle 2, Session 2

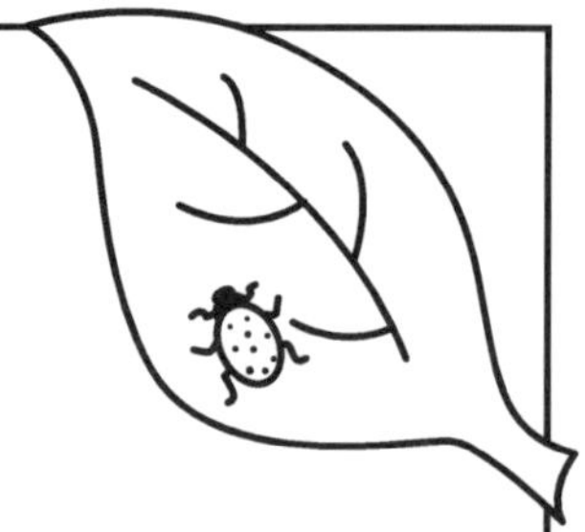

Theme: Animals

Description: Completing activities relating to bugs

Exemplars: [child's name]'s, ladybug's, leaf's

Materials:

The Grouchy Ladybug by Eric Carle
Photocopies of leaves (see pages 285–286 for directions and a pattern; 1 per child)
Child-safe scissors
Crayons or markers
Tape
Red dot stickers
Black markers

BOOK ACTIVITY

Book: *The Grouchy Ladybug* by Eric Carle

Instructions: Reread the book with children, emphasizing possessives. When possessive forms do not occur, discuss the story emphasizing them (e.g., "That is the **ladybug's** leaf").

Suggested Theme-Related Supplemental Books:
The Very Quiet Cricket by Eric Carle
The Very Lonely Firefly by Eric Carle
Froggy Goes to School
by Paulette Bourgeois and Brenda Clark (illustrator)

Transition

EDUCATOR: Remember how the ladybug in our story liked to crawl on leaves? Today we are going to make some leaves for our ladybugs to crawl on.

FOCUSED STIMULATION ACTIVITY

Description: Coloring and cutting out leaves

Skill Used: Fine motor

Instructions: For sessions with an individual child, use *ladybug* as the name onto which possessive *'s* is affixed as opposed to children's names.

Example Script

EDUCATOR: Look at this picture. *[Present book cover and point to leaves]* These are the **ladybug's** leaves. *[Give children photocopies of leaves, child-safe scissors, and crayons or markers; have children cut out and color the leaves]*

EDUCATOR: These are **Jane's** scissors.

EDUCATOR: **Maria's** leaves are green.

EDUCATOR: **John's** leaves are yellow.

EDUCATOR: That's the **leaf's** stem.

EDUCATOR: **Jake's** leaves are big.

EDUCATOR: These look like the **ladybug's** leaves. Maybe we should put some bugs on our leaves.

[Continue in a similar manner until numerous models of possessives have been provided.]

Transition

EDUCATOR: We made lots of leaves, but we need something to put on them. I thought we could put some ladybugs on them, just like in our story.

ELICITED PRODUCTION ACTIVITY

Description: Making ladybugs to put on leaves

Skills Used: Fine motor and gross motor

Goal: 10 productions of possessives per child

Level of Educator Support: Cloze task (____> indicates educator's pause for child to fill in the blank)

Instructions: Tape the leaves (made in the focused stimulation activity) to the wall prior to the activity. For sessions with an individual child, have a stuffed animal or puppet "participate" to create natural opportunities to use possessives.

Example Script

EDUCATOR: Now that we each have some stickers, we need to use these markers to put spots on our ladybugs!

EDUCATOR: Whose marker is this? It is ____>

CHILD: **Miguel's.**

EDUCATOR: He is going to put spots on his bug. Whose bug is it? It is ____>

CHILD: **John's.**

EDUCATOR: I like this ladybug. It has nice spots. Whose ladybug is it? It is ____>

CHILD: **Sally's.**

EDUCATOR: I am going to take a turn and make spots on my ladybug. Now who wants a turn? It is ____>

CHILD: **Jake's** turn.

EDUCATOR: Someone has red ladybugs. Whose ladybugs are these? They are ____>

CHILD: **Jane's.**

EDUCATOR: Look who has red ladybugs. These bugs are ____>

CHILD: **John's.**

EDUCATOR: Whose ladybug has lots of spots?

CHILD: **Sally's** does!

EDUCATOR: Now that we all have made ladybugs we need to put them on these leaves. *[Point to leaves taped to wall]*

EDUCATOR: Whose leaf is this?

CHILD: The **ladybug's!**

[Continue in a similar manner until each child has had at least 10 opportunities to use possessives.]

Transition

EDUCATOR: Our ladybugs crawled all over the leaves we made for them! It's time to sing our ladybug song.

SONG ACTIVITY

Instructions: Sing to the tune of "Mary Had a Little Lamb," emphasizing possessives. Consider using a leaf (live or artificial) as a visual aid for the song.

Ladybug's Leaf

This is the **ladybug's** leaf, **ladybug's** leaf, **ladybug's** leaf.
This is the **ladybug's** leaf. See how it grows.

This is the **ladybug's** leaf, **ladybug's** leaf, **ladybug's** leaf.
This is the **ladybug's** leaf. See how it blows.

Weekly Family Letter

For: ______________________________ **Date:** ______________

Theme

Our theme for language intervention this week is *animals.*

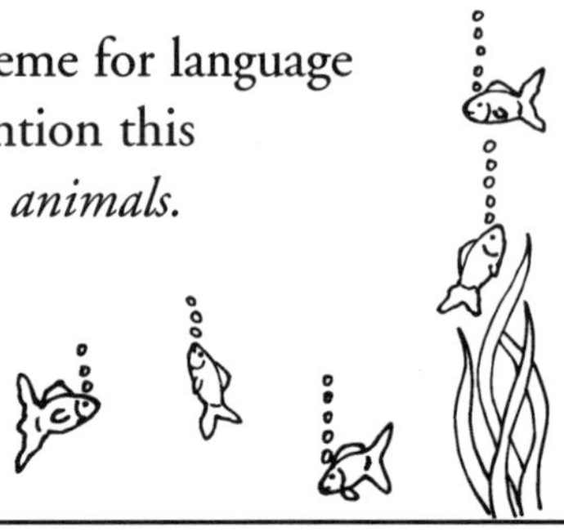

Target

Our target language structures are *pronouns.* Pronouns take the place of proper names. Examples include:

- **I** tickled **my** baby brother.
- **We** played outside.
- **They** cleaned the kitchen for **her.**

Book

Our book for the week is *The Rainbow Fish* by Marcus Pfister.

Here are some related books you could read at home: *One Fish, Two Fish, Red Fish, Blue Fish* by Dr. Seuss; *Swimmy* by Leo Lionni; and *Froggy Gets Dressed* by Jonathan London and Frank Remkiewicz (illustrator).

Song

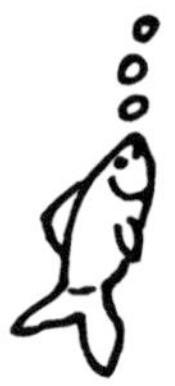

Little Fish, Little Fish
(Tune: "Little Bunny Foo Foo")

Little fish, little fish, **he** moved in the water.
Little fish, little fish, **he** jumped in the waves.

Little fish, little fish, **he** moved in the water.
Little fish, little fish, **he** chased **his** friend away.

Little fish, little fish, **he** moved in the water.
Little fish, little fish, **he** played all day long!

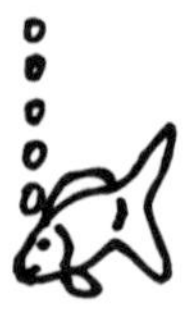

Activities

Our planned activities for the week include:

- Discussing events in the book using pronouns
- Making a paper plate fish
- Having crackers that look like fish
- Going on a pretend fishing trip

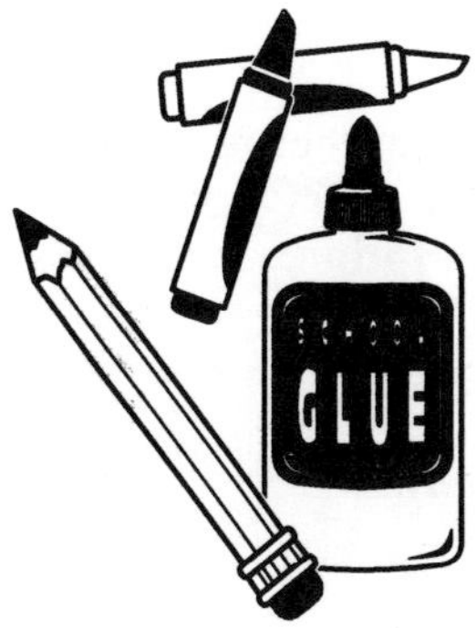

Follow-Up

Suggested follow-up activities for home include:

- Have your child retell *The Rainbow Fish* story using pronouns such as *he, she,* and *they.*
- Make a pile of small things owned by you and another pile of things owned by your child. Mix the piles together and discuss each item as you sort, for example:

  I see **my** comb.

  Do **you** see **your** cup?

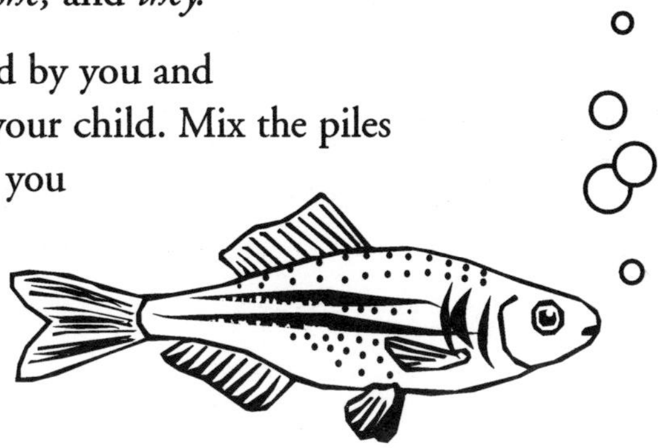

Thank You Very Much for your participation!

Phone Number

Email

Signature

Pronouns

Cycle 2, Session 1

Theme: Animals

Description: Completing activities relating to fish

Exemplars: he, her, him, his, I, it, our, she, them, they, us, we, you

Materials:

The Rainbow Fish by Marcus Pfister
Completed Rainbow Fish (see page 287 for directions)
Stuffed animal or puppet
Rainbow Fish bodies (see page 287 for directions; 1 per child)
Sequins
Glue
Aluminum foil

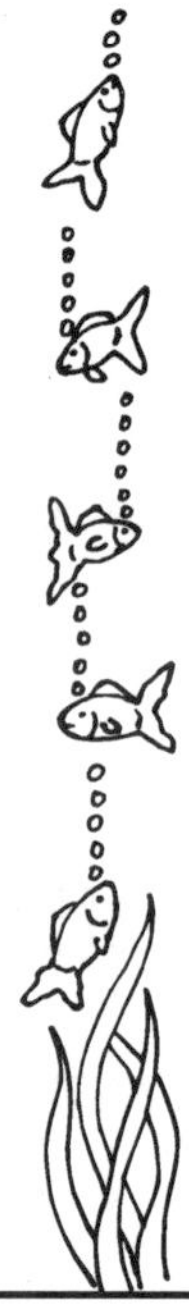

INTRODUCTION TO THEME

EDUCATOR: Last week, **we** talked a bit about ladybugs. This week **we**'re going to talk about fish. Let**'s** read **our** story about fish.

BOOK ACTIVITY

Book: *The Rainbow Fish* by Marcus Pfister

Instructions: Read the book with children, emphasizing pronouns.

Suggested Theme-Related Supplemental Books:
One Fish, Two Fish, Red Fish, Blue Fish by Dr. Seuss
Swimmy by Leo Lionni
Froggy Gets Dressed
by Jonathan London and Frank Remkiewicz (illustrator)

Transition

EDUCATOR: That was such a nice story. Let**'s** talk a little bit about the Rainbow Fish and look at the pictures in **our** book.

FOCUSED STIMULATION ACTIVITY

Description: Discussing the story and pictures using pronouns

Skills Used: Narrative, sequencing, and describing

Example Script

EDUCATOR:	This is the Rainbow Fish. *[Point to a picture]* **He** lived in the sea.
EDUCATOR:	Look at the other fish. **They** followed **him** wherever **he** went!
EDUCATOR:	Rainbow Fish liked the way **his** scales looked.
EDUCATOR:	Rainbow Fish didn't share **his** scales. **He** turned and swam away!
EDUCATOR:	This is the octopus. **She** talked to Rainbow Fish.
EDUCATOR:	**She** helped **him** make friends.
EDUCATOR:	Look, the octopus disappeared!
EDUCATOR:	What happened next?
CHILD:	**She** touched Rainbow Fish.
CHILD:	**She** wanted to be **his** friend.
EDUCATOR:	Rainbow Fish shared one of **his** beautiful scales.
EDUCATOR:	Rainbow fish shared all **his** beautiful scales. **He** shared with all the fish.
EDUCATOR:	**They** all laughed and played together.
EDUCATOR:	**They** became friends because Rainbow Fish shared with **them.**

[Continue in a similar manner until numerous models of pronouns have been provided.]

Transition

EDUCATOR: What a nice story that was. Today **we** will make a Rainbow Fish for **you** to take home. Look at this pretty Rainbow Fish. *[Present model]* Let**'s** make one just like **it.**

ELICITED PRODUCTION ACTIVITY

Description: Making paper plate Rainbow Fish

Goal: 10 productions of pronouns per child

Level of Educator Support: Cloze task (____> indicates educator's pause for child to fill in the blank)

Instructions: Prepare a Rainbow Fish prior to the activity to serve as a model. Discuss with children what was done to make the fish, targeting pronouns. For sessions with an individual child, have a stuffed animal or puppet "participate" to create natural opportunities to use the pronouns *he/his/him* or *she/hers/her.* Or focus on the pronouns *you/your/yours, we/our/ours,* and *you/your/yours* instead.

Example Script

EDUCATOR: Look at this Rainbow Fish **I** made. *[Present model]* How do you think **I** made **it**? After **we** figure out how to make **it**, **you** are going to make one like **it** to take home!

EDUCATOR: How did **I** get these pretty things *[sequins]* to stay on? ____> *[Point to glue on foil]*

CHILD: **You** glued **them** on.

EDUCATOR: Yes, **I** did. **I** glued lots of shiny stuff on the fish.

EDUCATOR: See, **I** folded the shiny stuff on the back like this. *[Demonstrate]*

EDUCATOR: Now **it**'s **your** turn. **I** gave some shiny stuff to ____>

CHILD: **Him**.

EDUCATOR: Who folded **it**? ____>

CHILD: **He** did!

EDUCATOR: Who glued colors on **him**? ____>

CHILD: **She** did.

EDUCATOR: Sally gave **her** colors to ____>

CHILD: **You**.

EDUCATOR: Yes, **I** glued the colors on the fish. *[Have children complete the activity]*

EDUCATOR: Now let**'s** tell the puppet how **we** made **our** fish. First ____>

CHILD: **We** glued shiny stuff on.

EDUCATOR: Then ____>

CHILD: **We** folded the shiny stuff.

[Continue in a similar manner until each child has had at least 10 opportunities to use pronouns.]

Transition

Educator: Now that **we** each have a Rainbow Fish to take home, let**'s** sing a song about **our** fish!

SONG ACTIVITY

Instructions: Sing to the tune of "Little Bunny Foo Foo," emphasizing pronouns.

Little Fish, Little Fish

Little fish, little fish, **he** moved in the water.
Little fish, little fish, **he** jumped in the waves.

Little fish, little fish, **he** moved in the water.
Little fish, little fish, **he** chased **his** friend away.

Little fish, little fish, **he** moved in the water.
Little fish, little fish, **he** played all day long!

Pronouns

Cycle 2, Session 2

Theme: Animals

Description: Completing activities relating to fish

Exemplars: he, her, him, his, I, it, me, my, our, ours, she, them, they, us, we, you

Materials:

The Rainbow Fish by Marcus Pfister
Fish-shaped crackers
Napkins (1 per child)
Juice boxes (1 per child)
Blue blanket or rug
Fishing pole (see page 288 for directions)
Fish (see page 288–289 for directions and patterns)
Bucket
Puppet

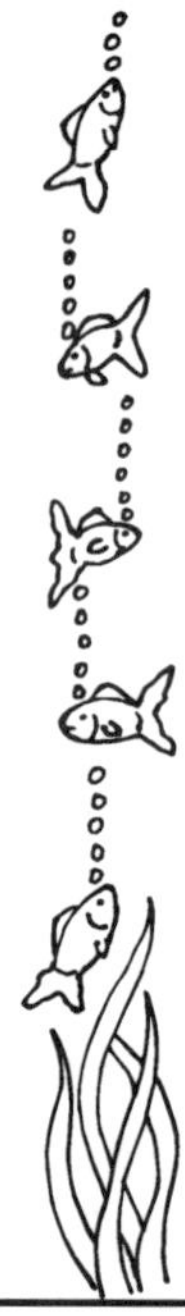

BOOK ACTIVITY

Book: *The Rainbow Fish* by Marcus Pfister

Instructions: Reread the book with the children, emphasizing pronouns.

Suggested Theme-Related Supplemental Books: *One Fish, Two Fish, Red Fish, Blue Fish* by Dr. Seuss
Swimmy by Leo Lionni
Froggy Gets Dressed
by Jonathan London and Frank Remkiewicz (illustrator)

Transition

EDUCATOR: Today **we** are going to have a snack that reminds **me** of the story **we** just read!

FOCUSED STIMULATION ACTIVITY

Description: Having a snack

Skills Used: Sharing and turn taking

Example Script

EDUCATOR: Is anybody hungry? **I** brought a fish snack for **us** today. Sally, can **you** look around? Do **you** see any fish snacks? Please get **them.**

EDUCATOR: See, **she** looked around and **she** got **them.**

EDUCATOR: John, please pass out these napkins. See, **he** passed out the napkins to **us.**

EDUCATOR: Jane, please pour some crackers on **her** napkin. **She** poured the fish out. **She** poured out lots of fish!

EDUCATOR: **I** tasted **my** fish.

EDUCATOR: **They** tasted good!

EDUCATOR: **I**'m thirsty. Sally, when **you** looked around, did **you** see some juice?

EDUCATOR: Please hand **it** to **me.**

EDUCATOR: **She** passed out the juice to all of **us.**

EDUCATOR: **I** like to sip **my** juice through **my** straw. Watch. See, **I** sipped **my** juice.

[Continue in a similar manner until numerous models of pronouns have been provided.]

Transition

EDUCATOR: That was a delicious snack. Let's clean up and get ready to do something new!

ELICITED PRODUCTION ACTIVITY

Description: Going fishing

Skills Used: Gross motor and dramatic play

Goal: 10 productions of pronouns per child

Level of Educator Support: Cloze task (____> indicates educator's pause for child to fill in the blank)

Instructions: Put the blanket or rug on the floor and tell children that it is the lake. Complete the fishing activity and then have children tell the puppet what they did using pronouns.

Example Script

EDUCATOR: Look what **I** brought for **us** to do today. **I** brought a fishing pole and some fish. **I** thought **we** could go fishing.

EDUCATOR: *[Untie the string from the pole]* Uh-oh, this pole is broken. Whose is **it**? **It** is ___>

CHILD: **Ours**!

EDUCATOR: Let's fix **it**. John can fix **it**. Who fixed **it**? ___>

CHILD: **He** did.

EDUCATOR: Yes, **he** fixed **it**. What did **he** do to the string? ___>

CHILD: **He** tied **it**.

EDUCATOR: **You**'re right, **he** tied **it** and that fixed **it**. Now **we** can go fishing.

EDUCATOR: **I** want to look in the lake to see **our** fish. Does anybody else want to see **them**? **You** want to see ___>

CHILD: **Them**.

EDUCATOR: **You** looked in and **you** saw lots of fish.

EDUCATOR: **I** need a helper to put these fish on the hook. *[Ask a child to help]*

EDUCATOR: What a good helper! Who helped? ___>

CHILD: **He** helped.

EDUCATOR: **I** got a fish! **I** dropped **him** into the bucket. *[Continue until each child has had a turn to fish]*

EDUCATOR: Now let'**s** tell the puppet what **we** did today. [Present puppet] First ____>

CHILD: **We** fixed **our** pole.

[Continue in a similar manner until each child has had at least 10 opportunities to use pronouns.]

Transition

Educator: **I** sure like to go fishing! Sometimes when **I** go fishing **I** sing songs. Let**'s** sing our song about the little fish!

SONG ACTIVITY

Instructions: Sing to the tune of "Little Bunny Foo Foo," emphasizing pronouns.

Little Fish, Little Fish

Little fish, little fish, **he** moved in the water.
Little fish, little fish, **he** jumped in the waves.

Little fish, little fish, **he** moved in the water.
Little fish, little fish, **he** chased **his** friend away.

Little fish, little fish, **he** moved in the water.
Little fish, little fish, **he** played all day long!

Weekly Family Letter

For: ______________________ **Date:** ____________

Theme

Our theme for language intervention this week is *animals.*

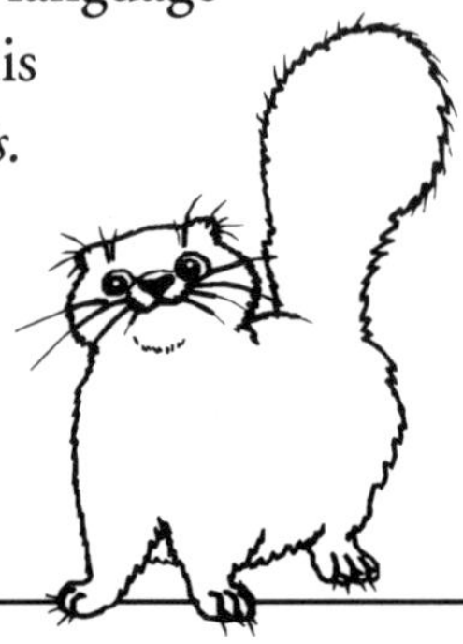

Target

Our target language structures are *auxiliary* be *verbs.* These are the verbs *am ('m), are ('re),* and *is ('s)* when used as "helping" verbs in a sentence. Generally, these verbs are used in front of verbs with *-ing* endings. Examples include:

- **I'm** going to sleep.
- The dog **is** barking.
- They **are** playing on the swings.

Book

The book we will read this week is *Have You Seen My Cat?* by Eric Carle.

Here is a related book you could read at home: *The Tale of Tom Kitten* abridged by Marian Hoffman.

Song

Kitty Is Sleeping
(Tune: "Where Is Thumbkin?")

Kitty **is** sleeping. Kitty **is** sleeping.
Yes he is! Yes he is!

He **is** sleeping. He **is** sleeping.
Yes he is! Yes he is!

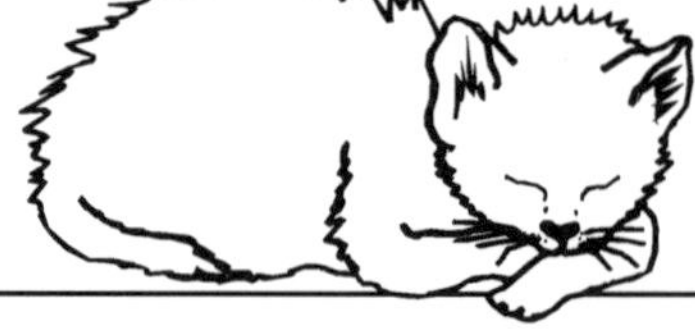

Activities

Our planned activities for the week include:

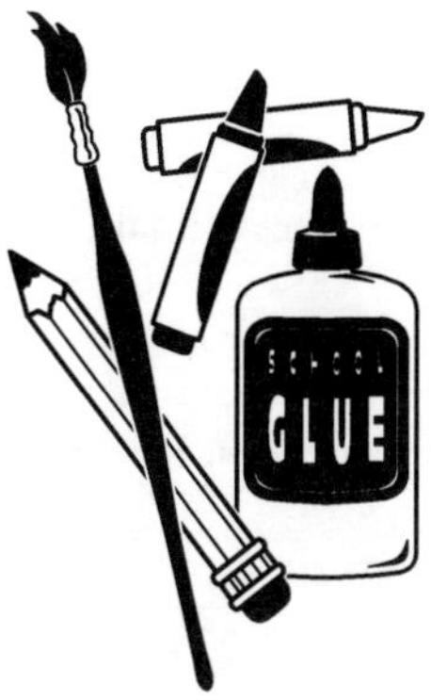

- Making a cat mask
- Playing show-and-tell using the cat mask
- Going on a "cat hunt" (searching for cat pictures)
- Making a category poster using pictures of cats and other animals

Follow-Up

Suggested follow-up activities for home include:

- Look through a book about animals or watch a television program about animals (preferably cats!), and take turns with your child "narrating" what is happening using auxiliary *be* verbs, for example:

  Look how fast that tiger**'s** running.

  These cats **are** licking their hair.

- Play a "back-and-forth" game with your child by making a body movement and describing it. Go back and forth, taking turns, for example:

  YOU: I **am** hopping.

  CHILD: I **am** running.

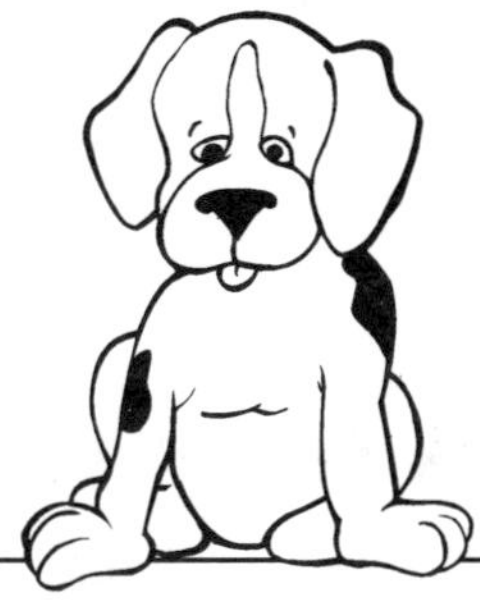

Thank You Very Much for your participation!

____
Phone Number

____
Email

____
Signature

Auxiliary *be*

Cycle 2, Session 1

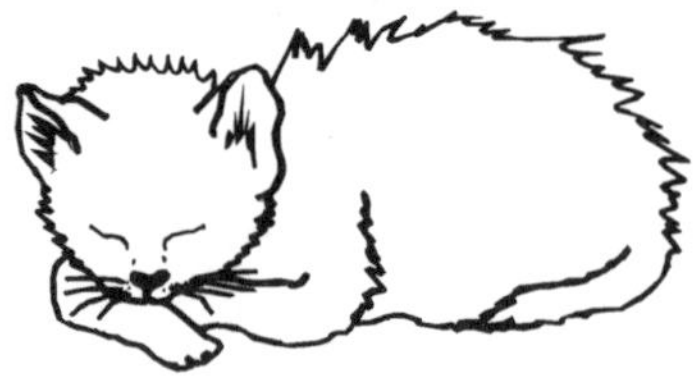

Theme: Animals

Description: Completing activities relating to cats

Exemplars: am ('m), are ('re), is ('s)

Materials:

- *Have You Seen My Cat?* by Eric Carle
- Completed cat ears and nose (see page 290 for directions)
- Glue
- Ears (see page 290 for directions; 1 pair per child)
- Pompons (1 per child)
- Paper cups (1 per child)
- 12" pieces of yarn (2 per child)
- 24" pieces of yarn (1 per child)
- 3" pipe cleaner pieces (2 per child)
- Stuffed animal or puppet (for individual sessions only)

INTRODUCTION TO THEME

EDUCATOR: We have been talking a lot about animals. We talked about fish, bugs, and bears. This week we **are** going to talk about another kind of animal that is a pet. This animal has whiskers, it purrs, and it meows. Can you guess what it is? *[Allow children to guess]* Yes! It's a cat! Let's read our story about cats.

BOOK ACTIVITY

Book: *Have You Seen My Cat?* by Eric Carle

Instructions: Read the book with children, emphasizing auxiliary *be* verbs. When auxiliary *be* verbs do not naturally occur in the story, go back and discuss events in the story using them.

Suggested Theme-Related Supplemental Book: *The Tale of Tom Kitten* abridged by Marian Hoffman

Transition

EDUCATOR: Our book was about a cat and today we **are** going to do an art project about cats.

FOCUSED STIMULATION ACTIVITY

Description: Making cat masks (ears and noses)

Skill Used: Fine motor

Instructions: Prepare a mask prior to the activity to serve as a model.

Example Script

EDUCATOR: I thought we could make some masks today. We can wear our masks and pretend to be cats, just like the cat in our book. *[Present model]*

EDUCATOR: Let's get our stuff out to make our ears and noses. See, Sally **is** finding stuff. I **am** helping. *[Pass out cups]*

EDUCATOR: Jane**'s** gluing ears on her cat.

EDUCATOR: Jake **is** coloring his cat's nose pink.

EDUCATOR: John **is** cutting string.

EDUCATOR: Jake**'s** making a big nose for his cat mask.

EDUCATOR: Sally **is** making a little whisker.

EDUCATOR: John **is** putting a green nose on his cat.

EDUCATOR: Jane **is** gluing the nose on.

[Continue in a similar manner until cat masks have been assembled and numerous models of auxiliary be *verbs have been provided.]*

Transition

EDUCATOR: You did such a nice job making your cat masks! Let's show each other what we made!

ELICITED PRODUCTION ACTIVITY

Description: Playing show-and-tell using cat masks

Skills Used: Describing, sharing, and turn taking

Goal: 10 productions of auxiliary *be* verbs per child

Level of Educator Support: Cloze task (_____> indicates educator's pause for child to fill in the blank)

Instructions: Have children perform various "cat" actions and talk about what they are doing. For sessions with an individual child, have a stuffed animal or puppet "participate" to create natural opportunities to use auxiliary *be* verbs.

Example Script

EDUCATOR: Miguel, please wear your mask. What **is** Miguel doing? He_____>

CHILD: **Is** wearing his mask.

EDUCATOR: Jane, can you make your cat meow for us? Sally, tell us what Jane's kitty **is** doing. Jane's kitty ____>

CHILD: **Is** meowing.

EDUCATOR: Miguel, have your cat pretend to drink some milk. Sally, what **is** Miguel's cat doing? He ___>

CHILD: **Is** drinking milk.

EDUCATOR: John **is** petting a kitty. I **am** watching. What **is** John doing? He ___>

CHILD: **Is** petting a kitty.

[Continue in a similar manner until each child has had at least 10 opportunities to use auxiliary be *verbs.]*

Transition

EDUCATOR: It was fun to talk about our cats. Let's clean up and then sing a song about a kitty!

SONG ACTIVITY

Instructions: Sing to the tune of "Where Is Thumbkin?" emphasizing auxiliary *be* verbs.

Kitty Is Sleeping

Kitty **is** sleeping. Kitty **is** sleeping.
Yes he is! Yes he is!

He **is** sleeping. He **is** sleeping.
Yes he is! Yes he is!

Auxiliary *be*

Cycle 2, Session 2

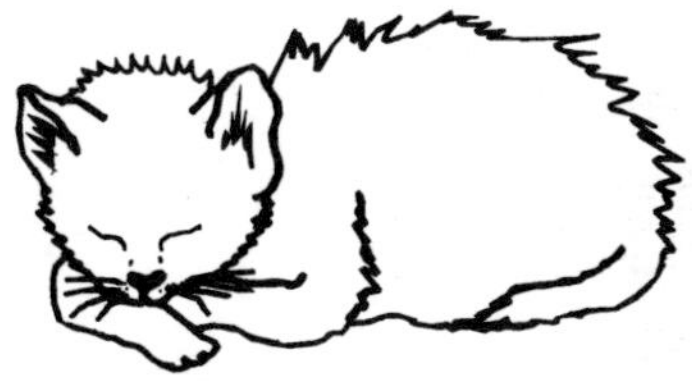

Theme: Animals

Description: Completing activities relating to cats

Exemplars: am ('m), are ('re), is ('s)

Materials:

Have You Seen My Cat? by Eric Carle
10 pictures of various animals (4 pictures that have cats and 4 pictures that do not; see pages 283–284 for directions and patterns)
Glue
Poster board

BOOK ACTIVITY

Book: *Have You Seen My Cat?* by Eric Carle

Instructions: Reread the book with children, emphasizing auxiliary *be* verbs. When auxiliary *be* verbs do not naturally occur in the story, go back and discuss the story using them.

Suggested Theme-Related Supplemental Book: *The Tale of Tom Kitten* abridged by Marian Hoffman

Transition

EDUCATOR: I think somebody has been hiding cats in our room. These cats are like the ones we read about in our story! Let's see if we can find them.

FOCUSED STIMULATION ACTIVITY

Description: Going on a cat hunt

Skills Used: Gross motor, searching and finding, and categorization

Instructions: Tape cat pictures back-to-back on other animal pictures. Hide animal pictures prior to the activity.

Example Script

EDUCATOR: We **are** going on a cat hunt. We **are** going to find lots of cats.

EDUCATOR: Jane **is** looking around the room, she **is** looking at a picture and she **is** pulling it off the wall.

EDUCATOR: John **is** looking behind the picture of the flamingo. It is not a cat!

EDUCATOR: Sally **is** looking behind the pigs. It is not a cat!

EDUCATOR: Jake **is** searching for the cat, but he **is** not finding it!

EDUCATOR: Jane **is** finding a cat!

EDUCATOR: Jane **is** finding lots of cats, but Sally **is** not finding any.

EDUCATOR: I **am** looking by the window for cats.

EDUCATOR: We **are** finding lots of cats!

[Continue in a similar manner until numerous models of auxiliary be *verbs have been provided.]*

Transition

EDUCATOR: We **are** going to do something with all the pictures we found. Everyone grab your pictures and get ready!

ELICITED PRODUCTION ACTIVITY

Description: Making a "cat" and "not a cat" category poster

Skills Used: Fine motor and categorization

Goal: 10 productions of auxiliary *be* verbs per child

Level of Educator Support: Cloze task (____> indicates educator's pause for child to fill in the blank)

Instructions: Draw a vertical line dividing the poster board into two halves: label one side "This is a cat" and the other side "This is not a cat." Glue the pictures found around the room, and extra copies of other animal pictures if desired, onto the appropriate side of the poster. For sessions with an individual child, have a stuffed animal or puppet "participate" to create natural opportunities to use auxiliary *be* verbs.

Example Script

EDUCATOR: Who **is** taping a cat on the poster? Jane___>

CHILD: **Is** taping it.

EDUCATOR: Who **is** taping a dog on the poster? John___>

CHILD: **Is** taping it.

EDUCATOR: Tell me what Sally**'s** doing. She**'s** taping or cutting? She__>

CHILD: **Is** taping.

EDUCATOR: I have a picture that is not a cat. Tell me what I **am** doing. I__>

CHILD: **Am** taping it.

EDUCATOR: Look at Jane. She__>

CHILD: **Is** ripping a picture.

EDUCATOR: Tell me about what Sally **is** doing. She __>

CHILD: **Is** looking for a cat.

[Continue in a similar manner until each child has had at least 10 opportunities to use auxiliary be *verbs.]*

Transition

EDUCATOR: You made a very nice picture with cats and other animals! Now let's clean up and sing our kitty song.

SONG ACTIVITY

Instructions: Sing to the tune of "Where Is Thumbkin?" emphasizing auxiliary *be* verbs.

Kitty Is Sleeping

Kitty **is** sleeping. Kitty **is** sleeping.
Yes he is! Yes he is!

He **is** sleeping. He **is** sleeping.
Yes he is! Yes he is!

Weekly Family Letter

For: ______________________________ **Date:** ______________

Theme

Our theme for language intervention this week is *food.*

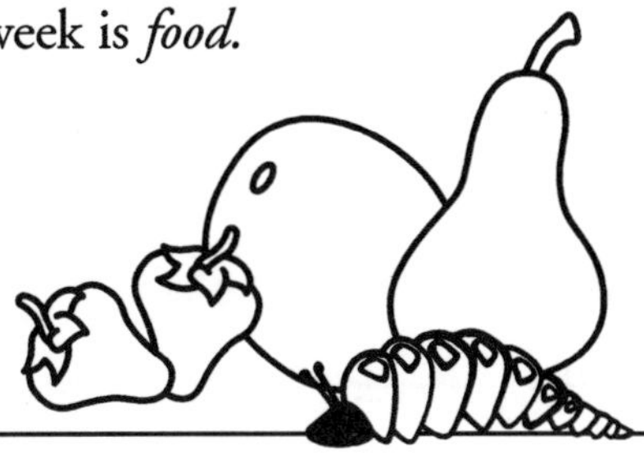

Target

Our target language structures are *regular plurals.* These are words ending in *-s* that indicate more than one of something. Examples include:

- I have two **dogs.**
- Sarah ate two **cookies.**
- My **friends** are neat.

Book

Our book for the week is *The Very Hungry Caterpillar* by Eric Carle.

Here is a related book you could read at home: *What's for Lunch?* by Eric Carle.

Song

The Hungry Caterpillar
(Tune: "Where Is Thumbkin?")

The hungry caterpillar ate his lunch. Yes he did, yes he did.

He ate **apples.** He ate **pears!** Yes he did, yes he did.

The hungry caterpillar ate his lunch. Yes he did, yes he did.
He ate **plums.** He ate **strawberries.** Yes he did, yes he did!

(Repeat for oranges and watermelons.)

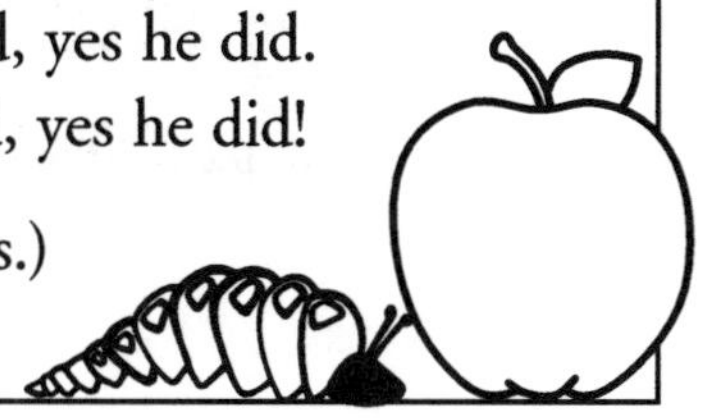

Activities

Our planned activities for the week include:

- Making a hungry caterpillar sock puppet
- Feeding food to the caterpillar puppet
- Cutting out pictures from magazines
- Making a food collage out of magazine pictures

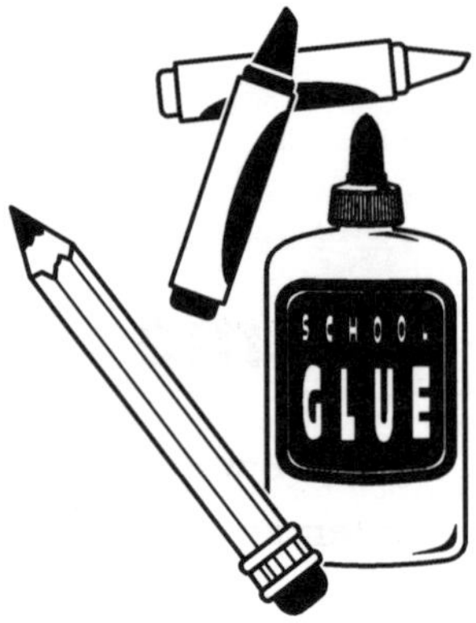

Follow-Up

Suggested follow-up activities for home include:

- Look around your kitchen and discuss the different kinds of food you see, emphasizing regular plurals, for example:

  We have lots of **eggs** in our refrigerator.

  I think Bobby ate all the **cookies!**

- Encourage your child to "fill in the blanks" as you count his or her toys, for example:

  I see five _____. *(blocks)*

  Here are three _____. *(puzzles)*

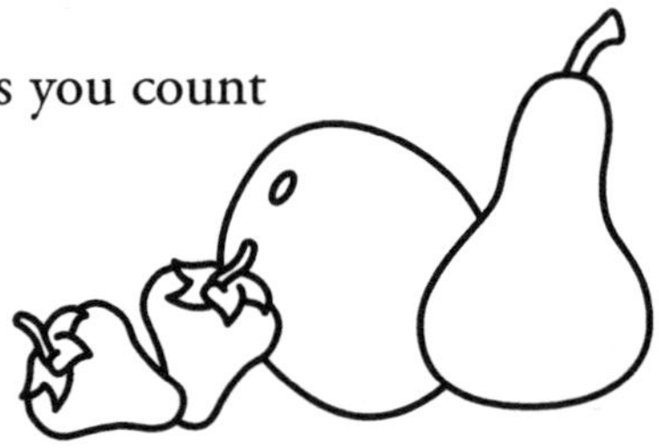

Thank You Very Much for your participation!

____
Phone Number

____
Email

____
Signature

Plurals

Cycle 3, Session 1

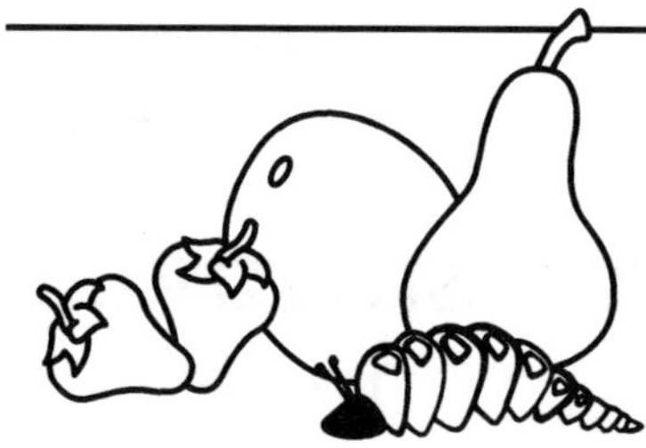

Theme: Food

Description: Completing activities relating to *The Very Hungry Caterpillar*

Exemplars: apples, beads, bugs, caterpillars, colors, cookies, dots, eyes, legs, lots, noses, oranges, pears, pieces, pies, plums, strawberries, things, watermelons

Materials:

- *The Very Hungry Caterpillar* by Eric Carle
- Completed caterpillar sock puppet (see page 297 for directions)
- Light-colored adult-sized socks (1 per child)
- Felt mouths (see page 297 for directions; 1 per child)
- Decorations (sequins, beads, etc.)
- Glue
- Markers
- Pipe cleaner (1 piece per child)
- Food (see pages 297–299 for directions and patterns; 1 set per child)
- Child-safe scissors

INTRODUCTION TO THEME

Educator: Do you know that **caterpillars** eat food? What are some **things** you think they like to eat? Today we'll read a book and find out what on very hungry caterpillar ate. Do you think it was **cookies? Pies? Bugs?** We'll find out!

BOOK ACTIVITY

Book: *The Very Hungry Caterpillar* by Eric Carle

Instructions: Read the book to children, emphasizing regular plurals.

Suggested Theme-Related Supplemental Book: *What's for Lunch?* by Eric Carle

Transition

Educator: That caterpillar sure ate **lots** of food! I thought it would be fun to make **caterpillars,** just like the one in our story.

FOCUSED STIMULATION ACTIVITY

Description: Making hungry caterpillar sock puppets

Skill Used: Fine motor and direction following

Example Script

Educator:	You are each going to make a caterpillar puppet today. You will make your puppet with a sock. *[Present sock]* You can use all these things to decorate your **puppets.** *[Present decorations]* When you are done, your puppet should look something like this. *[Present completed model]* Let's get started and see what our **caterpillars** will look like.
Educator:	I like these **eyes.** Let's talk about the **caterpillars** we are making. This caterpillar has blue **eyes.**
Educator:	John wants two **eyes.**
Educator:	Maria's caterpillar has two **noses!**
Educator:	I need three **pieces** of string.
Educator:	Jake has five **colors** on his caterpillar.
Educator:	This caterpillar has ten **legs!**
Educator:	I see two big **caterpillars.**
Educator:	John put four **dots** on his caterpillar.
Educator:	Jake used **beads** for his caterpillar's **eyes.**

[Continue in a similar manner until caterpillars have been made and numerous models of regular plurals have been provided.]

Transition

Educator: Now we all have **caterpillars.** Remember what the caterpillar in our story did? That's right. He ate **lots** of food. What should we do with our caterpillar? Let's feed him!

ELICITED PRODUCTION ACTIVITY

Description: Feeding caterpillars food (consult the story for order)

Skills Used: Narrative, gross motor, dramatic play, and sequencing

Goal: 10 productions of regular plurals per child

Level of Educator Support: Preparatory set

Example Script

EDUCATOR: Remember the caterpillar in our story? *[Children respond]* He was very hungry so he ate lots of **things.** First he ate an apple. Then he ate two **pears.** What did he do next? *[Present picture in story if necessary]*

CHILD: He ate three **plums.**

EDUCATOR: Let's feed our **caterpillars.** What did he eat first? *[Consult book; feed child's caterpillar or have child feed educator's caterpillar]*

CHILD: An apple!

EDUCATOR: OK, so put one apple in his mouth.

EDUCATOR: Jane, tell John what the caterpillar eats next.

CHILD: Two **pears.**

EDUCATOR: Yes, two **pears.** Next, the caterpillar eats what?

CHILD: Three **plums.**

EDUCATOR: He's a hungry caterpillar.

EDUCATOR: Look! What does he do now?

CHILD: He eats some **oranges!**

[Continue in a similar manner until all items have been "eaten" and each child has had at least 10 opportunities to use regular plurals.]

Transition

EDUCATOR: Our **caterpillars** sure ate **lots** of food! Now it's time to sing a song about a hungry caterpillar who eats **lots** of food. Do you want to hear it?

SONG ACTIVITY

Instructions: Sing to the tune of "Where Is Thumbkin?" emphasizing plural forms. Felt food items may be held up as children sing about them.

The Hungry Caterpillar

The hungry caterpillar ate his lunch.
Yes he did, yes he did.

He ate **apples.** He ate **pears!**
Yes he did, yes he did.

The hungry caterpillar ate his lunch.
Yes he did, yes he did.
He ate **plums.** He ate **strawberries.**
Yes he did, yes he did!

(Repeat for the oranges and watermelons.)

Plurals

Cycle 3, Session 2

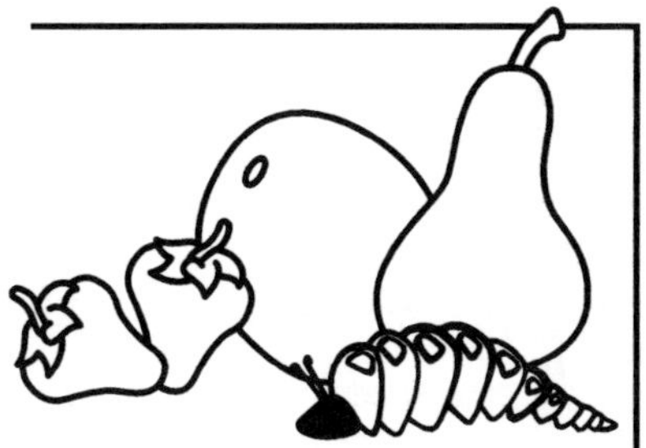

Theme: Food

Description: Completing activities relating to *The Very Hungry Caterpillar*

Exemplars: apples, cakes, cats, cookies, grapes, hot dogs, ice-cream cones, lots, magazines, oranges, pears, pictures, pieces, strawberries, things, watermelons

Materials:

The Very Hungry Caterpillar by Eric Carle
Magazines containing food pictures
Child-safe scissors
Glue
Construction paper

BOOK ACTIVITY

Book: *The Very Hungry Caterpillar* by Eric Carle

Instructions: Reread the book with children, emphasizing regular plurals.

Suggested Theme-Related Supplemental Book: *What's for Lunch?* by Eric Carle

Transition

EDUCATOR: That caterpillar sure ate a lot of food! Today we are going to cut out **pictures** of food in these **magazines** *[present magazines and child-safe scissors]* and make a project with them. Let's get started.

FOCUSED STIMULATION ACTIVITY

Description: Cutting out food pictures from magazines

Skills Used: Categorization and fine motor

Instructions: Remind children about the food theme, and ask them to cut or tear out food pictures from magazines.

Example Script

EDUCATOR:	Jane found **lots** of food **pictures.**
EDUCATOR:	Sally has three **cookies** in her picture.
EDUCATOR:	I see four **cakes!**
EDUCATOR:	I need some **oranges.**
EDUCATOR:	Jake has five **grapes** in his picture.
EDUCATOR:	Those **hot dogs** look yummy!
EDUCATOR:	I see three **apples!**
EDUCATOR:	We have **lots** of food **pictures.**
EDUCATOR:	Those are **cats,** they aren't food!

[Continue in a similar manner until many food pictures have been cut out and numerous models of regular plurals have been provided.]

Transition

EDUCATOR: We have all these great food **pictures.** I thought we could glue them on this paper and make a pretty food picture.

ELICITED PRODUCTION ACTIVITY

Description: Making food collages

Skill Used: Fine motor

Goal: 10 productions of regular plurals per child

Level of Educator Support: Preparatory set

Instructions: Have children glue pictures on construction paper.

Example Script

EDUCATOR:	John found **pictures** of cake. Tell me about what Jake found.
CHILD:	He found **grapes.**
EDUCATOR:	Yes, he did. How about Maria? What was in her **pictures?**
CHILD:	**Oranges.**
EDUCATOR:	John, tell me what you have on your paper.

Example Script—*Continued*

CHILD:	Two **pears.**
EDUCATOR:	What should we glue onto our picture next?
CHILD:	Some **pieces** of bread.
EDUCATOR:	That sounds good.
EDUCATOR:	Look at all these funny **things.** Tell me what they are.
CHILD:	**Ice-cream cones!**
EDUCATOR:	We have so many yummy **things** on our food **pictures!**

[Continue in a similar manner until all pictures have been glued on and each child has had at least 10 opportunities to use regular plurals.]

Transition

EDUCATOR: You all did a great job making your food **pictures.** Now it's time to clean up and sing a song about food.

SONG ACTIVITY

Instructions: Sing to the tune of "Where Is Thumbkin?" emphasizing plural forms. Felt food items may be held up as the children sing about them.

The Hungry Caterpillar

The hungry caterpillar ate his lunch.
Yes he did, yes he did.
He ate **apples.** He ate **pears!**
Yes he did, yes he did.

The hungry caterpillar ate his lunch.
Yes he did, yes he did.
He ate **plums.** He ate **strawberries.**
Yes he did, yes he did!

(Repeat for oranges and watermelons.)

Weekly Family Letter

For: ______________________________ **Date:** ______________

Theme

Our theme for language intervention this week is *food.*

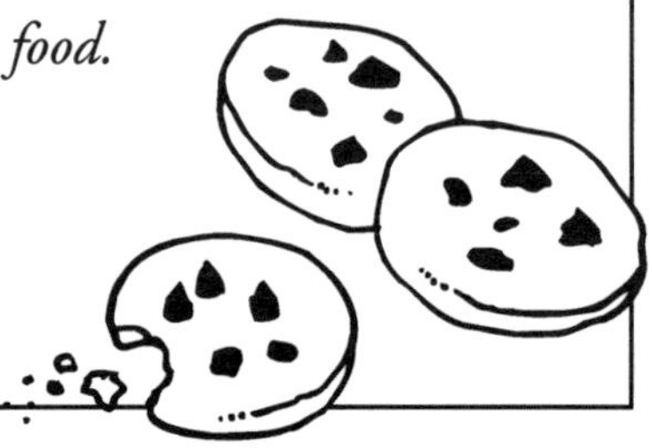

Target

Our target language structures are *possessives.* Possessives indicate ownership and usually have an *'s* ending. Examples include:

- I like **mom's** apple pie.
- **Jenny's** dog has lots of spots.
- It is **Bob's** turn to go next.

Book

Our book for the week is *If You Give a Mouse a Cookie* by Laura Joffe Numeroff and Felicia Bond (illustrator).

Here are some related books you could read at home: *If You Give a Moose a Muffin* by Laura Joffe Numeroff and Felicia Bond (illustrator) and *If You Give a Pig a Pancake* by Laura Joffe Numeroff and Felicia Bond (illustrator).

Song

The Mouse and the Cookie
(Tune: "Mary Had a Little Lamb")

The **mouse's** cookie is eaten up, eaten up, eaten up.
The **mouse's** cookie is eaten up. Now he's all done!

The **mouse's** milk is all sipped up, all sipped up, all sipped up.
The **mouse's** milk is all sipped up. Now it's all gone!

The **mouse's** house is all cleaned up,
all cleaned up, all cleaned up.
The **mouse's** house is all cleaned up.
Now it's time for bed!

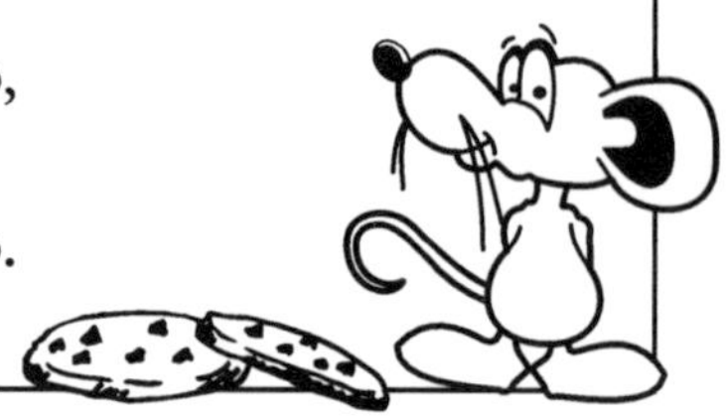

Activities

Our planned activities for the week include:

- Making construction paper cookies and feeding them to a mouse puppet
- Making felt mice to use in a story reenactment
- Reenacting the story *If You Give a Mouse a Cookie*

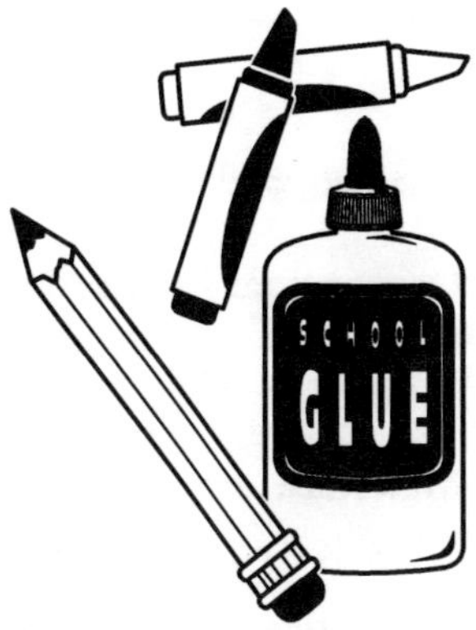

Follow-Up

Suggested follow-up activities for home include:

- Discuss different features of family members' food at the dinner table, for example:

  Bobby's spaghetti is all gone!

  Mom's juice looks good!

  Dad's bread fell on the ground.

- Look through a family photo album and talk about the pictures, for example:

  Daddy's hair was long.

  Lee's shirt was pretty.

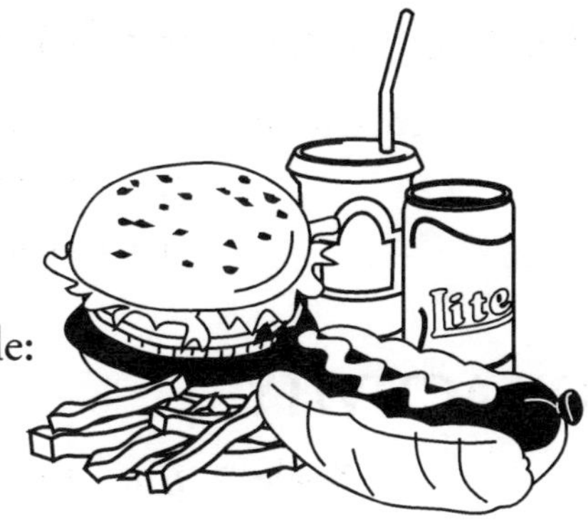

Thank You Very Much for your participation!

Phone Number

Email

Signature

Possessives

Cycle 3, Session 1

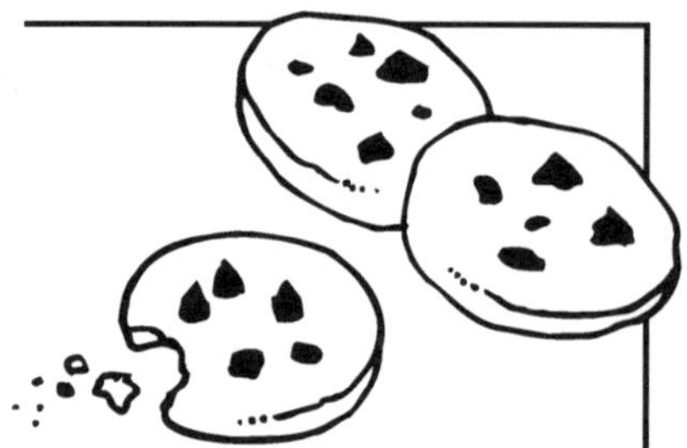

Theme: Food

Description: Completing activities relating to cookies

Exemplars: [child's name]'s, mouse's

Materials:

If You Give a Mouse a Cookie by Laura Joffe Numeroff and Felicia Bond (illustrator)
Stuffed animal or puppet (for individual sessions only)
Cookies (see page 291 for directions)
Cookie decorations (see page 291 for directions)
Glue
Milk carton mouse (see pages 291–292 for directions and a pattern)

INTRODUCTION TO THEME

Educator: We have been talking about food. Last week we talked about the hungry caterpillar who ate lots of food, and today we are going to talk about a mouse who likes cookies!

BOOK ACTIVITY

Book: *If You Give a Mouse a Cookie* by Laura Joffe Numeroff and Felicia Bond (illustrator)

Instructions: Read the book with children. Then go back and discuss using possessives.

Suggested Theme-Related Supplemental Books:
If You Give a Moose a Muffin
by Laura Joffe Numeroff and Felicia Bond (illustrator)
If You Give a Pig a Pancake
by Laura Joffe Numeroff and Felicia Bond (illustrator)

Transition

Educator: That was a great story. Now let's make some cookies like the ones in our story.

FOCUSED STIMULATION ACTIVITY

Description: Decorating paper cookies

Skill Used: Fine motor

Instructions: Glue construction paper cookie decorations onto construction paper cookies. For sessions with an individual child, have a stuffed animal or puppet "participate" to create natural opportunities to use possessives.

Example Script

EDUCATOR: Let's make some cookies like the ones in the story. I have lots of things we can use to make cookies. Let's see what we have.

EDUCATOR: **Jake's** cookies are big.

EDUCATOR: **Jane's** glue is open.

EDUCATOR: **John's** chocolate chips are falling on the floor.

EDUCATOR: Now **Jane's** glue is closed.

EDUCATOR: John puts **Maria's** chips on his cookie.

EDUCATOR: John uses **Jane's** glue for his chip.

EDUCATOR: Sally sticks **Jake's** chip on the cookie.

EDUCATOR: Sally uses **Jane's** glue again.

EDUCATOR: Now it's **Miguel's** turn to make a cookie.

EDUCATOR: **Jane's** cookie is very pretty!

EDUCATOR: **Jake's** cookie has three chips on it.

EDUCATOR: **Sally's** cookie looks very yummy!

[Continue in a similar manner until numerous models of possessives have been provided.]

Transition

EDUCATOR: Look at all these yummy cookies we made! Remember the mouse in our story? He liked to eat cookies. Let's feed our cookies to this mouse! *[Present milk carton mouse]*

ELICITED PRODUCTION ACTIVITY

Description: Feeding cookies to the milk carton mouse

Skills Used: Gross motor and dramatic play

Goal: 10 productions of possessives per child

Level of Educator Support: Preparatory set

Instructions: Prepare the milk carton mouse prior to the activity. For sessions with an individual child, have a stuffed animal or puppet "participate" to create natural opportunities to produce possessives.

Example Script

EDUCATOR: We have all these cookies. The mouse wants to eat them! Watch. The mouse opens his mouth and eats my cookies! Whose turn is it?

CHILD: **Jane's!**

EDUCATOR: Jane, give him your cookie.

EDUCATOR: Whose cookie did the mouse eat?

CHILD: **Jane's.**

EDUCATOR: Now he wants someone **else's** cookie. Whose is it?

CHILD: **Sally's** cookie!

EDUCATOR: Yes, he wants **Sally's.**

EDUCATOR: Now whose turn is it?

CHILD: It's **John's** turn.

EDUCATOR: OK, go ahead and give the mouse your cookie, John.

EDUCATOR: Whose cookie did the mouse eat?

CHILD: **John's.**

[Continue in a similar manner until each child has had at least 10 opportunities to use possessives.]

Transition

Educator: Our mouse sure was hungry! Let's sing a song about our hungry little mouse!

SONG ACTIVITY

Instructions: Sing to the tune of "Mary Had a Little Lamb," emphasizing possessives.

The Mouse and the Cookie

The **mouse's** cookie is eaten up, eaten up, eaten up.
The **mouse's** cookie is eaten up. Now he's all done!

The **mouse's** milk is all sipped up, all sipped up, all sipped up.
The **mouse's** milk is all sipped up. Now it's all gone!

The **mouse's** house is all cleaned up, all cleaned up, all cleaned up.
The **mouse's** house is all cleaned up. Now it's time for bed!

Possessives

Cycle 3, Session 2

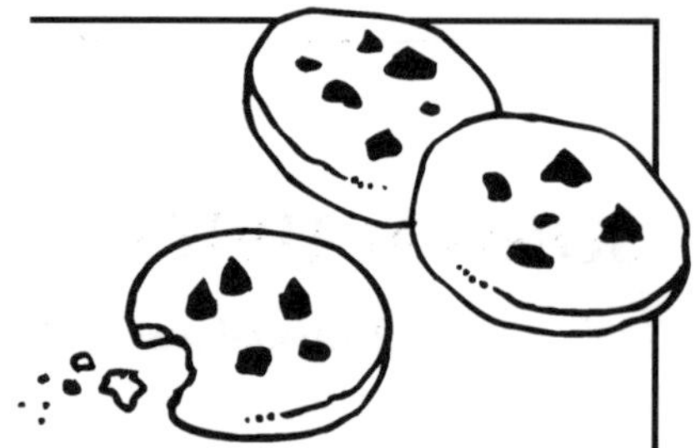

Theme: Food

Description: Completing activities relating to cookies

Exemplars: boy's, [child's name]'s, mouse's

Materials:

If You Give a Mouse a Cookie by Laura Joffe Numeroff and Felicia Bond (illustrator)
Completed felt mouse (see pages 293–294 for directions and patterns)
Glue
Felt mouse cutouts (see pages 293–294 for directions and patterns; 1 set per child)
Felt mouse story cutouts (see pages 293 and 295–296 for directions and patterns; 1 set)
Felt board

BOOK ACTIVITY

Book: *If You Give a Mouse a Cookie*
by Laura Joffe Numeroff and Felicia Bond (illustrator)

Instructions: Reread the book with children. Then go back and discuss using possessives.

Suggested Theme-Related Supplemental Books: *If You Give a Moose a Muffin*
by Laura Joffe Numeroff and Felicia Bond (illustrator)
If You Give a Pig a Pancake
by Laura Joffe Numeroff and Felicia Bond (illustrator)

Transition

EDUCATOR: Today we are each going to make a mouse like the one in our story.

FOCUSED STIMULATION ACTIVITY

Description: Decorating felt mice

Skill Used: Fine motor

Instructions: Each child will decorate (i.e., put on a face and clothing) a felt mouse. Make a mouse prior to the activity to serve as a model. For sessions with an individual child, use the mouse or other items as the subjects of sentences to create natural opportunities to use possessives.

Example Script

EDUCATOR: Let's make a mouse like the one in our story. I have some things we can use to make our mouse look like the one in our story. When we are all done, we can have our mouse eat cookies!

EDUCATOR: I see **Sally's** glue.

EDUCATOR: The **mouse's** pants have pockets on them.

EDUCATOR: The **mouse's** nose is pink.

EDUCATOR: Now it's **John's** turn. He likes the **mouse's** pink nose.

EDUCATOR: **John's** mouse eyes are being glued on.

EDUCATOR: **Jane's** mouse is very cute!

EDUCATOR: **Sally's** mouse is little and **Jake's** mouse is big.

EDUCATOR: I like how **Jane's** mouse has a red shirt.

[Continue in a similar manner until mice have been decorated and numerous models of possessives have been provided.]

Transition

EDUCATOR: Now each person has a mouse that is like the one in the story. Let's look at our book and make our own story on this. *[Present felt board]* Let's see what happens after our mouse eats a cookie.

ELICITED PRODUCTION ACTIVITY

Description: Reenacting the events in *If You Give a Mouse a Cookie*

Skills Used: Narrative, fine motor, and sequencing

Goal: 10 productions of possessives per child

Level of Educator Support: Preparatory set

Special Instructions: Put one child's felt mouse on the felt board and have children add felt pieces in the order they appeared in the story.

Example Script

EDUCATOR: Let's look at our book. Whose cookie is this?

CHILD: The **mouse's.**

EDUCATOR: Great, let's put our cookie on the board. Whose milk is this?

CHILD: The **boy's.**

EDUCATOR: Put the milk on the board. Tell me whose scissors these are.

CHILD: The **boy's.**

EDUCATOR: Look at our story. Whose broom is this?

CHILD: The **mouse's.**

[Continue in a similar manner until all items in the story have been discussed and each child has had at least 10 opportunities to use possessives.]

Transition

EDUCATOR: It was fun to retell the story! Now it's time to clean up and sing our mouse song!

SONG ACTIVITY

Instructions: Sing to the tune of "Mary Had a Little Lamb," emphasizing possessives.

The Mouse and the Cookie

The **mouse's** cookie is eaten up, eaten up, eaten up.
The **mouse's** cookie is eaten up. Now it's all gone!

The **mouse's** milk is all sipped up, all sipped up, all sipped up.
The **mouse's** milk is all sipped up. Now it's all gone!

The **mouse's** house is all cleaned up, all cleaned up, all cleaned up.
The **mouse's** house is all cleaned up. Now it's time for bed!

Weekly Family Letter

For: ______________________________ **Date:** ______________

Theme

Our theme for language intervention this week is *food.*

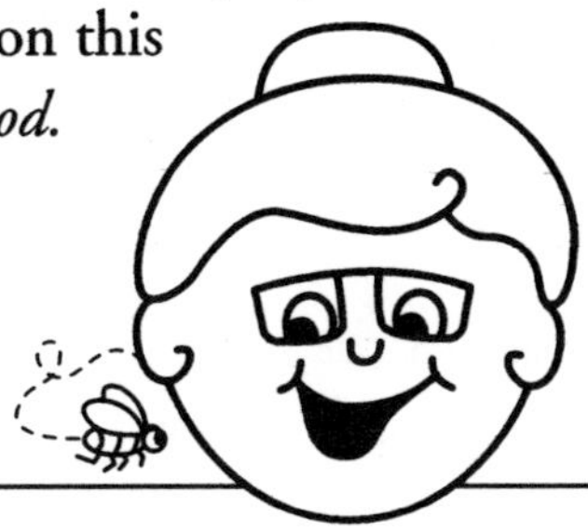

Target

Our target language structures are *pronouns.* Pronouns take the place of proper names. Examples include:

- **She** swallowed a fly.
- It wiggled inside **her.**
- **He** gave the old lady a spider.

Book

Our book for the week is *There Was an Old Lady Who Swallowed a Fly* by Pam Adams (illustrator).

Here is a related book you could read at home: *Golly Gump Swallowed a Fly* by Joanna Cole and Bari Weissman (illustrator).

Song

There Was an Old Lady Who Swallowed a Fly
(Chant)

There was an old lady. **She** swallowed a fly.
I don't know why **she** swallowed the fly.

I don't know why.

There was an old lady. **She** swallowed a spider.
It wiggled and wiggled and jiggled inside **her.**

She swallowed the spider to catch the fly.
But **I** don't know why **she** swallowed the fly.

I don't know why!

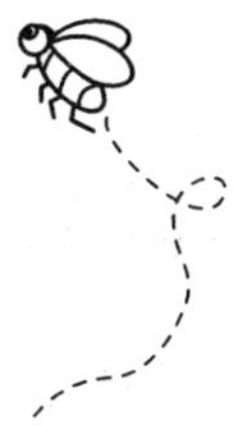

(Continue with the verses for the bird, cat, dog, cow, and horse.)

Activities

Our planned activities for the week include:

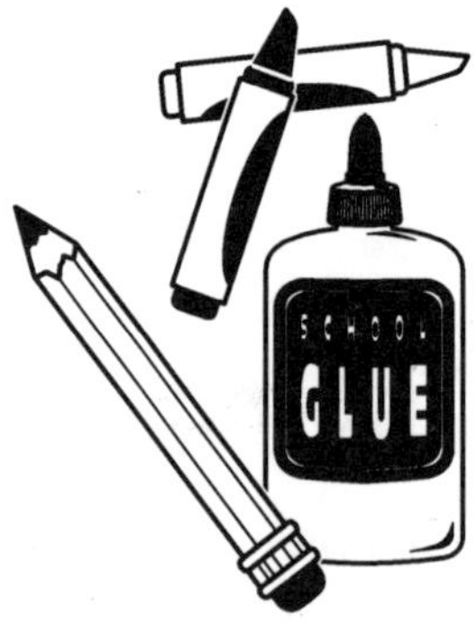

- Making "food" for an old lady puppet to eat
- Feeding food to the Old Lady
- Making a paper plate Old Lady

Follow-Up

Suggested follow-up activities for home include:

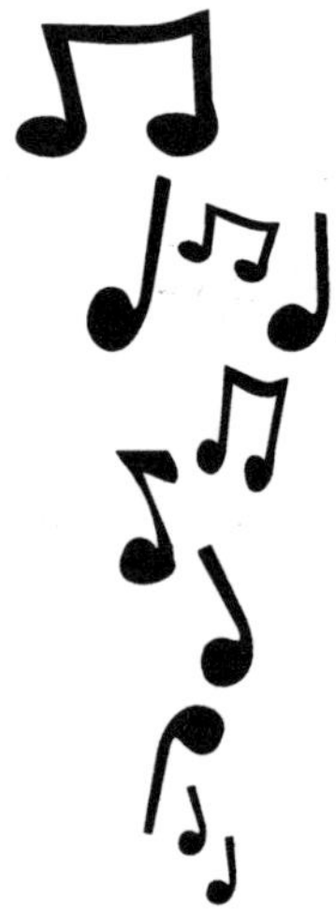

- Sing the song or read the book and discuss the funny things the Old Lady did, focusing on pronouns, for example:

  She swallowed a fly.

  She ate a spider.

- Collect pictures drawn by your child and pictures drawn by a sibling or friend. Sort them as you emphasize pronouns, for example:

  You drew this picture of **your** cat.

  He made a picture of **his** bike.

Thank You Very Much for your participation!

____
Phone Number

____
Email

____
Signature

Pronouns

Cycle 3, Session 1

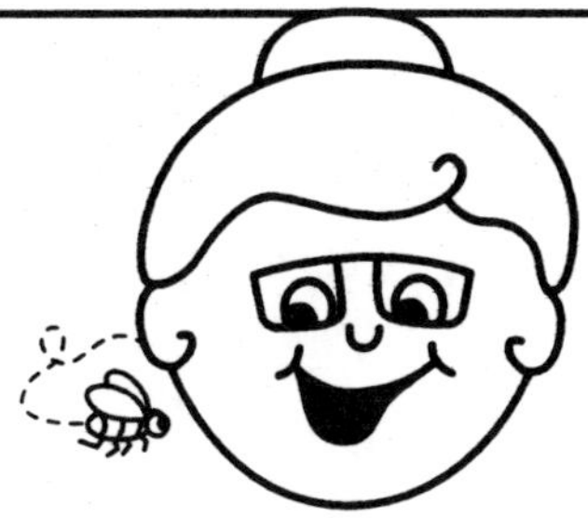

Theme: Food

Description: Completing activities relating to *There Was an Old Lady Who Swallowed a Fly*

Exemplars: he, her, his, I, it, mine, my, our, she, us, we, your

Materials:

There Was an Old Lady Who Swallowed a Fly by Pam Adams (illustrator)
Old Lady jar (see pages 300–301 for directions and a pattern)
Stuffed animal or puppet (for individual sessions only)
Old Lady food (see pages 300 and 302 for directions and patterns; 1 set)
Glue
Decorations (sequins, beads, glitter, etc.)
Crayons or markers

INTRODUCTION TO THEME

EDUCATOR: Last week **we** talked about a mouse who was very hungry. When **he** was hungry, what did **he** do? *[Allow children to respond]* That's right, **he** ate food! Today **we** are going to talk about an old lady who was hungry like **our** mouse. **She** was so hungry that **she** swallowed a fly and lots of other silly things!

BOOK ACTIVITY

Book: *There Was an Old Lady Who Swallowed a Fly* by Pam Adams (illustrator)

Instructions: Read the book with children, emphasizing pronouns.

Suggested Theme-Related Supplemental Book: *Golly Gump Swallowed a Fly* by Joanna Cole and Bari Weissman (illustrator)

Transition

EDUCATOR: Today **we** are going to make some food for **our** Old Lady to eat! *[Present Old Lady jar]* **We** need to look in **our** story to see what kinds of food to make.

FOCUSED STIMULATION ACTIVITY

Description: Coloring "food" (animals) for the Old Lady to eat

Skill Used: Fine motor

Instructions: Have each child color and decorate 2–3 animals. For sessions with an individual child, have a stuffed animal or puppet "participate" to create natural opportunities to use *he/his/him* or *she/hers/her.* Or focus on the pronouns *you/your/yours, we/our/ours,* or *me/mine/my* instead.

Example Script

EDUCATOR: Let's see what that Old Lady ate first. *[Look in the book]* First, **she** swallowed a fly. Let's make a fly.

EDUCATOR: Look at Jane. **She** has lots of wings on **her** fly.

EDUCATOR: Next, **she** swallowed a spider so let's make a spider.

EDUCATOR: **I** see John's spider. **He** colored lots of legs on **it.**

EDUCATOR: Next, **she** swallowed a bird.

EDUCATOR: Look at Jane. **She** colored **her** bird blue.

EDUCATOR: Now look at the Old Lady. **She** gobbled up a cat!

EDUCATOR: Let's see what Jake did. **He** glued eyes on **his** cat. Then **he** colored a big smile.

EDUCATOR: Look at the silly Old Lady! **She** swallowed a dog!

EDUCATOR: **I** am going to put long ears on **my** dog.

EDUCATOR: It looks like **you** are going to put red hair on **your** dog.

EDUCATOR: Jane, Maria doesn't have a dog. Please give one to **her.**

[Continue in a similar manner until all animals have been colored and decorated and numerous models of pronouns have been provided.]

Transition

EDUCATOR: We have all this food for the Old Lady. Now **she** wants to eat **it!**

ELICITED PRODUCTION ACTIVITY

Description: Feeding the Old Lady

Skills Used: Fine motor and dramatic play

Goal: 10 productions of pronouns per child

Level of Educator Support: Preparatory set

Instructions: Prepare the Old Lady jar prior to the activity. Have children feed the Old Lady jar.

Example Script

EDUCATOR: The old lady in **our** story swallowed lots of things. After **we** talk about what **she** swallowed, **we** can feed **her. We** will be able to see all the things that **she** swallowed when **we** are done! **I**'ll start *[modeling]:* **I** know an old lady, **she** swallowed a fly. Now it's **your** turn, Jane.

CHILD: **She** swallowed a spider.

EDUCATOR: Yes, and **I** bet **he** crawled inside **her!** What happened next, John?

CHILD: **She** swallowed a bird!

EDUCATOR: How absurd! What happened next?

CHILD: **She** swallowed a cow.

EDUCATOR: Whose cow should **she** eat?

CHILD: **Mine!**

EDUCATOR: Someone needs a cat. Who should **I** give the cat to?

CHILD: **Her!**

EDUCATOR: Look, **she** gobbled up a cat!

EDUCATOR: Then what happened?

CHILD: **She** gobbled a horse.

EDUCATOR: Then **she** nibbled on a dog!

[Continue in a similar manner until all items have been eaten and each child has had at least 10 opportunities to use pronouns.]

Transition

EDUCATOR: The Old Lady ate all the food! Let**'s** clean up and sing a song about the Old Lady who swallowed a fly!

SONG ACTIVITY

Instructions: Chant while emphasizing pronouns. Food items may be held up as children sing about them.

There Was an Old Lady Who Swallowed a Fly

There was an old lady, **she** swallowed a fly.
I don't know why **she** swallowed the fly.

I don't know why.

There was an old lady. **She** swallowed a spider.
It wiggled and wiggled and jiggled inside **her.**

She swallowed the spider to catch the fly.
But **I** don't know why **she** swallowed the fly.

I don't know why!

(Continue with the verses for the bird, cat, dog, cow, and horse.)

Pronouns

Cycle 3, Session 2

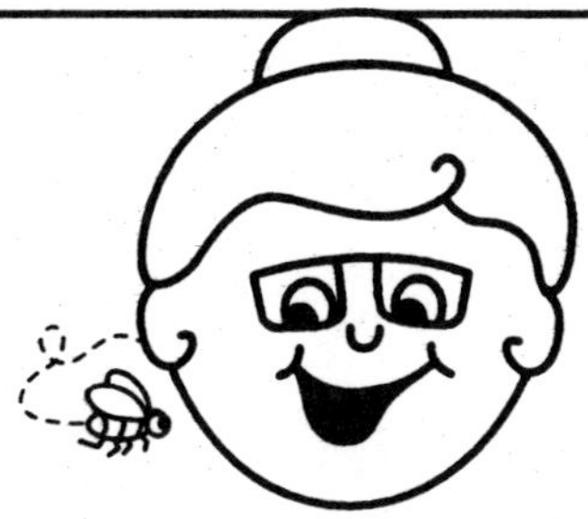

Theme: Food

Description: Completing activities relating to *There Was an Old Lady Who Swallowed a Fly*

Exemplars: he, her, his, I, my, it, our, she, them, us, we, us, you, your

Materials:

There Was an Old Lady Who Swallowed a Fly by Pam Adams (illustrator)
Old Lady animals (see pages 303 and 305–308 directions and patterns; 1 set per child)
Crayons or markers
Old Lady plates (see pages 303–304 for directions and patterns; 1 per child)
Completed Old Lady (see pages 303–308 directions and patterns)
Glue

BOOK ACTIVITY

Book: *There Was an Old Lady Who Swallowed a Fly* by Pam Adams (illustrator)

Instructions: Reread the book with children, emphasizing pronouns.

Suggested Theme-Related Supplemental Book: *Golly Gump Swallowed a Fly* by Joanna Cole and Bari Weissman (illustrator)

Transition

EDUCATOR: The Old Lady is still hungry, so **we** need to make some more food for **her! We** will color these circles that have animals on **them.** When **we** are done, **we** will feed **them** to the Old Lady so **we** can see everything **she** ate.

FOCUSED STIMULATION ACTIVITY

Description: Coloring "food" (animals) for the Old Lady to eat

Skills Used: Fine motor and sequencing

Instructions: Have each child color every animal in his or her set.

Example Script

EDUCATOR: Let'**s** see what the Old Lady did first. *[Look in the book]* **I** think **she** swallowed a fly. Let's color **our** flies.

EDUCATOR: Look what Jane did. **She** made wings on **her** fly.

EDUCATOR: See the Old Lady? Now **she** swallowed a spider.

EDUCATOR: John colored lots of legs on **his** spider.

EDUCATOR: That funny Old Lady! Now **she** swallowed a bird.

EDUCATOR: **I** colored **my** bird blue.

EDUCATOR: **You** colored **your** bird green!

EDUCATOR: Now **it** looks like **she** swallowed a cat!

EDUCATOR: Did **you** see what Jake did? **He** made eyes on **his** cat.

EDUCATOR: Now look at the Old Lady. **I** think **she** swallowed a dog!

EDUCATOR: **Our** dogs have tails on **them.**

EDUCATOR: Sally colored **her** dog yellow.

EDUCATOR: It looks like John colored **his** dog green.

EDUCATOR: Look at Jane's goat. **She** colored **it** purple!

[Continue in a similar manner until all animals have been colored and numerous models of pronouns have been provided.]

Transition

EDUCATOR: **Our** food pictures look so nice. Now **we** are going to put all these pictures in the Old Lady's tummy so that **we** can see all the things **she** ate!

ELICITED PRODUCTION ACTIVITY

Description: Gluing animals (from largest to smallest) on a paper plate

Skills Used: Fine motor and sequencing

Goal: 10 productions of pronouns per child

Level of Educator Support: Preparatory set

Instructions: Prepare an Old Lady plate prior to the activity to serve as a model.

Example Script

EDUCATOR: **Our** old lady swallowed lots of things. Now **we** are going to glue all the things **she** swallowed on this plate like this. *[Present model]* Before **we** glue each thing on, **I** want **you** to tell **me** what **she** swallowed. **I**'ll go first. **I** know an old lady. **She** swallowed a horse. Now **it**'s **your** turn John. **We** are going to glue on the biggest animals first.

CHILD: **She** swallowed a cow.

EDUCATOR: Yes **she** did. **I** like how **he** glued **his** cow on top of the horse.

EDUCATOR: Jane, tell **us** what **he** did.

CHILD: **He** glued the horse.

EDUCATOR: Yes. What do **you** think the old lady did next?

CHILD: **She** swallowed a dog!

EDUCATOR: Yes, **she** swallowed a whole dog! Tell **us** what Sally did to the dog.

CHILD: **She** glued it on the lady's tummy!

EDUCATOR: Yes, **she** glued it! Who did **she** glue **it** on?

CHILD: On **her**!

[Continue in a similar manner until all items have been "eaten" and each child has had at least 10 opportunities to use pronouns.]

Transition

EDUCATOR: Let's sing **our** song about the Old Lady who swallowed all those animals!

SONG ACTIVITY

Instructions: Chant while emphasizing pronouns. Food items may be held up as children sing about them.

There Was an Old Lady Who Swallowed a Fly

There was an old lady. **She** swallowed a fly.
I don't know why **she** swallowed the fly.

I don't know why.

There was an old lady. **She** swallowed a spider.
It wiggled and wiggled and jiggled inside **her.**

She swallowed the spider to catch the fly.
But **I** don't know why **she** swallowed the fly.

I don't know why!

(Continue with the verses for the bird, cat, dog, cow, and horse.)

Weekly Family Letter

For: ______________________________ **Date:** ______________

Theme

Our theme for language intervention this week is *food.*

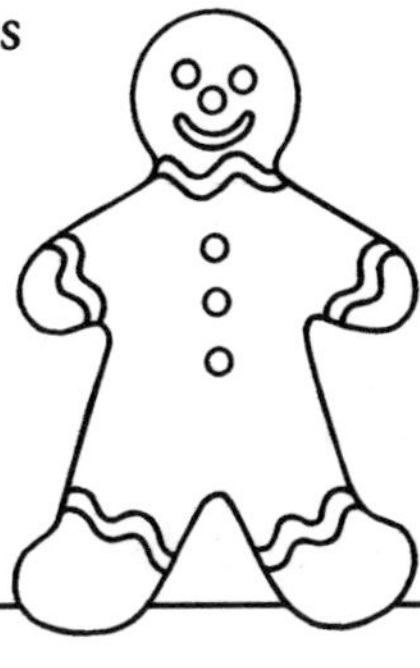

Target

Our target language structures are *auxiliary* be *verbs.* These are the verbs *am ('m), are ('re),* and *is ('s)* when used as "helping" verbs in a sentence. Generally, these verbs are used in front of verbs with *-ing* endings. Examples include:

- They **are** skiing.
- She**'s** crying.
- I **am** cooking dinner.

Book

Our book for the week is *The Gingerbread Man* by Karen Schmidt (illustrator).

Here are some related books you could read at home: *Whiff, Sniff, Nibble, and Chew: The Gingerbread Boy Retold* by Charlotte Pomerantz and Monica Incisa (illustrator) and *The Runaway Pancake* by P.C. Asbjorsen, Jorgen Moe, and Otto Svend (illustrator).

Song

The Gingerbread Man
(Tune: "Row, Row, Row Your Boat")

Gingerbread man, gingerbread man (or woman)
is running all day.

Faster, faster, faster, faster,
now he**'s** getting away!

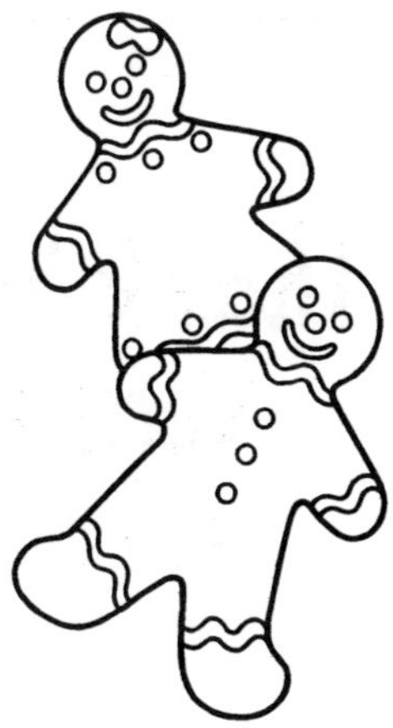

Activities

Our planned activities for the week include:

- Making a gingerbread person stick puppet
- Playing show-and-tell with the stick puppet
- Having a race with the stick puppet
- Decorating and eating gingerbread people cookies

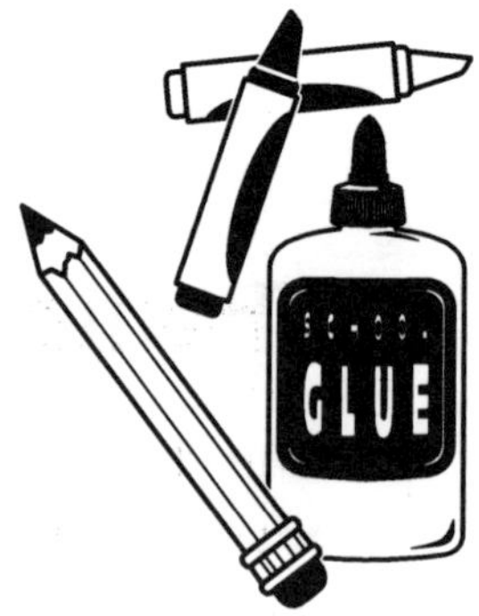

Follow-Up

Suggested follow-up activities for home include:

- Decorate gingerbread boy or girl cookies and discuss the steps as they are completed, for example:

  We **are** stirring up the flour and milk.

  You **are** cutting the dough.

  I **am** putting frosting on the cookie.

- Have your child tell you the story of the Gingerbread Man using auxiliary *be* verbs.

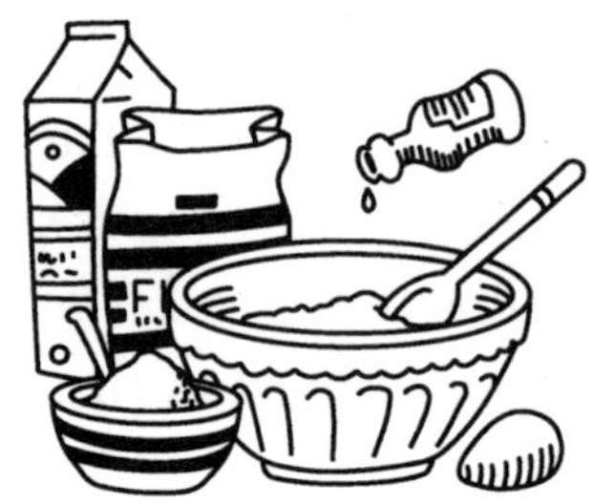

Thank You Very Much for your participation!

Phone Number

Email

Signature

Auxiliary *be*

Cycle 3, Session 1

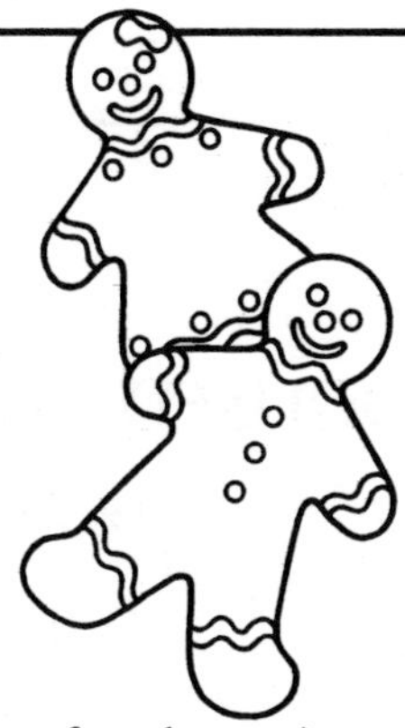

Theme: Food

Description: Completing activities relating to gingerbread people

Exemplars: am ('m), are ('re), is ('s)

Materials:

The Gingerbread Man by Karen Schmidt (illustrator)
Gingerbread people cutouts
(see pages 309–310 for directions and patterns; 1 set per child; 1 set for educator)
Completed gingerbread person stick puppet (see pages 309–310 for directions and patterns)
Single hole punch
Brass fasteners (2 per child; 2 for educator)
Decorations (glitter, google eyes, beads, etc.)
Glue
Child-safe scissors
Crayons or markers
Craft sticks (1 per child)
Hand puppet (for individual sessions only)

INTRODUCTION TO THEME

Educator: We'**re** going to talk about a special kind of cookie today. Do you like cookies? I do! I'**m** thinking of a kind of cookie that looks like a little girl or boy after it's decorated. This book will tell us more. Let's read it!

BOOK ACTIVITY

Book: *The Gingerbread Man* by Karen Schmidt (illustrator)

Instructions: Read the book with children, emphasizing auxiliary *be* verbs.

Suggested Theme-Related Supplemental Books:

Whiff, Sniff, Nibble, and Chew: The Gingerbread Boy Retold by Charlotte Pomerantz and Monica Incisa (illustrator)

The Runaway Pancake by P.C. Asbjorsen, Jorgen Moe, and Otto Svend (illustrator)

Transition

EDUCATOR: Today we **are** going to make gingerbread people like the one in the book. When we are done, our gingerbread people will look like this. *[Present model]*

FOCUSED STIMULATION ACTIVITY

Description: Making gingerbread people stick puppets

Skill Used: Fine motor

Instructions: Show children the model gingerbread person and explain that they are going to make one.

Example Script

EDUCATOR: Today we **are** going to make gingerbread people like the one in the story. Look. Watch what I do. *[Self talk]*

EDUCATOR: I'**m** putting glitter on the legs.

EDUCATOR: I **am** punching holes for the fasteners.

EDUCATOR: I **am** attaching his legs.

EDUCATOR: I **am** picking out eyes for my gingerbread boy.

EDUCATOR: I **am** gluing the eyes on.

EDUCATOR: I **am** making a big mess!

EDUCATOR: Now I'**m** drawing his teeth.

EDUCATOR: I **am** going to glue this stick on his back so that he will be like a puppet. *[Continue in a similar manner, narrating for children as they complete the project].*

EDUCATOR: John **is** making a red gingerbread boy.

EDUCATOR: Miguel, you **are** making a happy gingerbread boy.

[Continue in a similar manner until numerous models of auxiliary be *verbs have been provided.]*

Transition

Educator: We made some really nice gingerbread people today. Now I thought we could tell each other about what we made. Then we can have race with our gingerbread people.

ELICITED PRODUCTION ACTIVITY

Description: Playing show-and-tell with gingerbread people having a race with gingerbread people

Skills Used: Describing, sharing, and gross motor

Goal: 10 productions of auxiliary *be* verbs per child

Level of Educator Support: Preparatory set

Instructions: For sessions with an individual child, have a puppet "participate" in the race.

Example Script

Educator: We have some very nice gingerbread people. I would like us to talk about them, and then we **are** going to have a race. Remember how the gingerbread boy in the story ran really fast? Well, that's what our gingerbread people **are** going to do.

Educator: John **is** holding his gingerbread boy. Sally, tell me what Jake **is** doing.

Child: He **is** holding his gingerbread boy, too.

Educator: Jane, tell us what your girl **is** doing.

Educator: She **is** resting. *[Continue in a similar manner for all children]*

Educator: Let's have a race with our gingerbread people puppets. Let's get started. *[Designate a starting and finishing point for the race, and have children hold their gingerbread people and run or walk]*

Educator: My boy **is** losing. Tell me about Sally's girl.

Child: She **is** winning.

Educator: Oh no, now I **am** going slow! Tell me about you, John.

Child: I **am** going fast!

[Continue in a similar manner until each child has had at least 10 opportunities to use auxiliary be *verbs.]*

Transition

EDUCATOR: Our gingerbread people were very fast! Let's sing a song about a gingerbread man now.

SONG ACTIVITY

Instructions: Sing to the tune of "Row, Row, Row Your Boat," emphasizing auxiliary *be* verbs.

The Gingerbread Man

Gingerbread man, gingerbread man (or woman)
Is running all day.

Faster, faster, faster, faster,
now he'**s** getting away!

Auxiliary *be*

Cycle 3, Session 2

Theme: Food

Description: Completing activities relating to gingerbread people

Exemplars: am ('m), are ('re), is ('s)

Materials:

The Gingerbread Man by Karen Schmidt (illustrator)
Gingerbread cookies
Decorations (candy, sprinkles, etc.)
Frosting
Napkins
Juice boxes

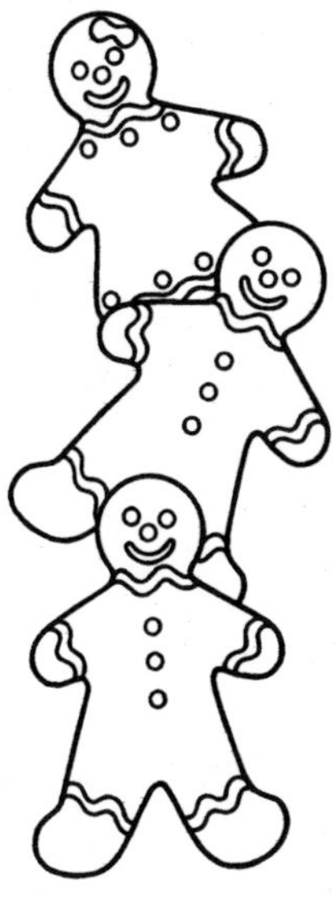

BOOK ACTIVITY

Book: *The Gingerbread Man* by Karen Schmidt (illustrator)

Instructions: Reread the book with children, emphasizing auxiliary *be* verbs.

Suggested Theme-Related Supplemental Books: *Whiff, Sniff, Nibble, and Chew: The Gingerbread Boy Retold* by Charlotte Pomerantz and Monica Incisa (illustrator)
The Runaway Pancake by P.C. Asbjorsen, Jorgen Moe, and Otto Svend (illustrator)

Transition

EDUCATOR: Remember in our story how the farmer and his wife wanted to eat the gingerbread man? Well, today I thought it would be fun if we made gingerbread people to eat!

FOCUSED STIMULATION ACTIVITY

Description: Decorating gingerbread people cookies

Skills Used: Describing and fine motor

Instructions: Bake or purchase gingerbread people cookies prior to the activity. Show children a decorated gingerbread person cookie, and explain that they are going to decorate their own.

Example Script

EDUCATOR: Today we **are** going to make gingerbread people to eat. See, here's mine. *[Present model]* He is little and he is yummy! He is a cookie! There are lots of things we can use to make our gingerbread people look good. Watch how I **am** decorating mine.

EDUCATOR: *[Present sprinkles]* I **am** sprinkling sugar on him.

EDUCATOR: *[Present candy]* I **am** putting candy on him.

EDUCATOR: I **am** putting eyes on him.

EDUCATOR: Let's see what Sally**'s** doing. She **is** putting licorice on the girl's arm.

EDUCATOR: Now she**'s** putting red candies on her shirt.

EDUCATOR: *[Present frosting]* This is frosting. I **am** spreading frosting on him.

EDUCATOR: This is messy. We need napkins. I **am** wiping up our mess.

[Continue in a similar manner until cookies have been decorated and numerous models of auxiliary be *verbs have been provided.]*

Transition

EDUCATOR: These gingerbread people **are** looking really good. They **are** looking good enough to eat! Is anybody hungry? I am! Let's eat our gingerbread people.

ELICITED PRODUCTION ACTIVITY

Description: Eating gingerbread people cookies and drinking juice

Skills Used: Sharing, turn taking, and describing

Goal: 10 productions of auxiliary *be* verbs per child

Level of Educator Support: Preparatory set

Example Script

EDUCATOR:	We all have very nice gingerbread people. I would like us to talk about them, and then we **are** going to eat them up.
EDUCATOR:	I **am** handing out napkins to everyone. John, tell us what I **am** doing.
CHILD:	She **is** handing out napkins.
EDUCATOR:	Excellent. Sally, tell us what I **am** doing now.
CHILD:	She **is** passing out juice. *[After items are handed out, eat cookies and have juice]*
EDUCATOR:	Sally, what **are** you doing?
CHILD:	I**'m** eating cookies.
EDUCATOR:	Who **is** drinking juice?
CHILD:	I **am.**
EDUCATOR:	Who **is** eating a gingerbread boy with green eyes?
CHILD:	John **is!**
EDUCATOR:	Who **is** eating a gingerbread girl with candy hair?
CHILD:	You **are!**

[Continue in a similar manner until each child has had at least 10 opportunities to use auxiliary be *verbs.]*

Transition

EDUCATOR: That snack sure was good! Now it's time to clean up and sing our gingerbread man song.

SONG ACTIVITY

Instructions: Sing to the tune of "Row, Row, Row Your Boat," emphasizing auxiliary *be* verbs.

The Gingerbread Man

Gingerbread man, gingerbread man (or woman)
is running all day.

Faster, faster, faster, faster,
now he**'s** getting away!

Appendices

WORKSHEET FOR GENERATING SCRIPTS FOR TARGETING MORPHEMES

Target: ______________________ **Theme:** ______________________

Cycle: ______________________ **Week:** ______________________

Auditory Awareness

Books (main and supplemental): ______________________

Song: ______________________

Sing to the tune of: ______________________

Lyrics: ______________________

____

____

____

Focused Stimulation Activity

Type of activity (check one):

❑ snack ❑ fine motor ❑ gross motor ❑ dramatic play ❑ other__________

Activity description: ______________________

Materials: ______________________

Exemplars: ______________________

Elicited Production Activity

Level of support (check one): ❑ Forced choice ❑ Cloze task ❑ Preparatory set

Type of activity (check one):

❑ snack ❑ fine motor ❑ gross motor ❑ dramatic play ❑ other__________

Materials: ______________________

Exemplars: ______________________

Photocopy this form and use the back for notes.

EXAMPLE LANGUAGE SAMPLE SCRIPT

Example language sample context: Playing with a toy house that has moveable windows and doors and accompanying accessories, including pets, family members, furniture, a boat, and a car.

Morpheme	Example Elicitations
Present progressive *-ing*	EDUCATOR: Look what this dog is doing! *CHILD:* **Barking!**
Preposition *in*	EDUCATOR: I wonder where I should put this table. *CHILD:* **In** the house.
Preposition *on*	EDUCATOR: I'm going to put this lamp under this table. *CHILD:* No! Put it **on** the table!
Regular plural *-s*	EDUCATOR: Look, this boy has a cat. I wonder if he has any other **pets.** *[There are two dogs]* *CHILD:* He has two **dogs.**
Irregular past tense	EDUCATOR: *[Unsnap a piece from the house]* Oh no! Look what happened! *CHILD:* It **broke!**
Possessive *'s*	EDUCATOR: I think this is the **mommy's** bed. *[Present crib/cradle]* *CHILD:* No, it's the **baby's!**
Uncontractible copula ***is, am, are, was, were*** (main verb)	EDUCATOR: Have the daddy ask the girl if she's hungry. *CHILD:* **Are** you hungry?
Articles ***a, an, the***	EDUCATOR: I want **a** bed for my room. I wonder what you would like for your room. *CHILD:* **A** chair.
Regular past *-ed*	EDUCATOR: *[Make a figurine jump on the bed]* The sister got in trouble. Daddy wants to know what she did. *CHILD:* She **jumped** on her bed!
Regular third person *-s*	EDUCATOR: This boy **runs** down the stairs. Look what his sister **does!** *CHILD:* She **eats** her dinner.
Irregular third person ***has, says, does***	EDUCATOR: This dog **has** a pretty yellow house. Tell me about the kitty. *CHILD:* She **has** a blue pillow.
Uncontractible auxiliary ***is, am, are, was, were*** (helping verb)	EDUCATOR: Have mommy ask daddy what he**'s** doing. *CHILD:* What **are** you doing?
Contractible copula ***is, am, are, was, were*** (main verb)	EDUCATOR: Look, he**'s** the daddy. Tell me about this guy. *CHILD:* He**'s** the baby.
Contractible auxiliary ***is, am, are, was, were*** (helping verb)	EDUCATOR: I think she**'s** running really fast! *CHILD:* No, she**'s** going slow!

Sources: Brown (1973); Miller and Chapman (1981)

Introductory Family Letter

Date: ______________________

For: ____

Dear family,

For the next several weeks, your child will be receiving language intervention to improve the way he or she uses various forms of grammar (for example, adding *-ed* to a word to make it past tense). Each week, a new grammatical form will be targeted. Activities designed to teach your child the weekly target will revolve around one of three main themes: water, animals, or food. The main focus of the activities will be to improve your child's language skills. However, other skills will also be worked on, including sharing, direction following, fine motor (like art activities), and gross motor (like playing a physical game). Each session will include the following components:

Book Activity
An age-appropriate and theme-related book will be read with your child. The books will either contain many examples of the target grammatical form, or the stories will be discussed using the target form.

Focused Stimulation Activity
These activities will provide your child with many opportunities to hear the target grammatical form being used in conversation. In these activities, your child will not be required to use the target form; he or she will be asked to listen to examples of the target form.

Elicited Production Activity
For these activities, your child will be asked to use the week's target grammatical form. There will be many opportunities for your child to practice using the target.

Song Activity
For further practice, a song will be used each week. This song will contain many examples of the target grammatical form. Singing songs is a fun way for children to practice using their newly learned grammatical forms!

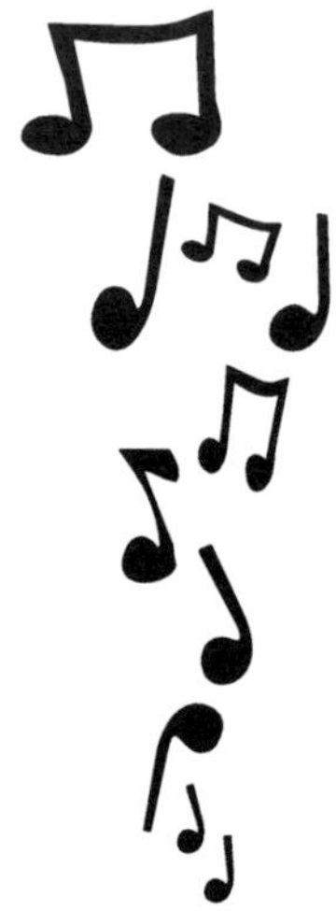

Family participation in the intervention process is very helpful and is encouraged. To provide you with ideas of how to help improve your child's language skills, weekly family letters will be sent home. In these letters, you will be told about the grammatical form your child will be working on for the week, the book that will be read, the song that will be sung, and the activities that will be completed. Suggestions for home practice will also be given.

Thank You Very Much
for your participation!

____
Phone Number

____
Email

____
Signature

Weekly Family Letter

For: ______________________ **Date:** __________

Theme

Our theme for language intervention this week is

____

Target

Our target language structures are

____

Examples include:

-
-
-

Book

Our book for the week is ______________________

Here are some related books you could read at home: ______________________

____

Song

Activities

Our planned activities for the week include:

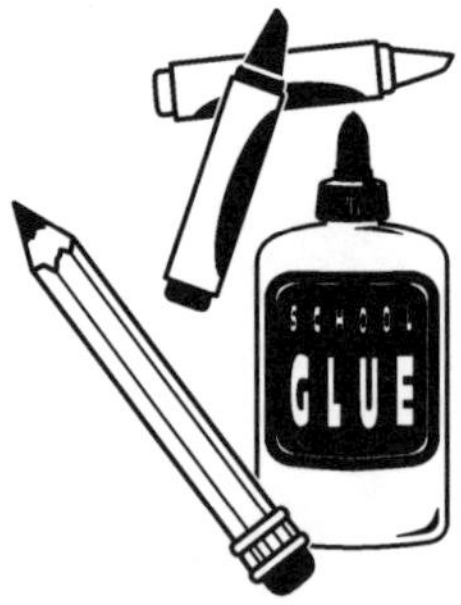

-
-
-

Follow-Up

Suggested follow-up activities for home include:

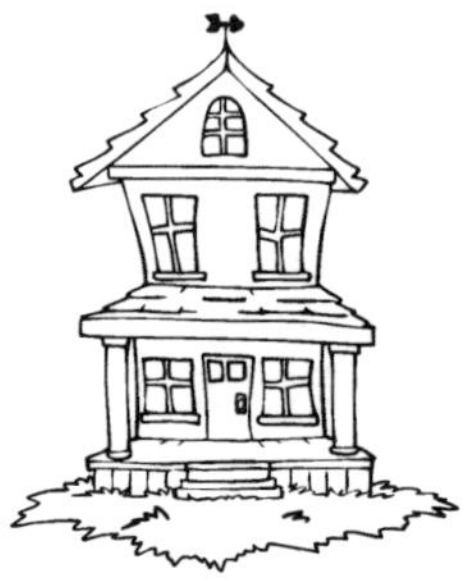

-
-

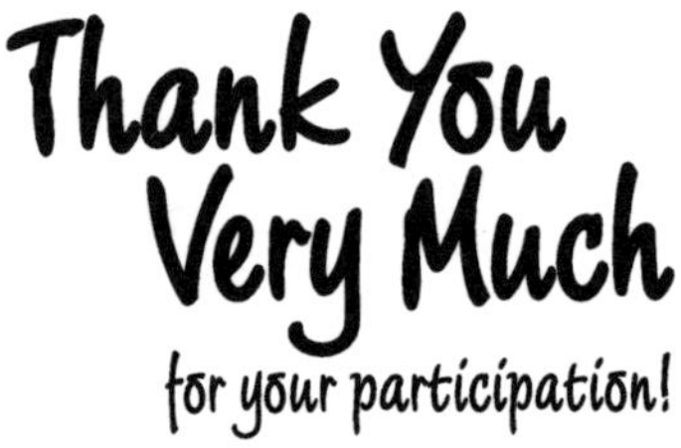

Phone Number

Email

Signature

BUBBLE SOAP

MATERIALS

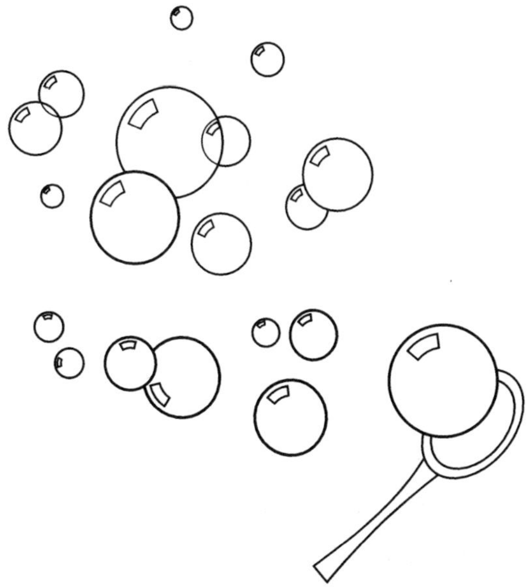

- Bowl (Part I only)
- Measuring cup
- Tablespoon
- Teaspoon
- Bottle of water
- Container of dish soap
- Bag of sugar
- Bag (Part I only)

RECIPE

- ½ cup water
- 3 tablespoons dish soap
- 2 teaspoons sugar

DIRECTIONS

Part I

1. Place the bowl, measuring cup, tablespoon, teaspoon, bottle of water, container of dish soap, and bag of sugar in the bag.
2. Have the bag of materials ready for use in the activity and make note of the recipe (above).

Part II

1. Have the materials ready for use in the activity and make note of the recipe (above).

SAILBOAT

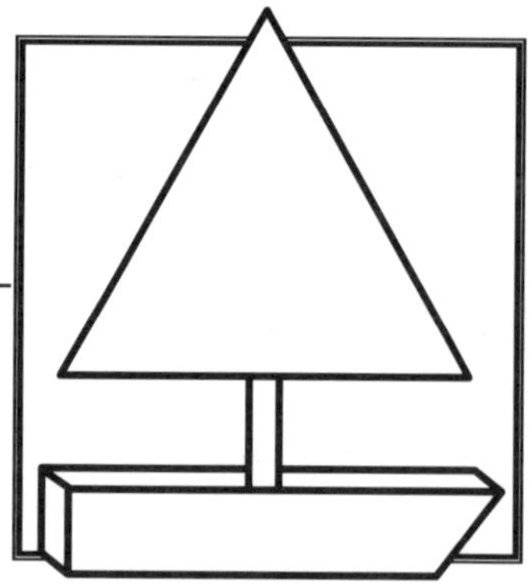

MATERIALS

- Scissors
- Decorations (glitter, stickers, etc.)
- Glue
- Milk carton
- Poster paint, construction paper, or wrapping paper
- Tape (if using construction paper or wrapping paper)
- Rubber cement
- Piece of Styrofoam (cut in 1 square inch)
- Craft stick

DIRECTIONS

1. Cut out 2 large (approximately 5" × 5") triangles to serve as sails.
2. Decorate the sails using glitter, stickers, etc.
3. Cut the milk carton in half lengthwise.
4. Paint one half of the milk carton or cover it in construction paper or wrapping paper. This will serve as the boat.
5. Using the rubber cement, stick the Styrofoam piece in the center of the boat. Allow 1 minute to dry.
6. Stick the craft stick in the center of the Styrofoam to create a mast.
7. Glue 1 sail on each side of the craft stick. Allow approximately 5 minutes for the glue to dry.
8. Have the model sailboat, triangle cutouts (2 per child), styrofoam pieces cut in 1 square inch pieces (1 per child), and milk cartons cut in half lengthwise (1 half per child) ready for use in the activity.

FACIAL FEATURES

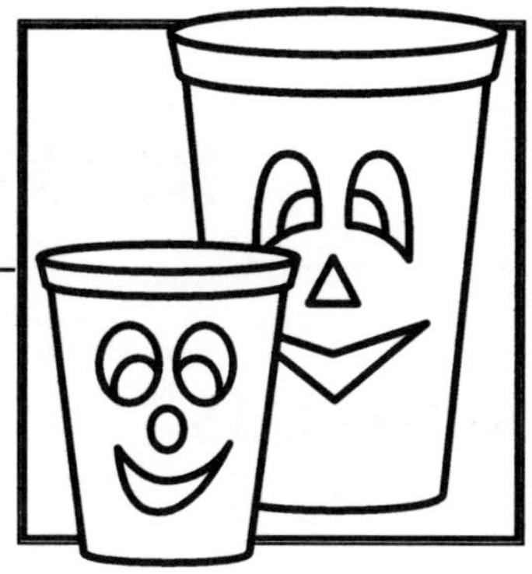

MATERIALS

- Colored paper

DIRECTIONS

1. Photocopy the *Facial Feature Patterns* onto colored paper. Enlarge or reduce the patterns as necessary to fit different sized cups.
2. Have photocopies of the facial features (1 per child) ready for use in the activity.

FACIAL FEATURE PATTERNS

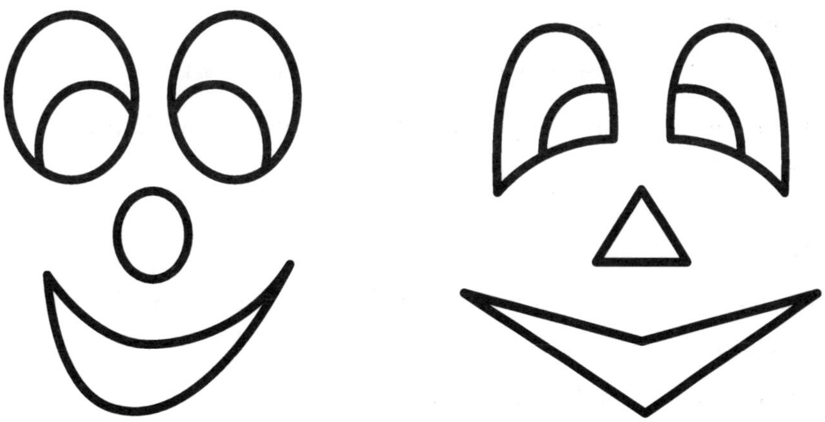

BROWN BEAR

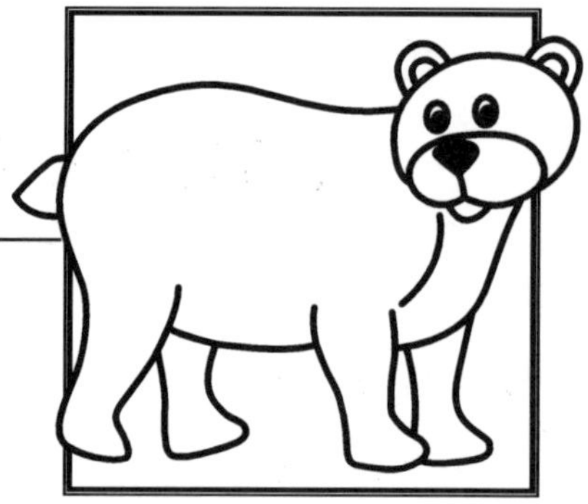

MATERIALS

Stick Puppet

- Construction paper in a variety of colors
- Scissors
- Decorations (sequins, beads, etc.)
- Glue
- Craft stick

Felt Animals

- Pencil or pen
- Felt in the following colors: red, blue, orange, white, black, yellow, green, and brown
- Scissors
- Glue

DIRECTIONS

Stick Puppet

1. Photocopy the *Brown Bear Pattern* on page 275 onto construction paper. Enlarge or reduce the pattern as necessary.
2. Cut the Brown Bear out.
3. Decorate the Brown Bear and glue the craft stick on its back.
4. Have the model Brown Bear puppet and Brown Bear cutouts (1 per child) ready for use in the activity.

Felt Animals

1. Photocopy the animal patterns on pages 276–282 to use as templates. Enlarge or reduce the patterns as necessary.
2. Trace the templates on the felt and cut the pieces out.
3. Glue the felt pieces together to create each animal.
4. Add detail lines (e.g., eyes and mouths) to the animals if desired.
5. Have felt animal cutouts (1 set) ready for use in the activity.

BROWN BEAR PATTERN

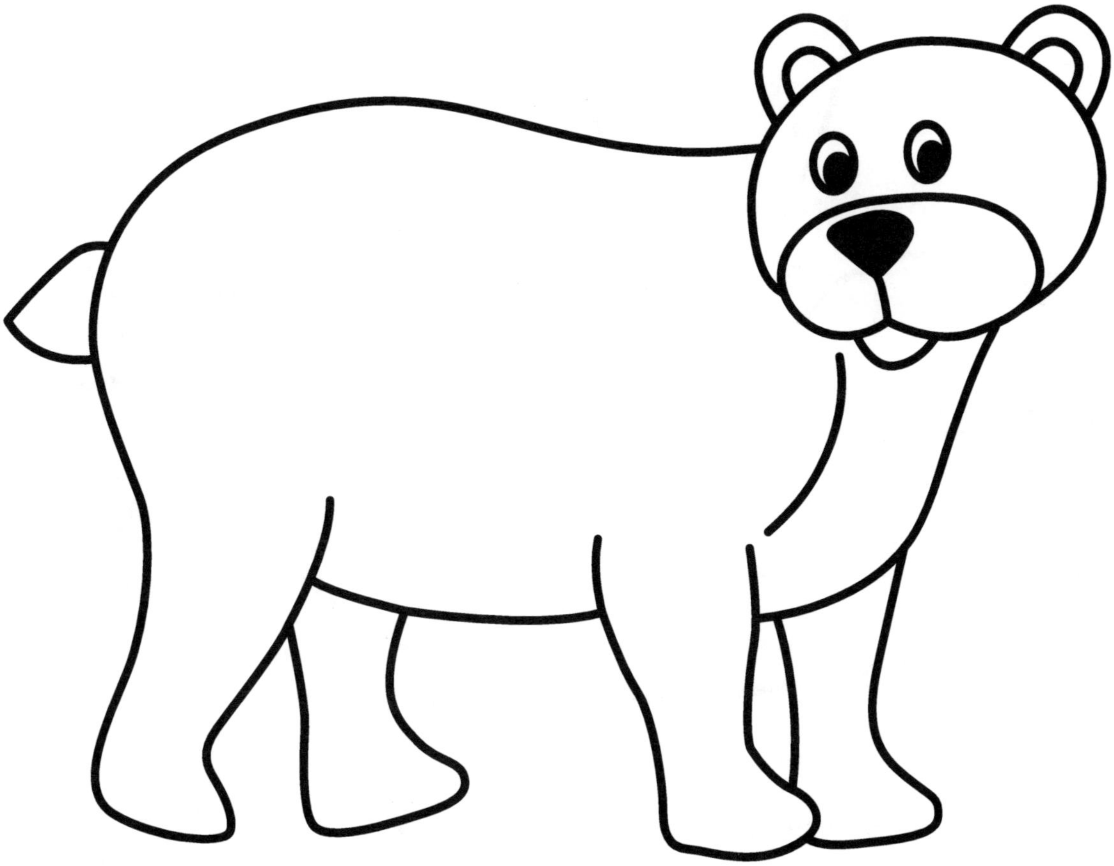

RED BIRD PATTERNS

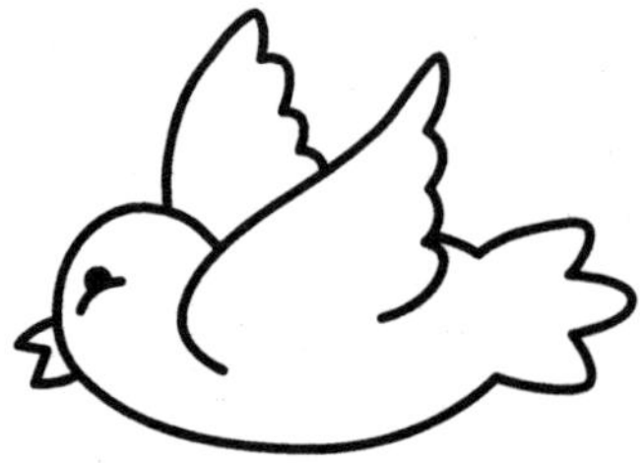

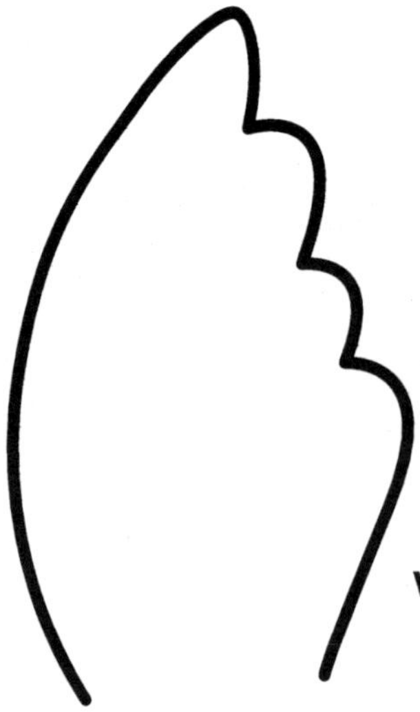

Wing

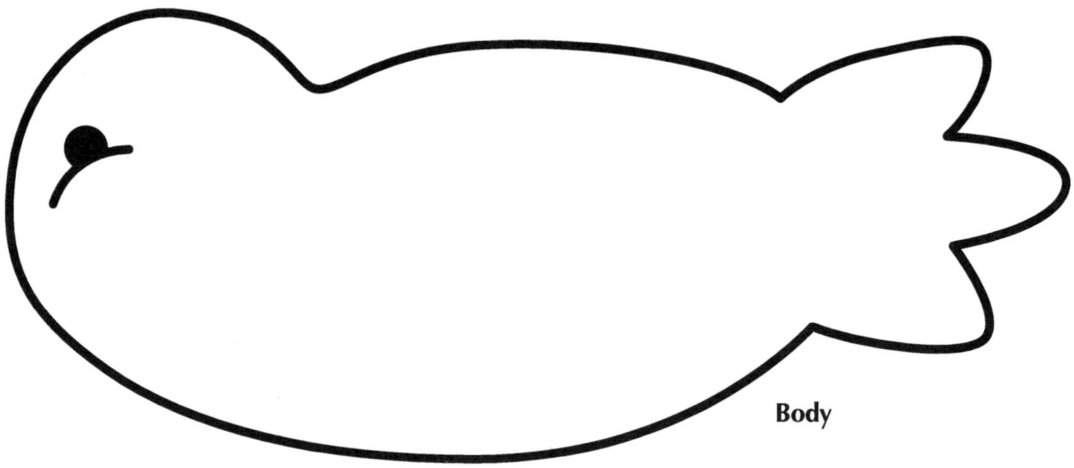

Body

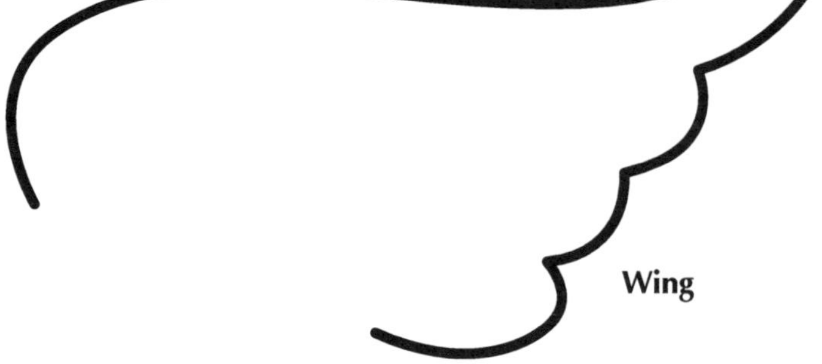

Wing

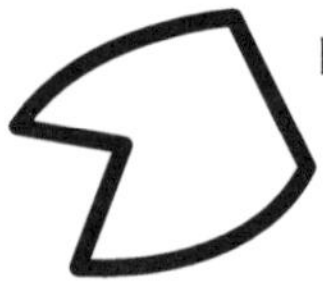

Beak

BLUE HORSE PATTERNS

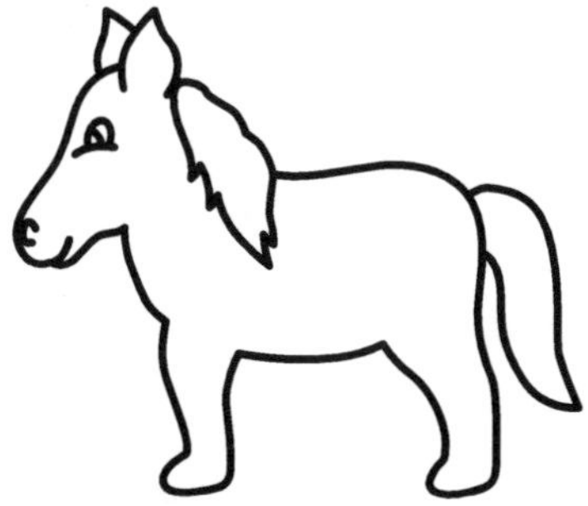

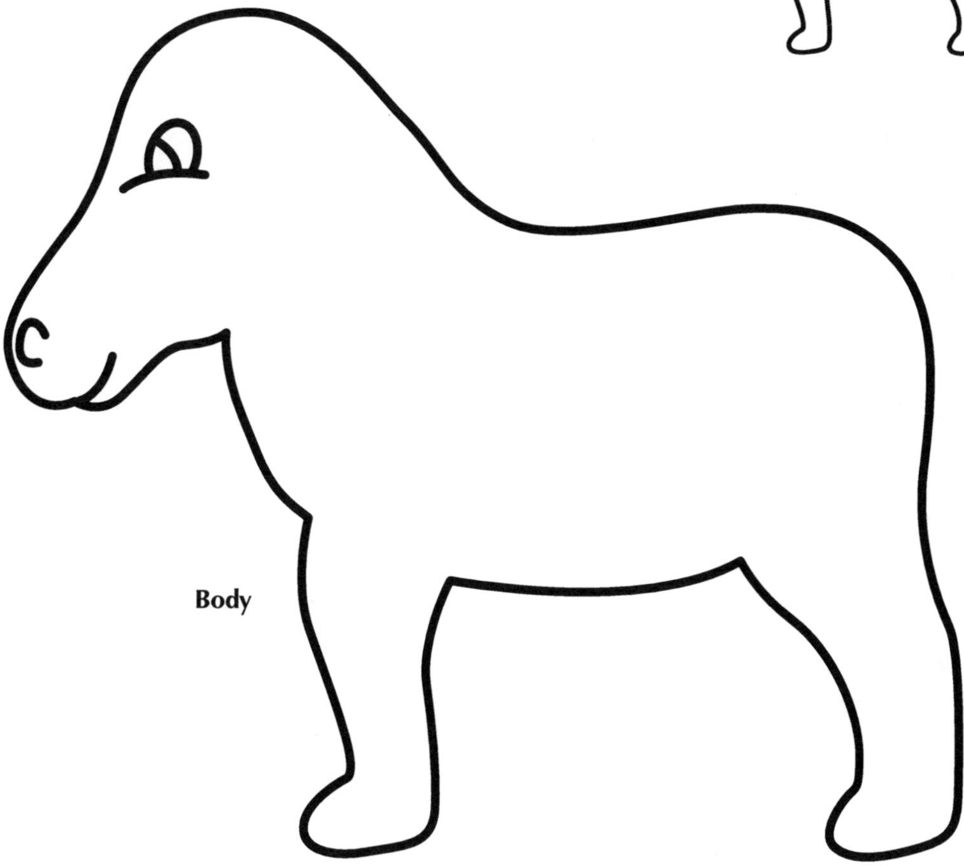

Body

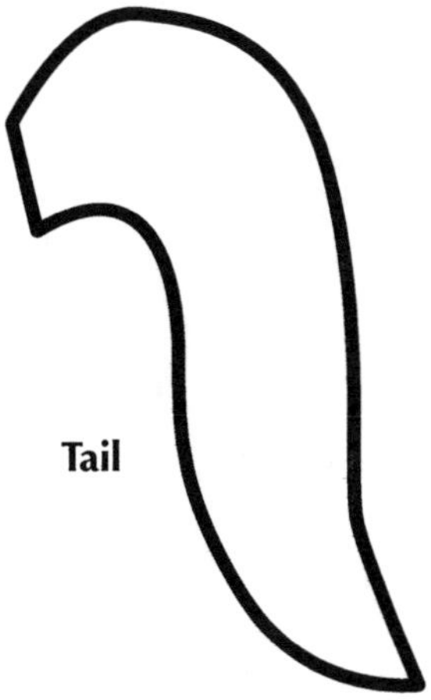

Tail

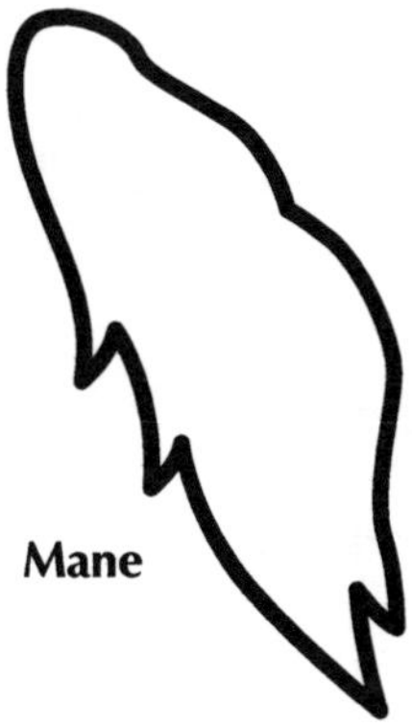

Mane

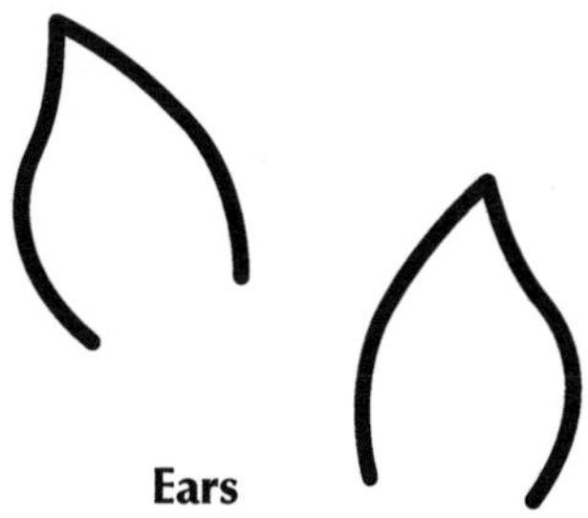

Ears

GOLDFISH PATTERNS

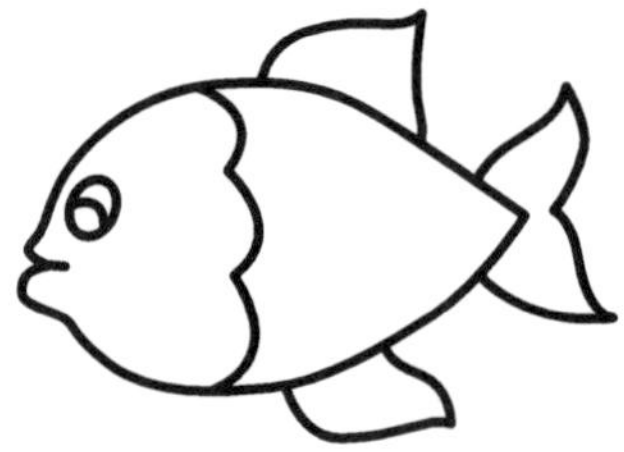

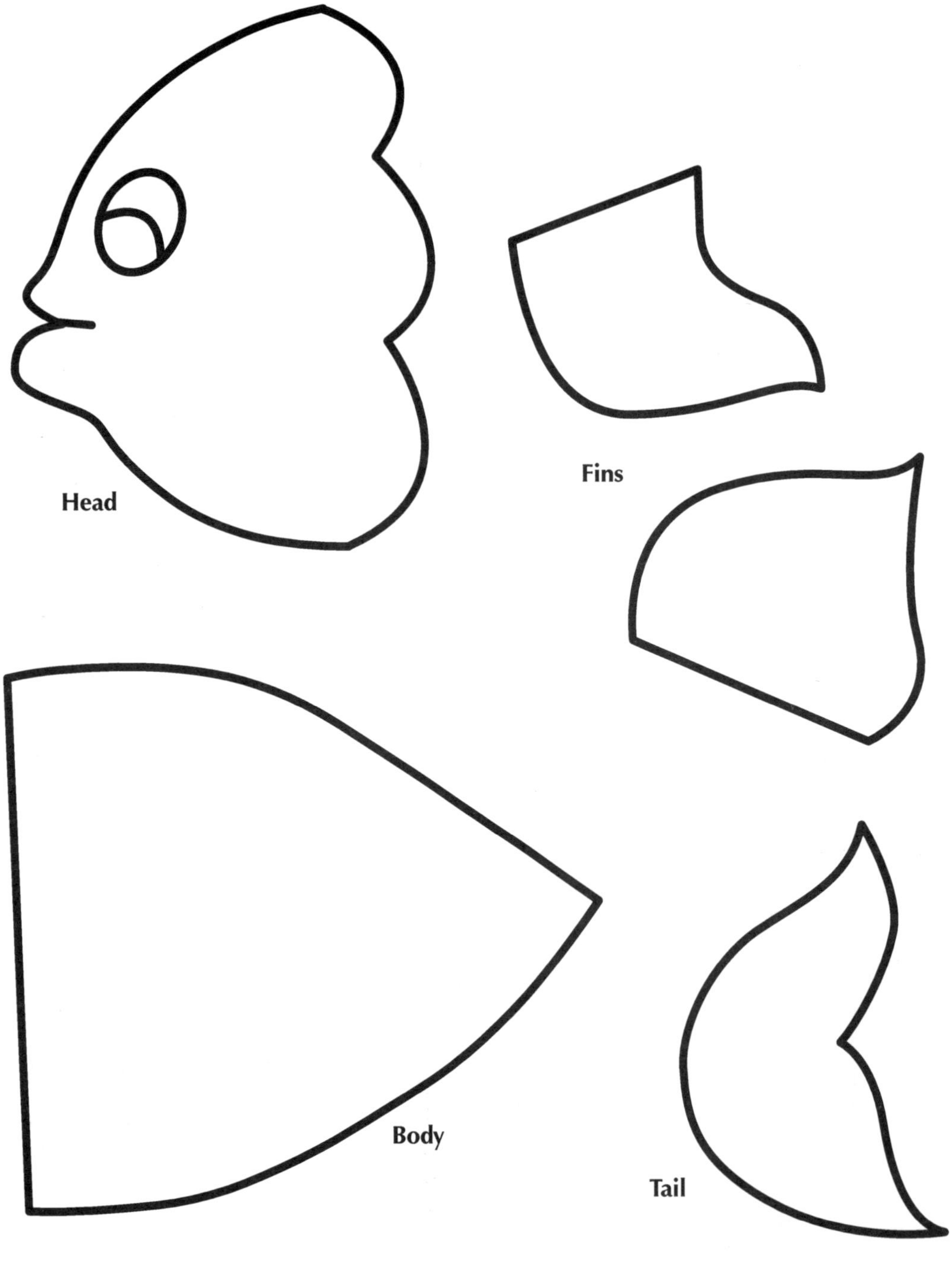

WHITE DOG PATTERNS

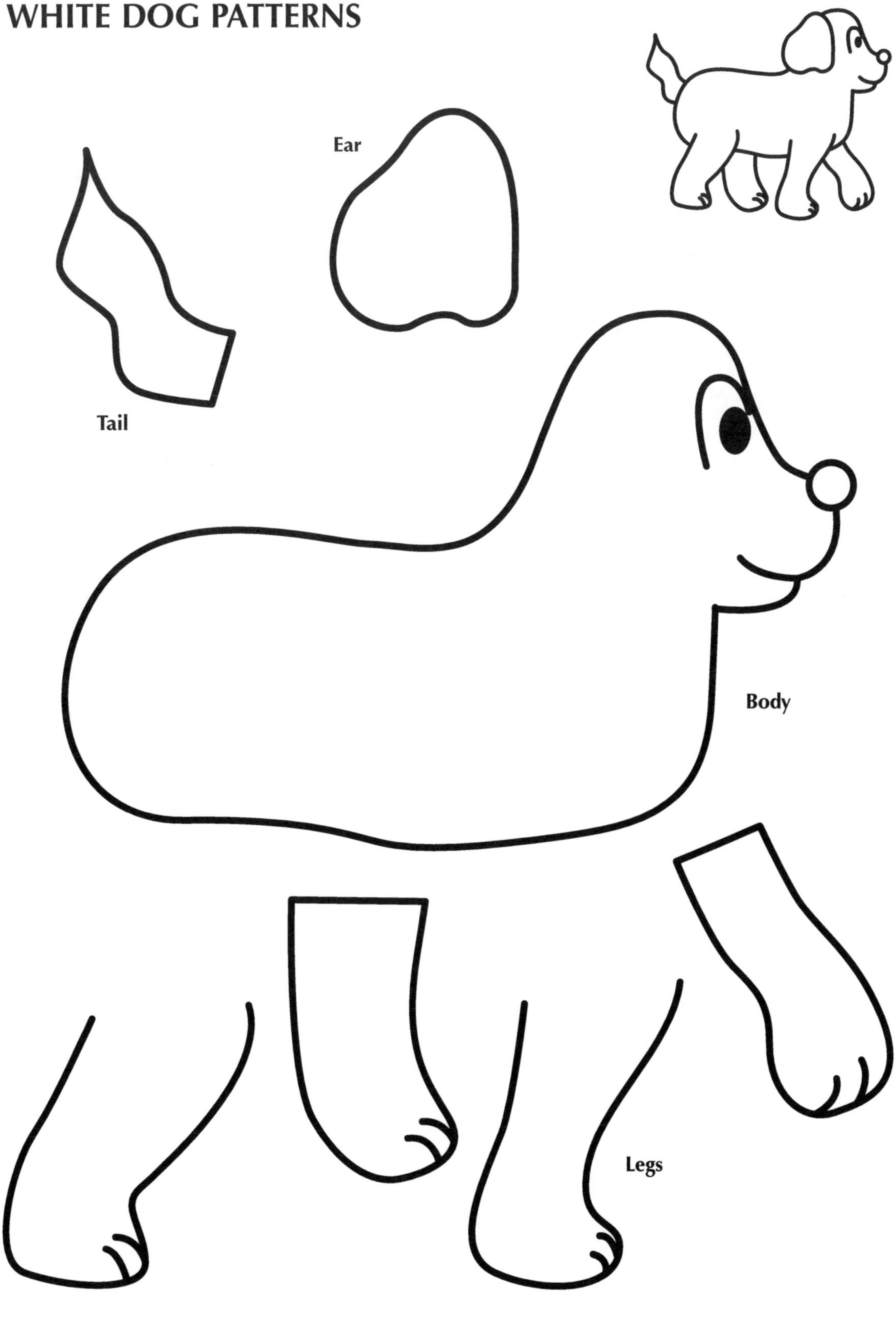

BLACK SHEEP PATTERNS

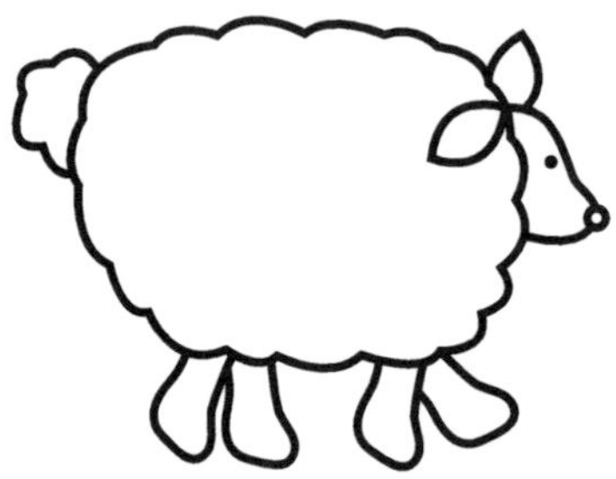

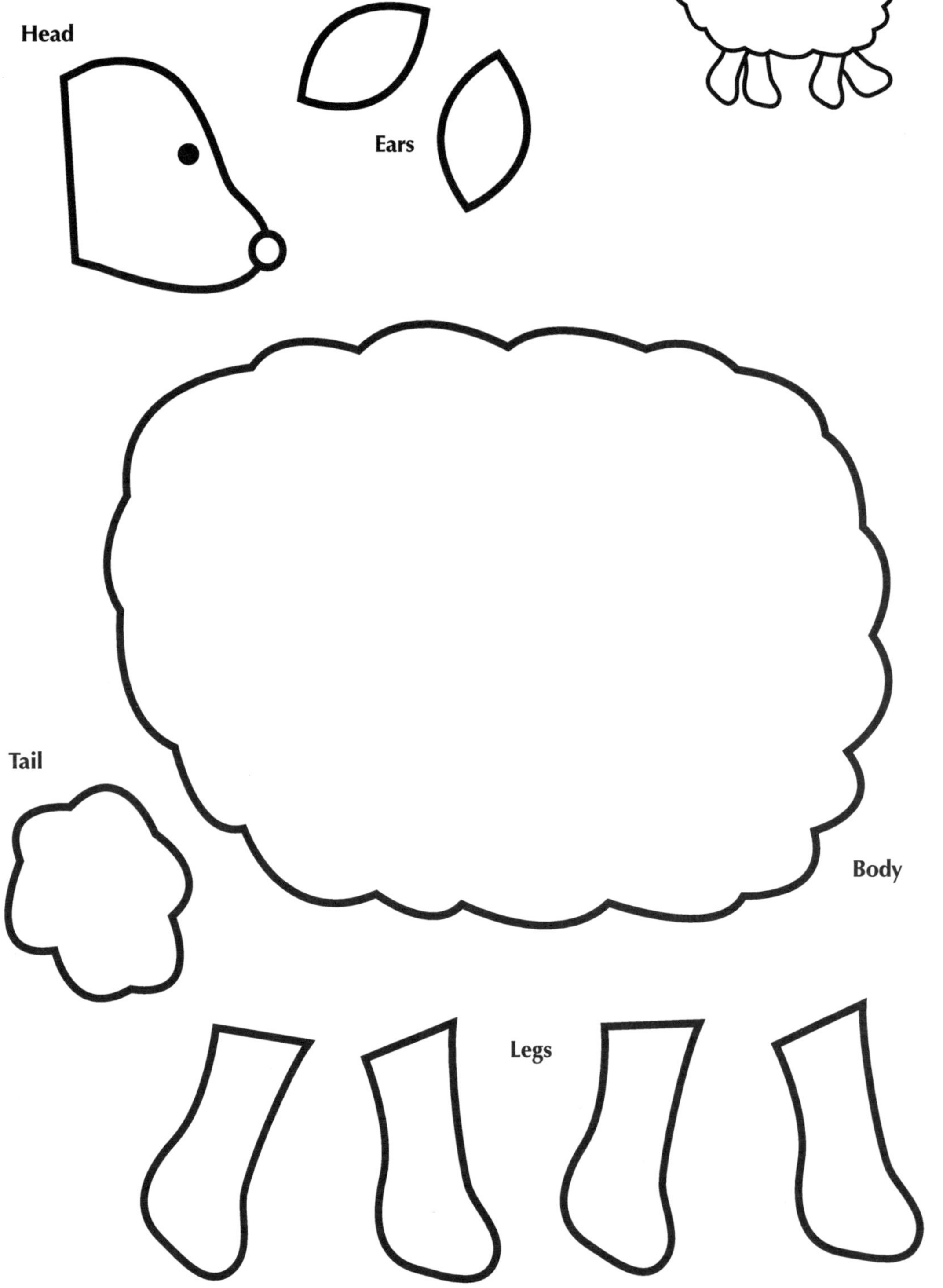

YELLOW DUCK PATTERNS

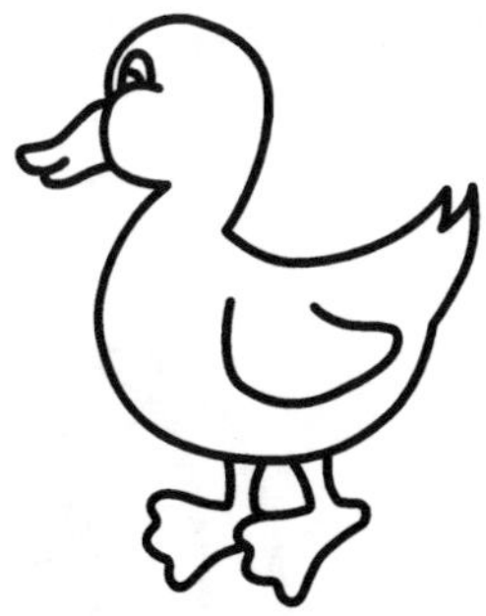

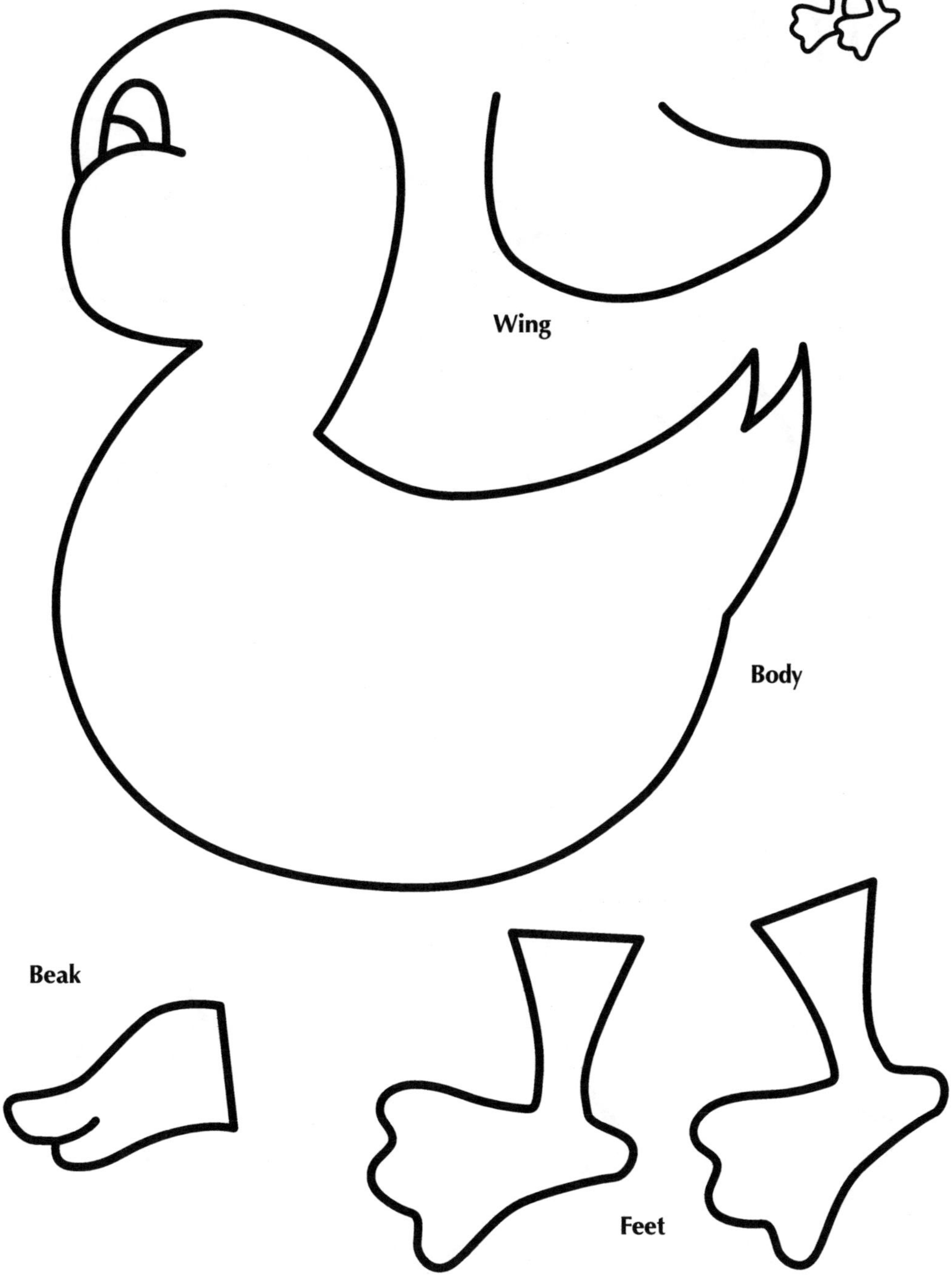

GREEN FROG PATTERNS

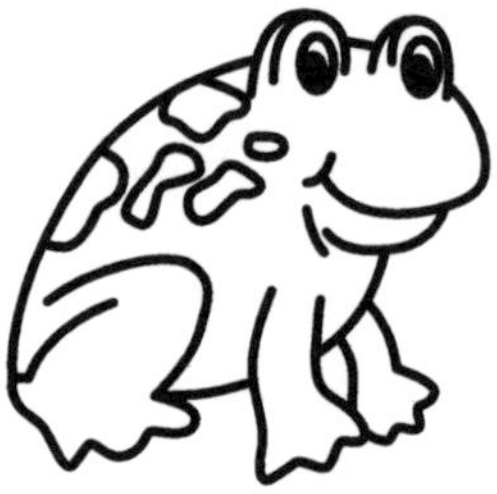

Eyes

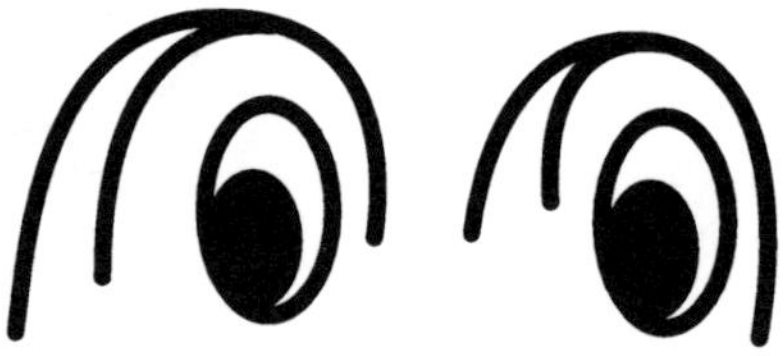

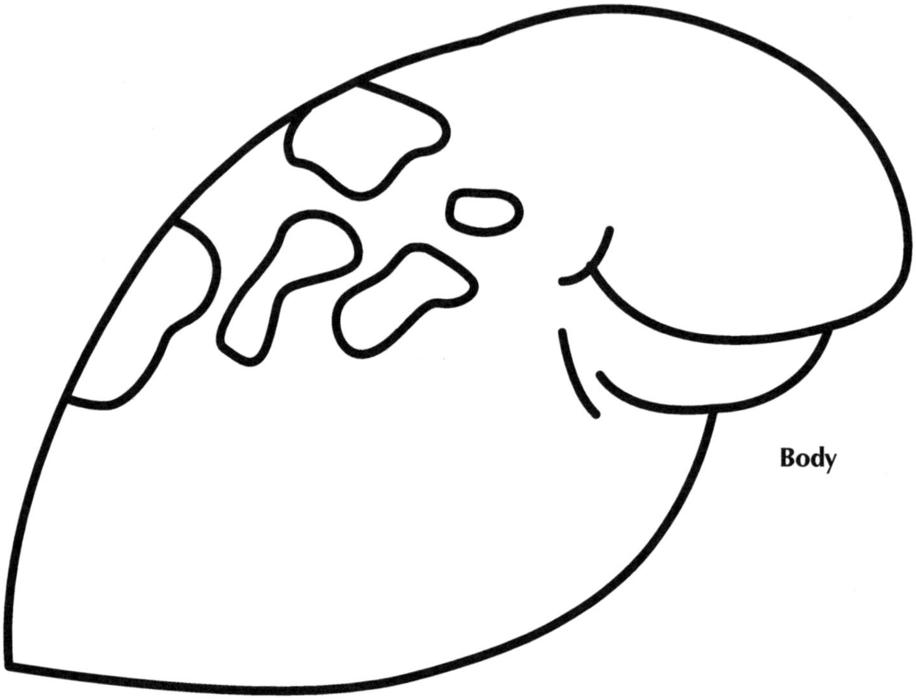

Body

Legs

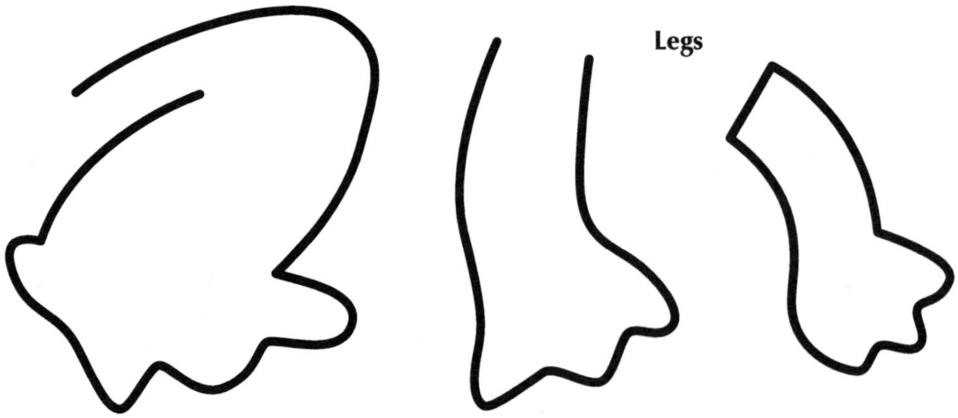

ANIMALS

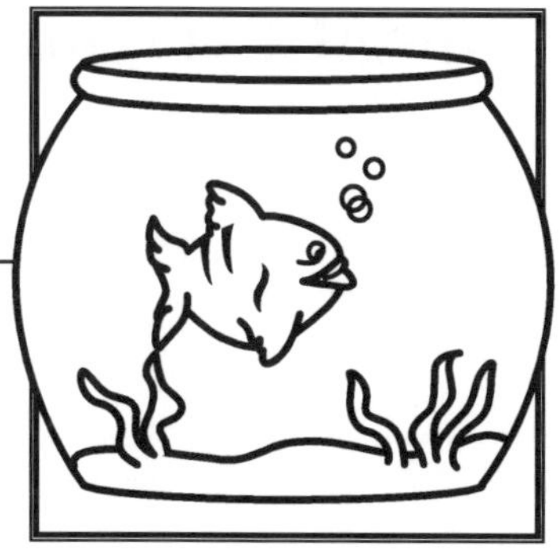

MATERIALS

- Paper
- Scissors
- Crayons or markers (optional)

DIRECTIONS

1. Photocopy the *Animal Patterns* below and on page 284. Enlarge or reduce the patterns as necessary.
2. Cut out the patterns and color if desired.

NOTE: For the cat hunt activity, multiple cats are needed.

ANIMAL PATTERNS

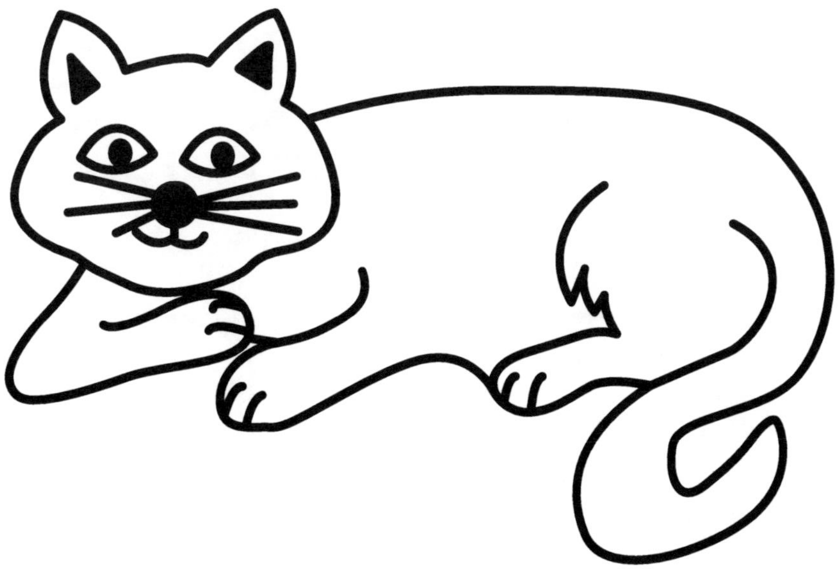

ANIMAL PATTERNS

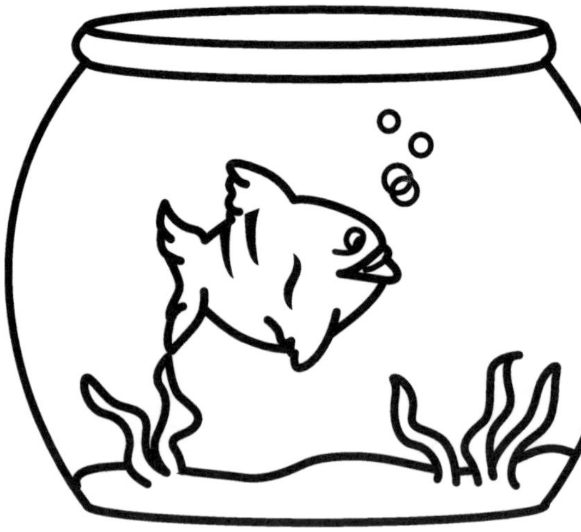

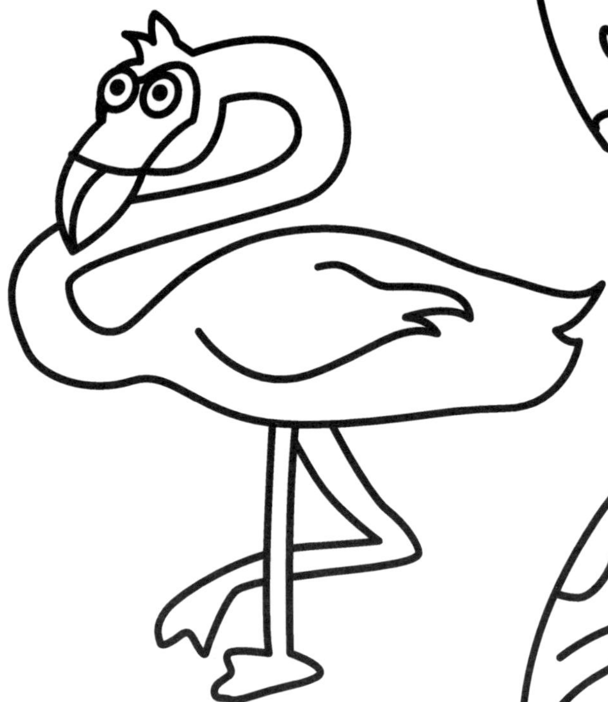

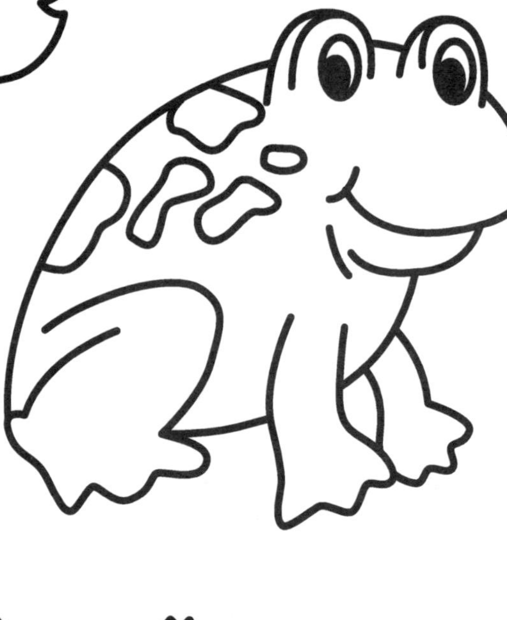

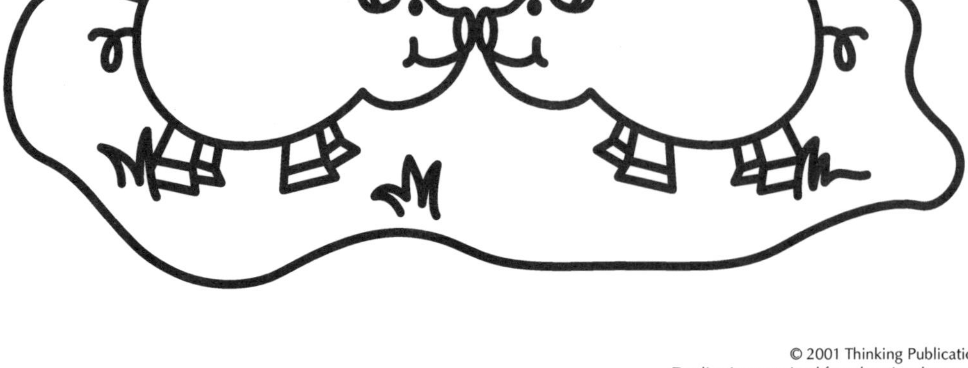

GROUCHY LADYBUG

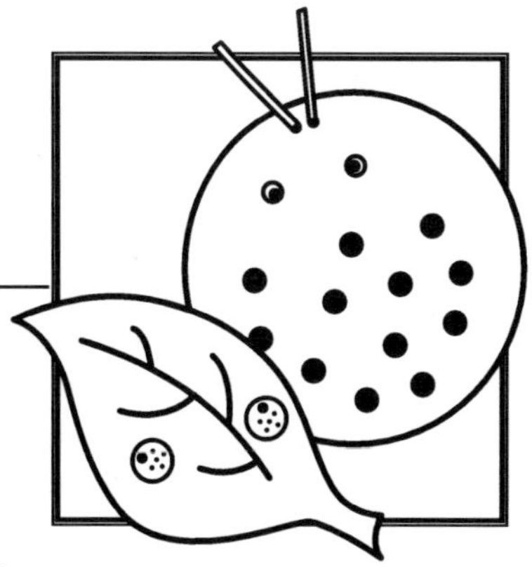

MATERIALS

Ladybug

- 12 black dot stickers
- 6" or 8" red plastic or paper plate
- Glue
- 2 google eyes
- Single hole punch
- Piece of pipe cleaner

Leaves

- Scissors
- Crayons or markers
- 12 red dot stickers
- Black marker or crayon

DIRECTIONS

Ladybug

1. Stick the 12 black dots on the plate.
2. Glue the google eyes on the plate.
3. Punch 2 holes close together above the google eyes.
4. Loop the pipe cleaner through the holes and twist. Curl the ends of the pipe cleaner to resemble antennae.
5. Have the model ladybug ready for use in the activity.

Leaves

1. Photocopy one sheet of the *Leaf Pattern* on page 286. Enlarge or reduce the pattern as necessary.
2. Cut out the leaves and color each using crayons or markers.
3. Draw spots on the 12 red dot stickers (ladybugs) with a black marker or crayon.
4. Stick the ladybugs on the leaves.
5. Have model leaves and photocopies of leaves (1 sheet per child) ready for use in the activity.

LEAF PATTERN

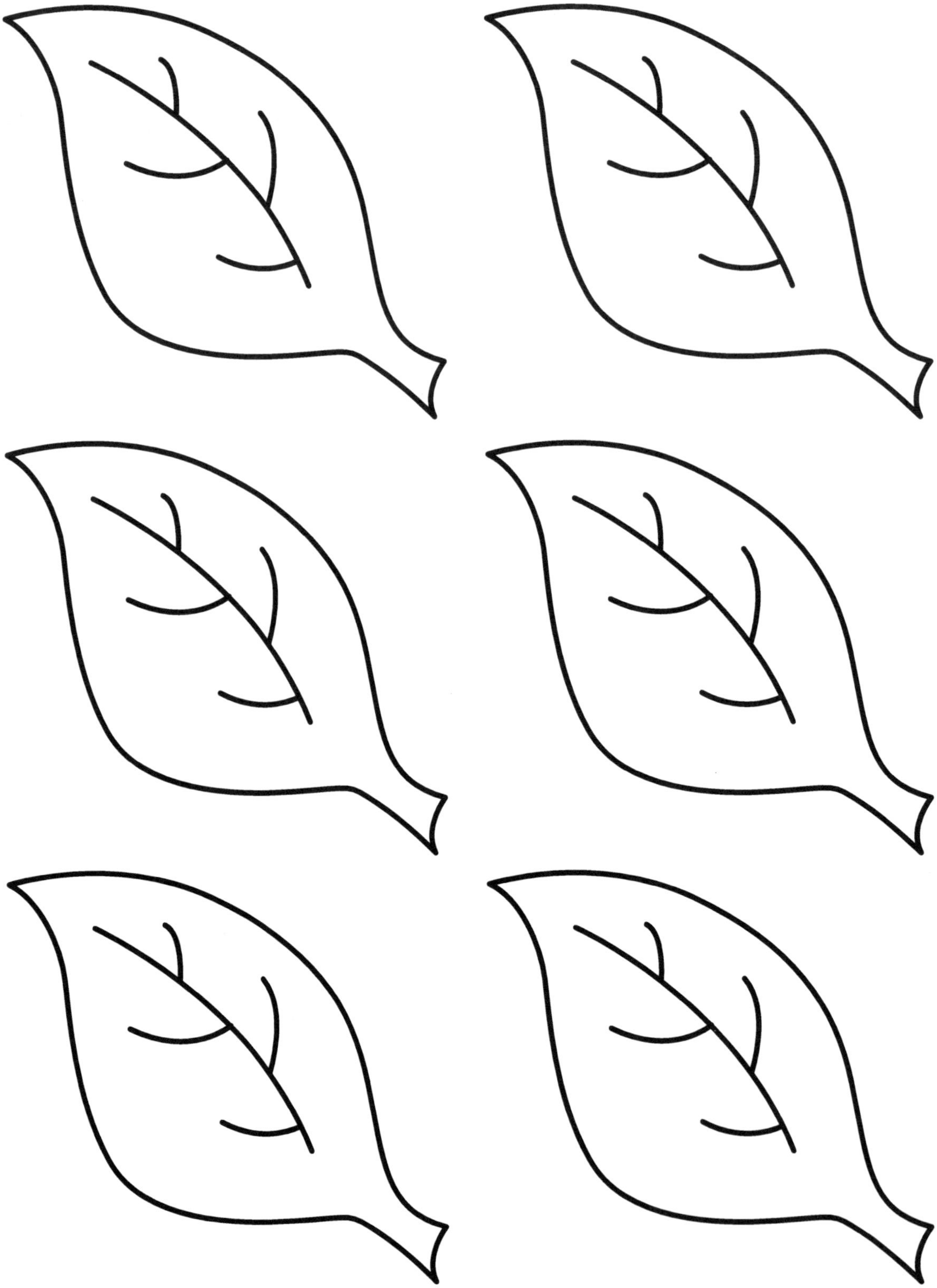

RAINBOW FISH

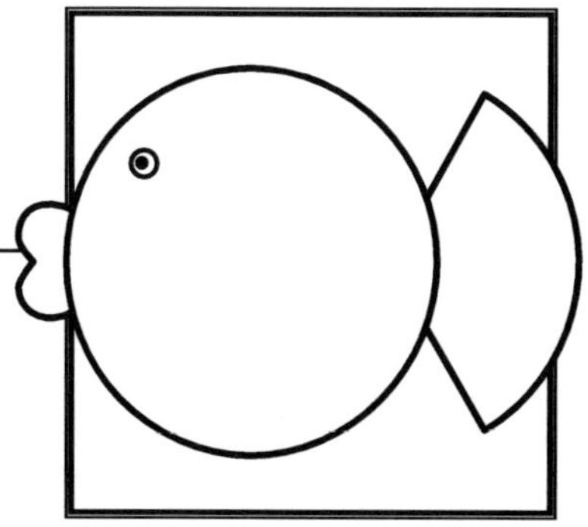

MATERIALS

- Scissors
- Construction paper
- Stapler
- One-third of a paper plate (triangle shape to function as fish tail)
- 6" or 8" round paper plate
- Aluminum foil
- Glue
- Decorations (beads, glitter, etc.)

DIRECTIONS

1. Cut a small heart shape (approximately 2" × 2") out of the construction paper.
2. Staple the one-third of a paper plate (i.e., fish tail) and the heart shape (i.e., fish lips) to the paper plate (i.e., fish body).
3. Cover the fish body and tail with aluminum foil; fold around the edges and glue onto the back side of the fish.
4. Add beads or glitter for scales and other decorations as desired.
5. Have the model Rainbow Fish and Rainbow Fish bodies (see #1–2 above; 1 per child) ready for use in the activity.

FISHING PROJECT

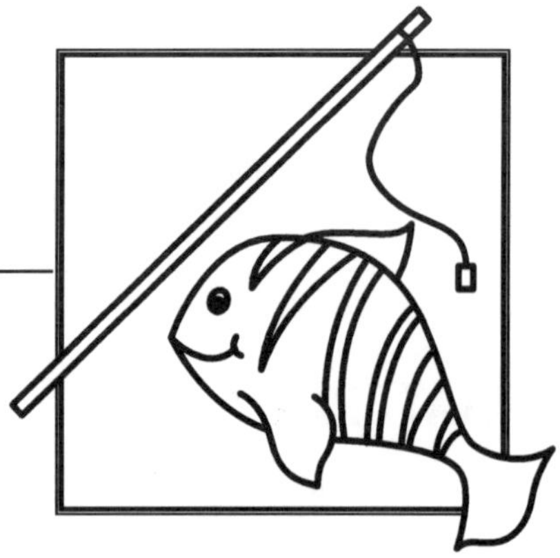

MATERIALS

Fishing Pole

- 3' piece of yarn
- Yard stick or 3' piece of wood (e.g., dowel)
- Tape
- Small magnet

Fish

- Scissors
- Decorations (beads, glitter, etc.)
- Metal paper clips

DIRECTIONS

Fishing Pole

1. Tie the yarn to the end of the yard stick or piece of wood.
2. Tape the small magnet to the end of the yarn to serve as the "hook."

Fish

1. Photocopy the *Fish Patterns* on page 289. Photocopy as many fish as needed. Enlarge or reduce the patterns as necessary.
2. Cut out the fish and decorate if desired.
3. Hook a paper clip into each fish.

FISH PATTERNS

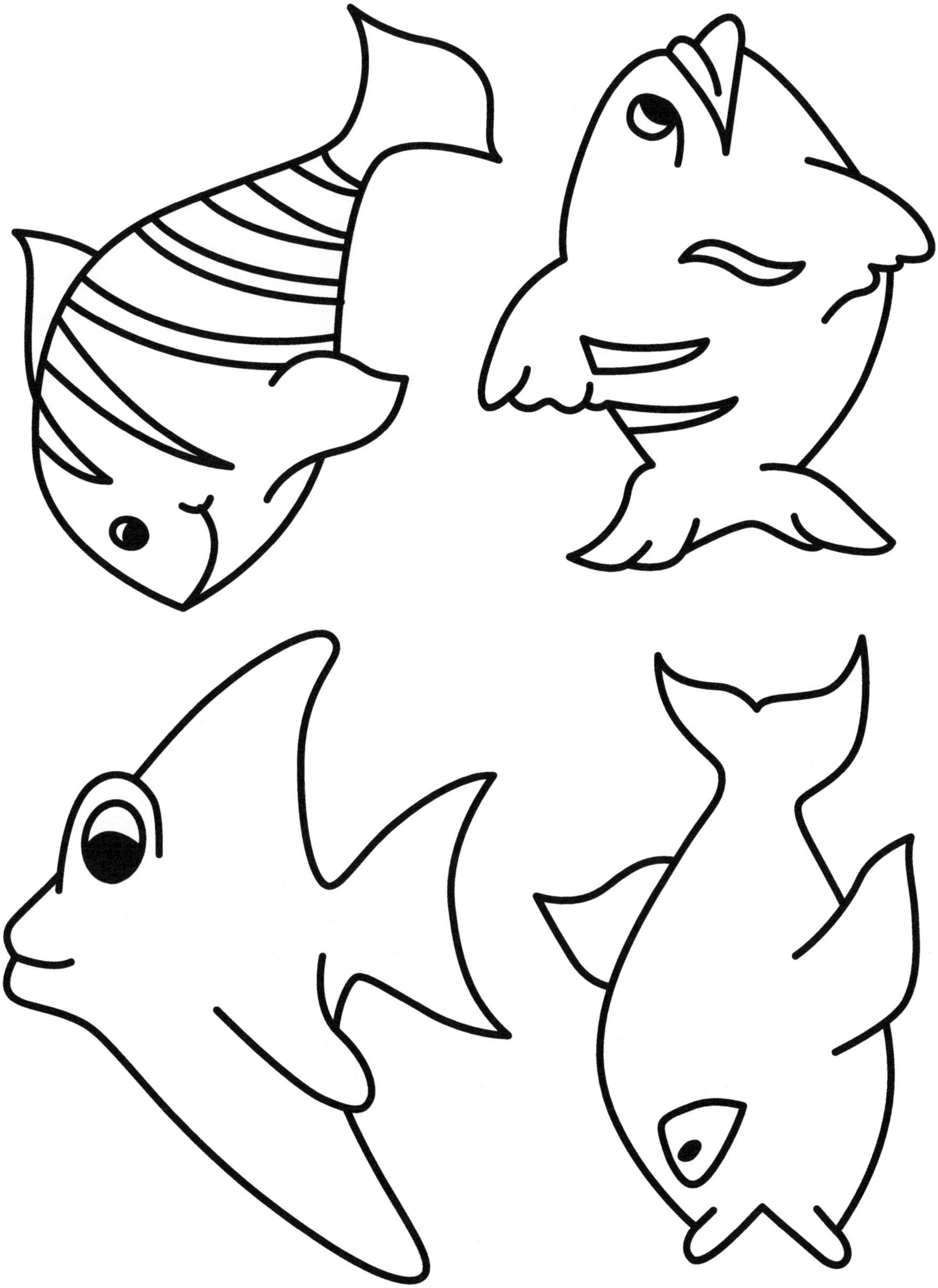

CAT EARS AND NOSES

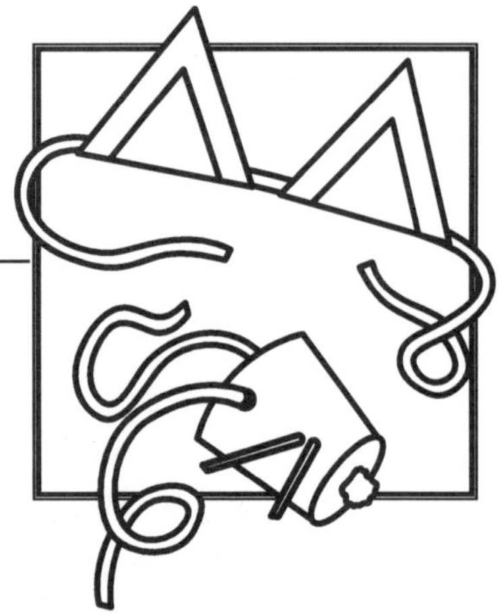

MATERIALS

Ears

- Scissors
- Felt in 2 contrasting colors
- Glue
- 24" piece of yarn

Noses

- Single hole punch
- Styrofoam cup
- 2, 12" pieces of yarn
- Pompon
- 4, 3" pipe cleaners

DIRECTIONS

Ears

1. Cut 2 small triangles (inner ears; approximately 2½" × 2½") and 2 large triangles (outer ears; approximately 4" × 4") out of felt. (Use one color for inner ears and the other for outer ears.)
2. Glue the inner ears in the middle of the outer ears.
3. Glue the ears, slightly spaced, onto the middle of the yarn. (Children will wear the ears as a "headband" and tie the ends of the yarn under their chins.)
4. Have the completed ears, small triangles and large triangles (2 each per child), and precut 24" pieces of yarn (1 per child) ready for use in the activity.

Noses

1. Punch 2 holes on opposite sides of the cup near the top opening.
2. Tie one 12" piece of yarn through each hole. (Children will tie the yarn around their head to secure the nose.)
3. Glue a pompon on the front of the cup (i.e., the bottom part of the cup).
4. Stick 2 pipe cleaners through each side of the cup for whiskers.
5. Have the completed nose, precut 12" pieces of yarn (2 per child), and precut 3" pipe cleaners (4 per child) ready for use in the activity.

COOKIES AND MILK CARTON MOUSE

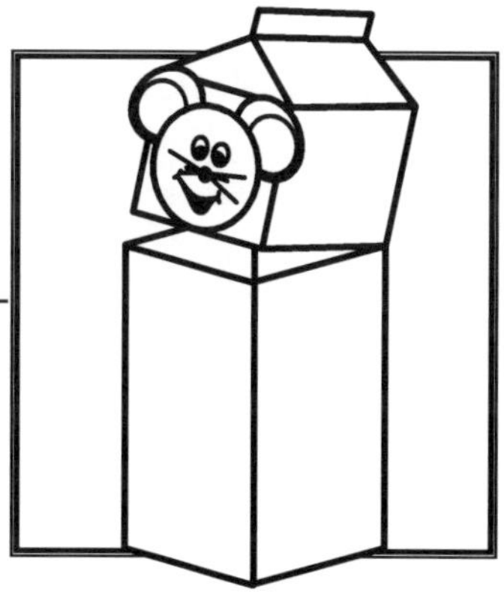

MATERIALS

Cookies

- Scissors
- Paper

Milk Carton Mouse

- Scissors
- Half-gallon milk carton
- Wrapping paper or poster paint
- Tape (if using wrapping paper)
- Glue

DIRECTIONS

Cookies

1. Cut several (6 per child) circles (approximately 3" in diameter) out of the paper.
2. Cut several (18–20 per child) triangles, squares, etc. (approximately ½" × ½") out of the paper.
3. Have cookies and shapes ready for use in the activity.

Milk Carton Mouse

1. Cut 3 sides of the milk carton as shown above.
2. Use the wrapping paper or the poster paint to cover the outside of the milk carton.
3. Photocopy the *Mouse Face Pattern* on page 292.
4. Cut out the mouse face and glue it on the top part of the milk carton.
5. Have the milk carton mouse ready for use in the activity.

MOUSE FACE PATTERN

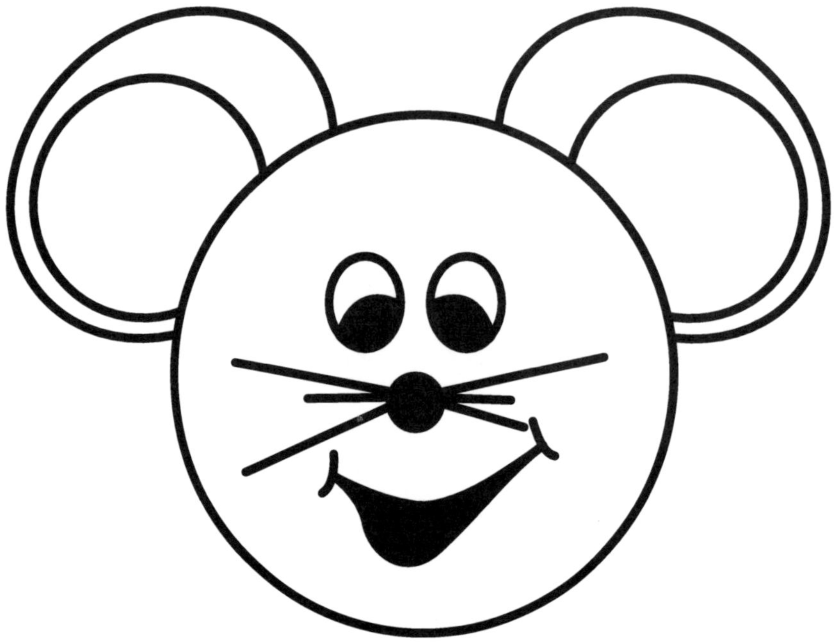

IF YOU GIVE A MOUSE A COOKIE FELT STORY

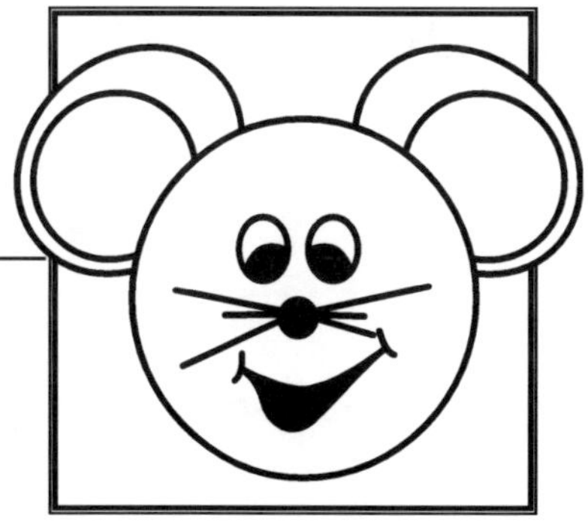

MATERIALS

Mouse and Story

- Pencil or pen
- Felt in a variety of colors
- Scissors
- Glue
- Markers (optional)

DIRECTIONS

Mouse

1. Photocopy the *Mouse Patterns* on page 294 to use as templates. Enlarge or reduce the patterns as necessary.
2. Trace the mouse templates on the felt and cut out.
3. Glue the mouse together.
4. Add detail lines (e.g., eyes and shirt stripes) to the mouse if desired.
5. Have the model mouse and sets of mouse cutouts (1 per child) ready for use in the activity.

Story

1. Photocopy the *Story Patterns* on pages 295–296 to use as templates.
2. Trace the story templates on the felt and cut out.
3. Add detail lines to the story cutouts if desired.
4. Have 1 set of story cutouts ready for use in the activity.

MOUSE PATTERNS

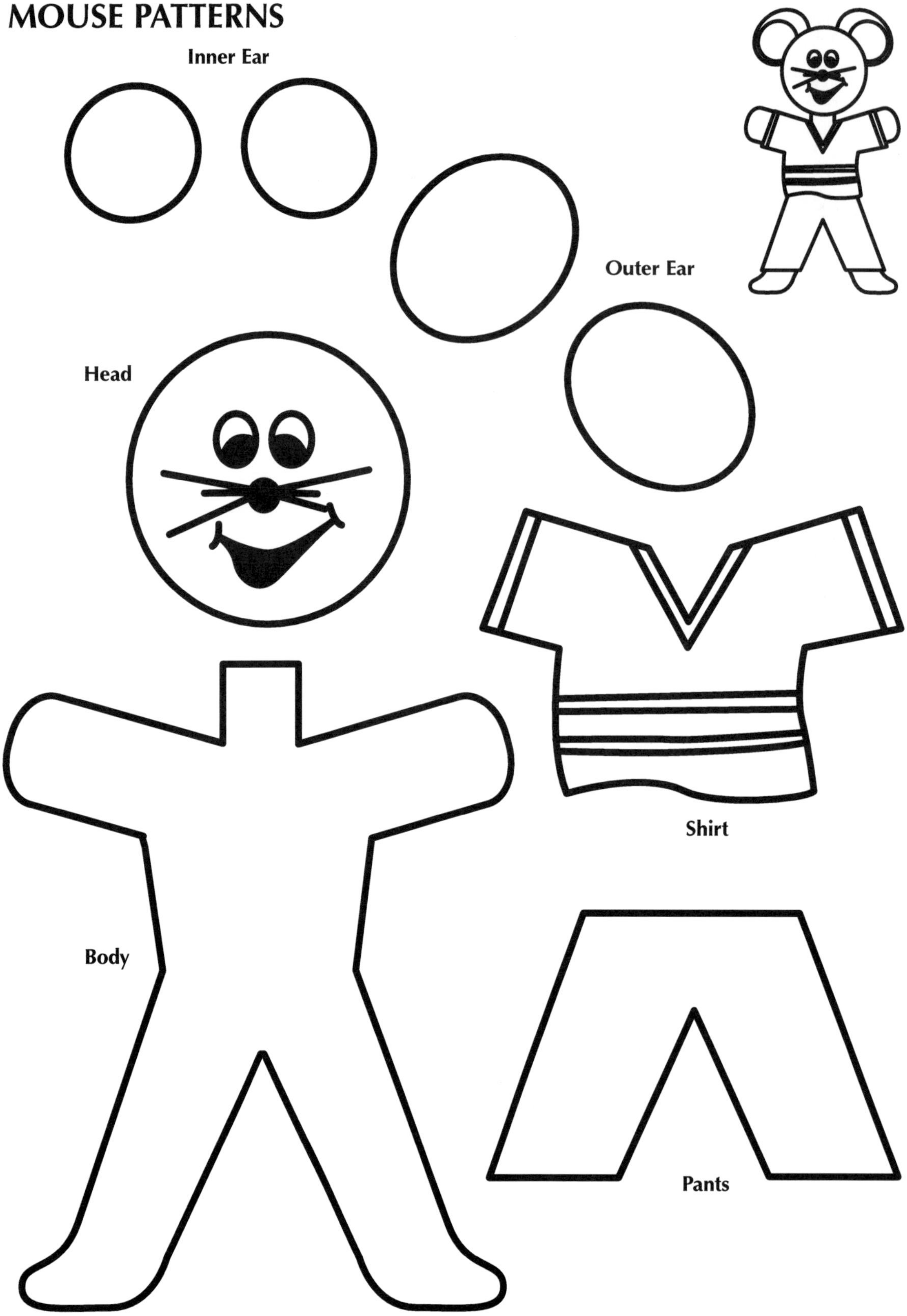

STORY PATTERNS

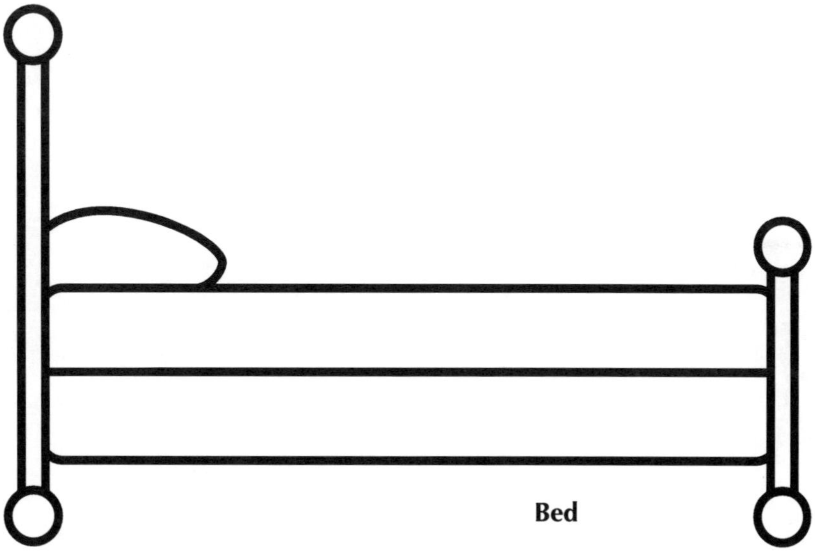

Bed

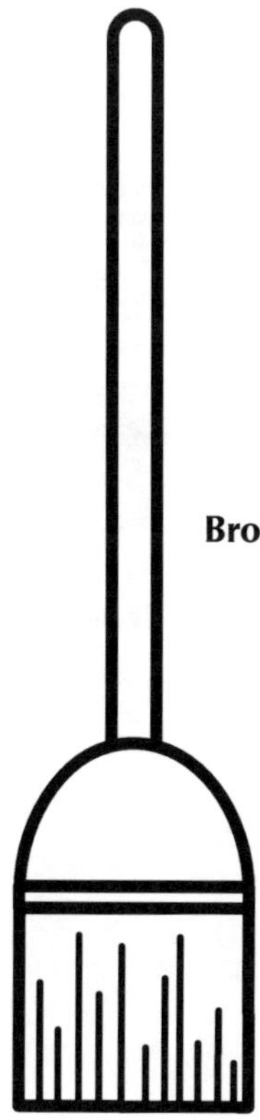

Broom

Book

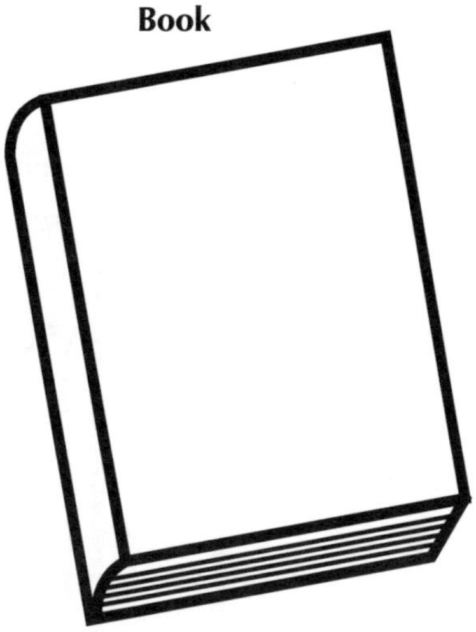

Napkin

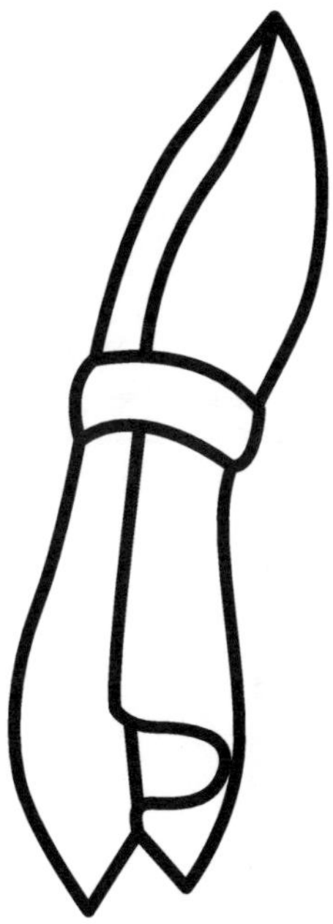

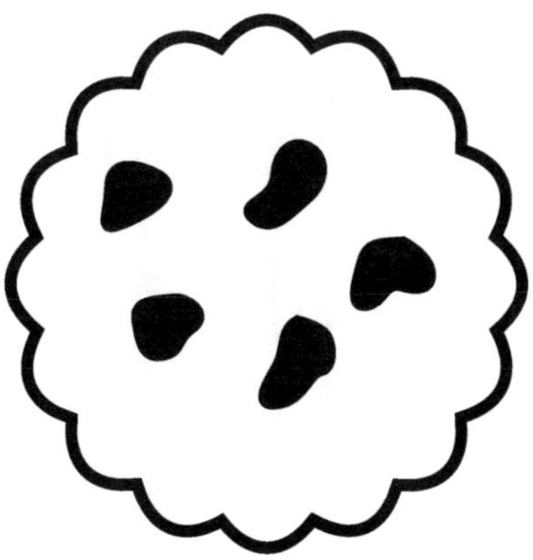

Cookie

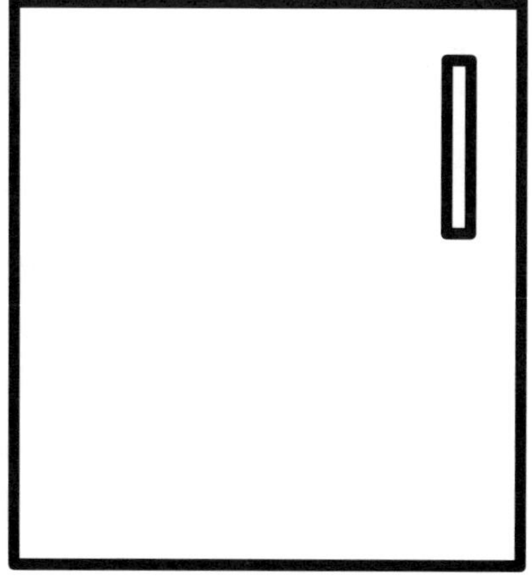

Refrigerator

STORY PATTERNS

Paper

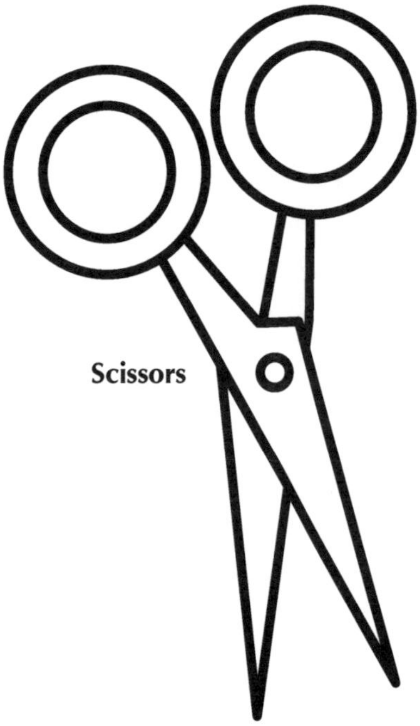

Scissors

Pencil

Straw

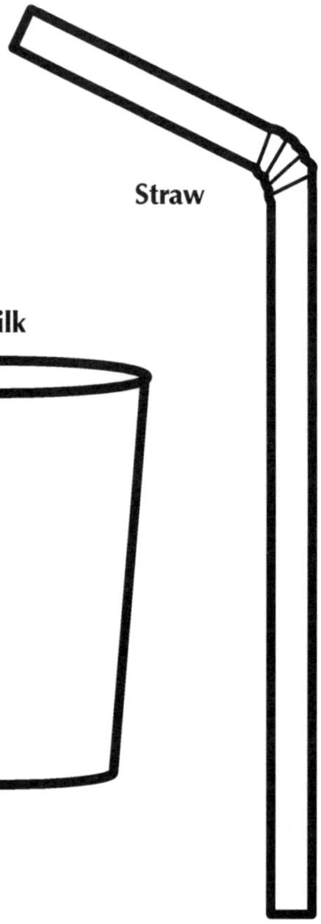

Mirror

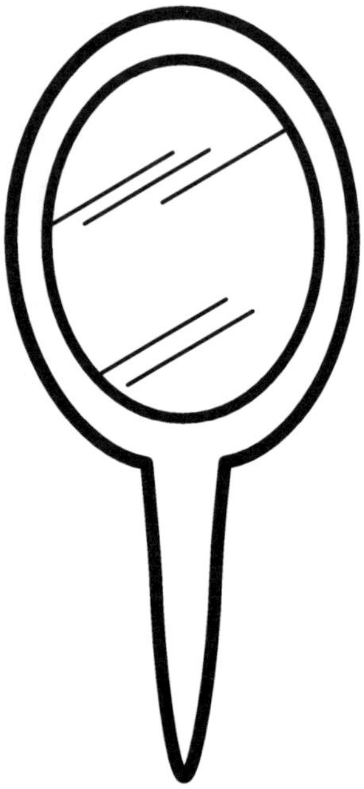

Milk

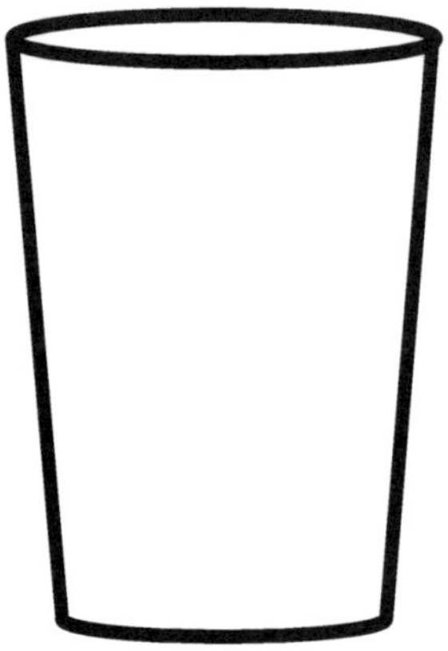

THE VERY HUNGRY CATERPILLAR SOCK PUPPET AND FOOD

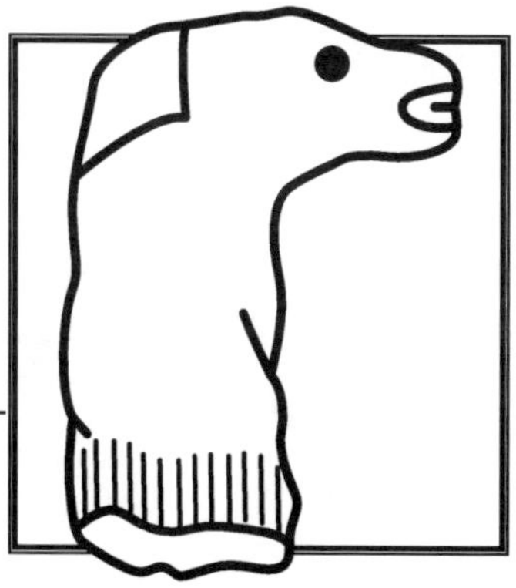

MATERIALS

Sock Puppet

- Scissors
- Red felt
- Light-colored adult-sized sock
- Glue
- Piece of pipe cleaner
- Decorations (beads, buttons, etc.)

Food

- Felt or construction paper in a variety of colors
- Pen or pencil
- Scissors

DIRECTIONS

Sock Puppet

1. Cut an oval shape (approximately 3" × 2") out of the red felt. This will be the caterpillar's mouth.
2. Glue the caterpillar mouth onto the toe part of sock.
3. Make 2 small holes in the sock and put the pipe cleaner through the sock for the antennae. Twist the ends to look like antennae.
4. Glue decorations on the caterpillar.
5. Have the completed caterpillar and oval shapes (1 per child) ready for use in the activity.

Food

1. Photocopy the *Food Patterns* on pages 298–299.
2. For felt food, trace the *Food Patterns* on the felt and cut them out. For construction paper food, cut out the *Food Patterns.*
3. Add detail lines (e.g., seeds) to the felt food if desired.
4. Have sets of food cutouts (1 per child) ready for use in the activity.

FOOD PATTERNS

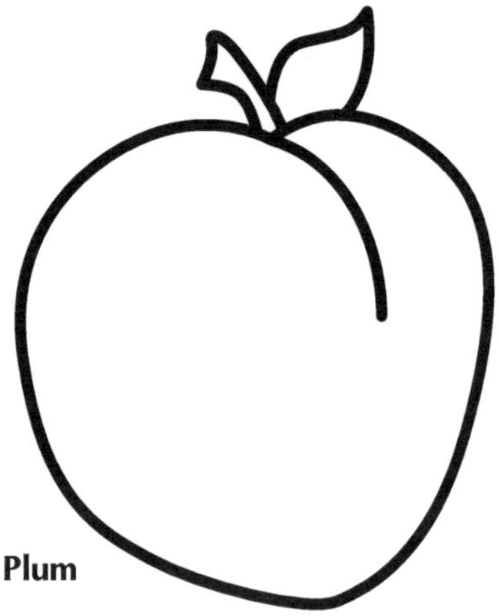

Plum

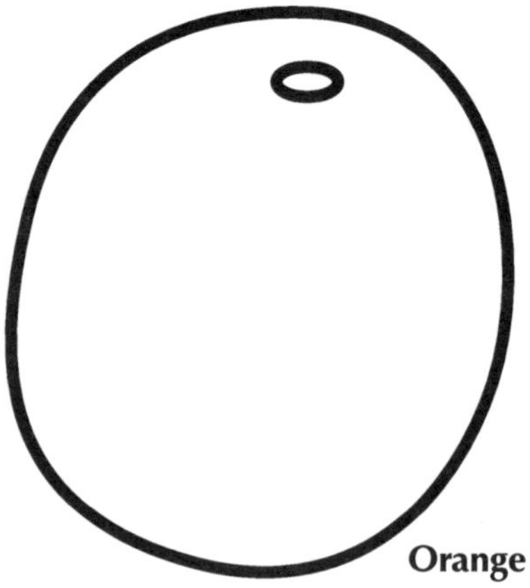

Orange

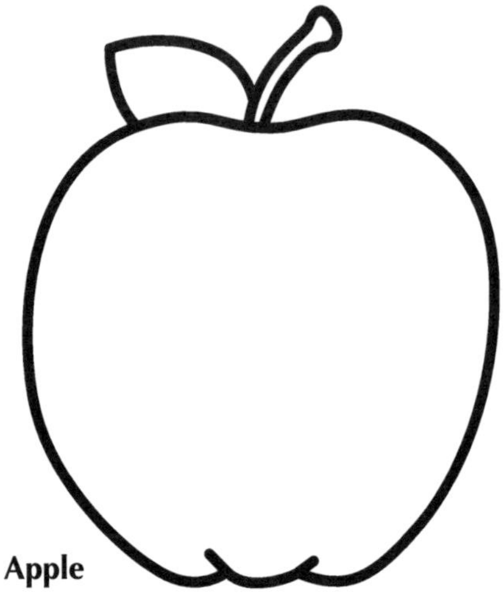

Apple

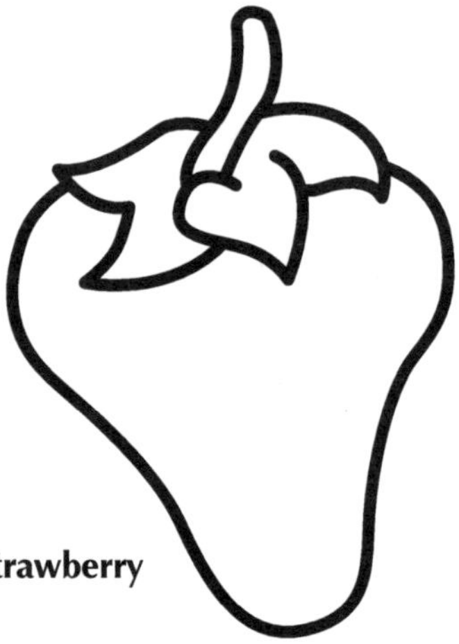

Strawberry

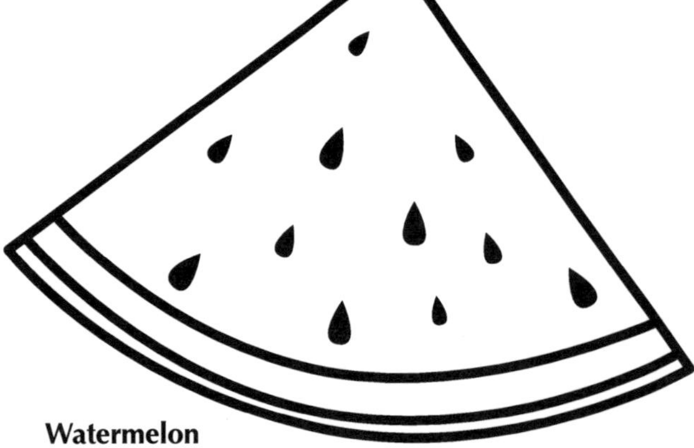

Watermelon

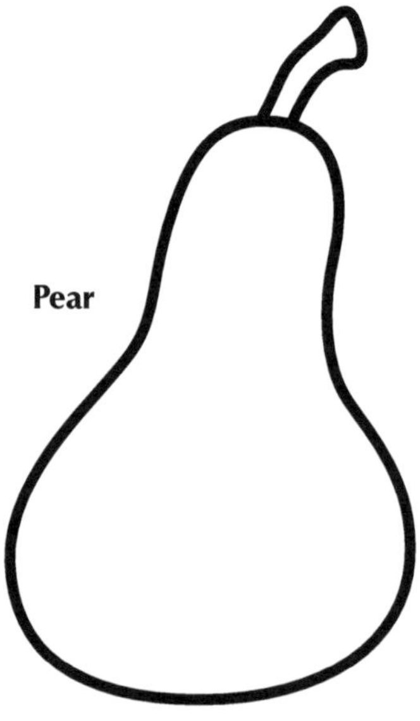

Pear

FOOD PATTERNS

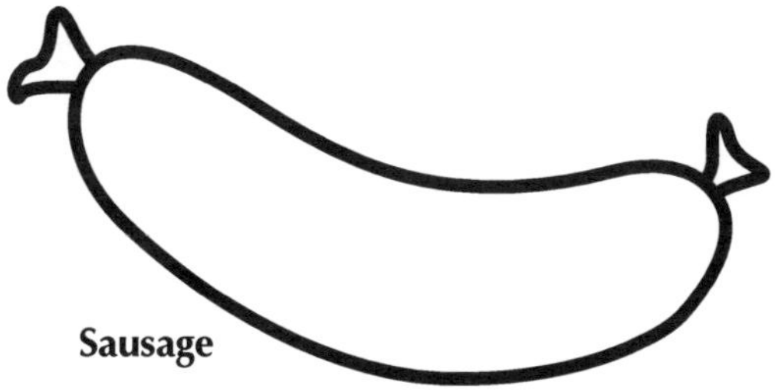

Sausage

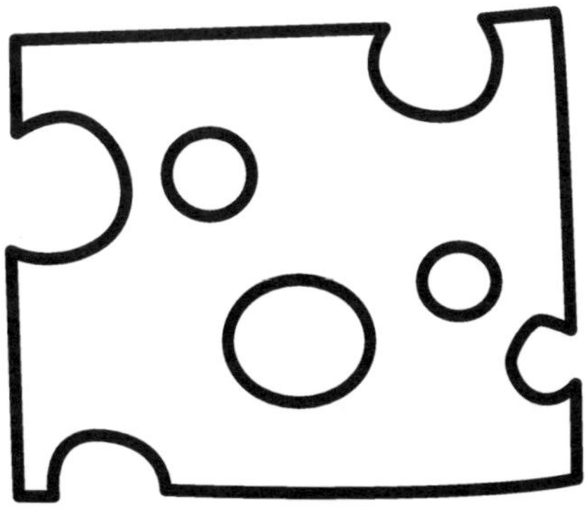

Cheese

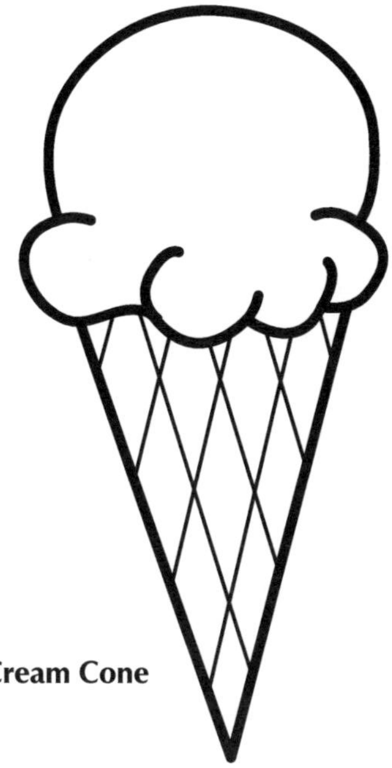

Ice-Cream Cone

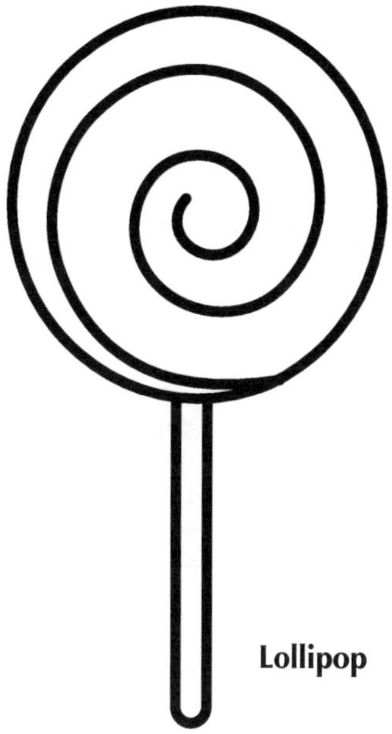

Lollipop

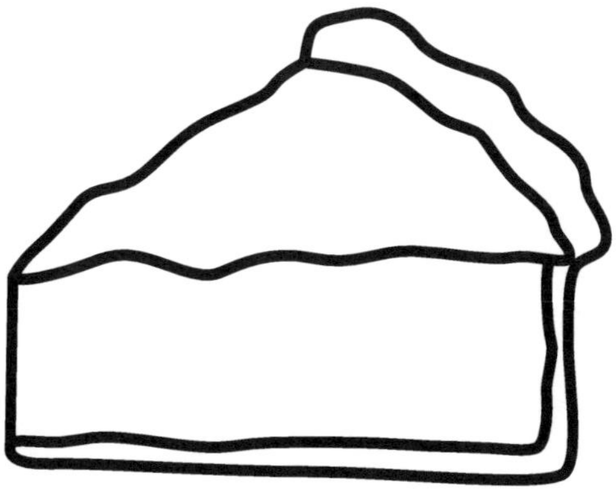

Pie

Muffin

OLD LADY JAR AND FOOD

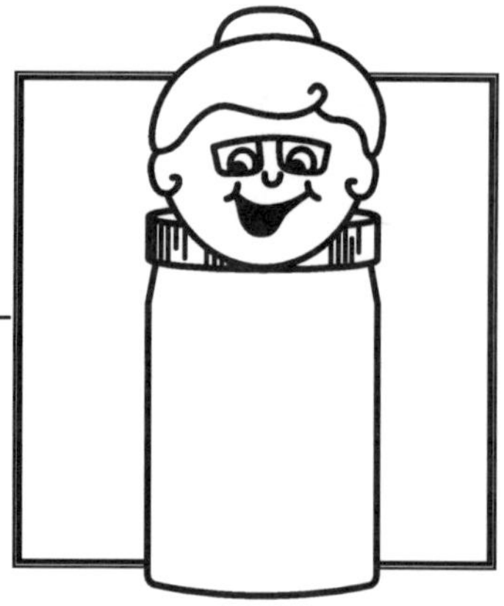

MATERIALS

Jar

- Crayons or markers
- Scissors
- Tape
- Glass jar (12–16 oz.)

Food

- Scissors

DIRECTIONS

Jar

1. Photocopy the *Old Lady Head Pattern* on page 301.
2. Cut out the *Old Lady Head* and color it.
3. Tape the *Old Lady Head* on the top part of the jar.
4. Have the Old Lady Jar ready for use in the activity.

Food

1. Make photocopies of the *Old Lady Food Patterns* on page 302.
2. Cut out the food pieces (1 set) and have them ready for use in the activity.

OLD LADY HEAD PATTERN

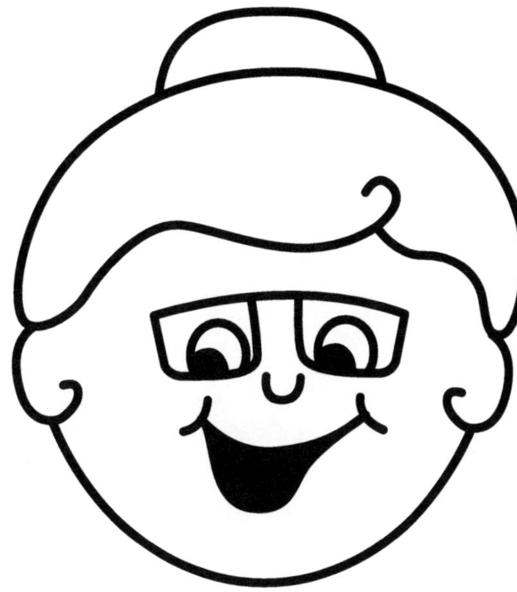

OLD LADY FOOD PATTERNS

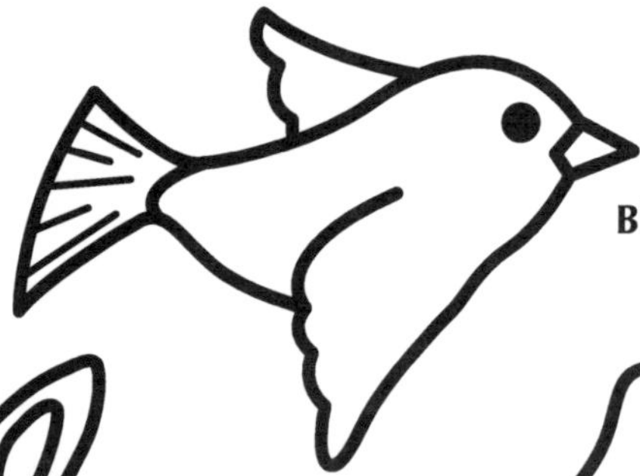

Bird

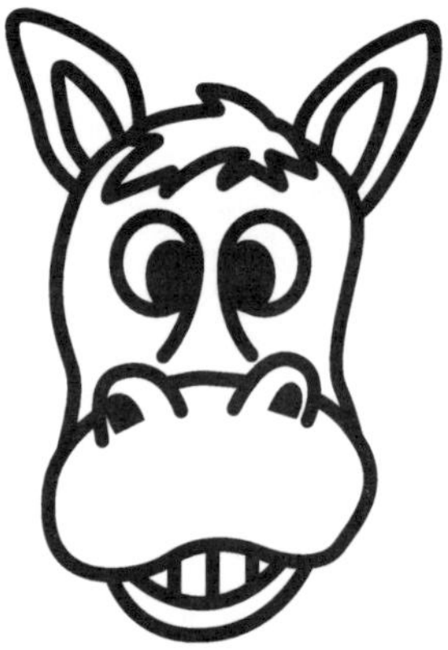

Horse

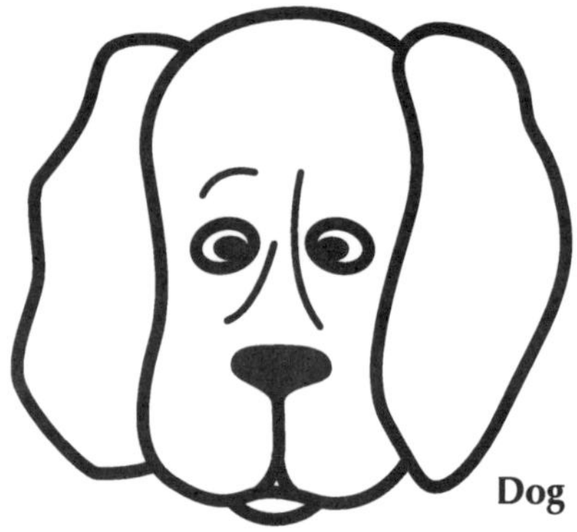

Dog

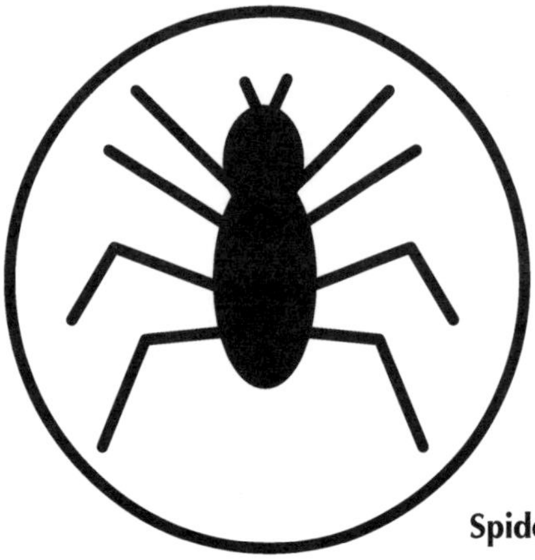

Spider

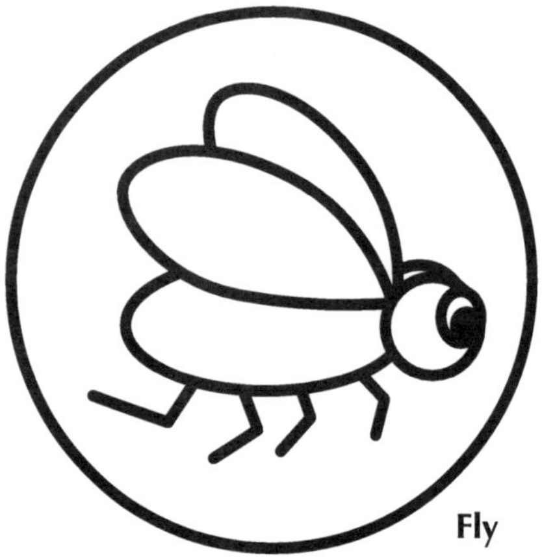

Fly

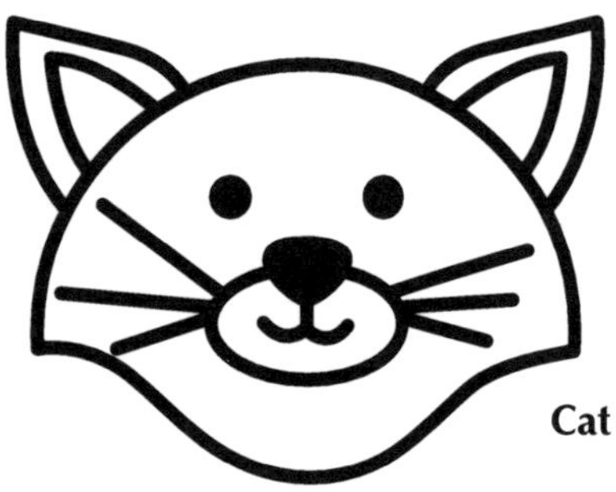

Cat

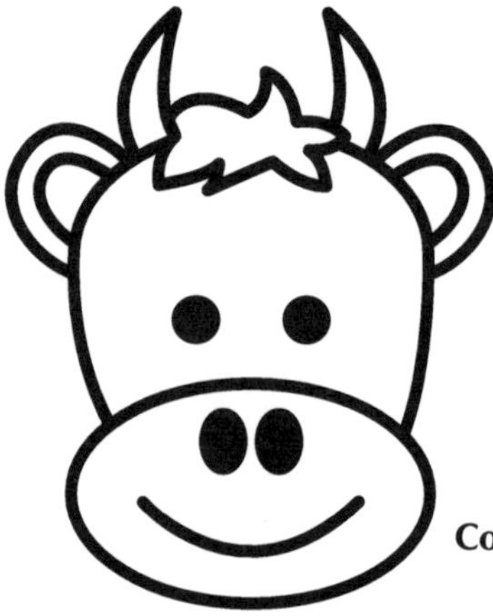

Cow

OLD LADY PLATE

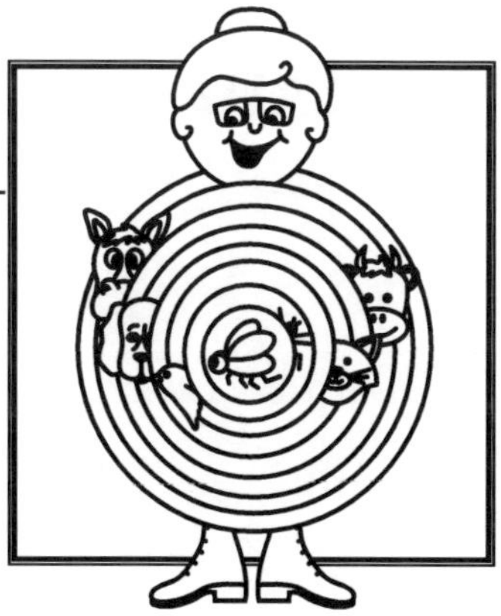

MATERIALS

- Scissors
- Glue
- 6" round paper plate
- Markers or crayons

DIRECTIONS

1. Photocopy the *Old Lady Plate Patterns* on page 304.
2. Cut out the patterns.
3. Glue the head on the top of the plate and the feet on the bottom.
4. Photocopy the *Old Lady Animal Patterns* on pages 305–308.
5. Cut out the patterns and color each animal's head (and, if desired, the circles).
6. Glue the animals on the Old Lady plate in the following order:
   Horse
   Cow
   Dog
   Cat
   Bird
   Spider
   Fly
7. Have the model Old Lady plate, plates with the *Old Lady Patterns* attached (1 per child), and sets of animal cutouts (1 per child) ready for use in the activity.

OLD LADY PLATE PATTERNS

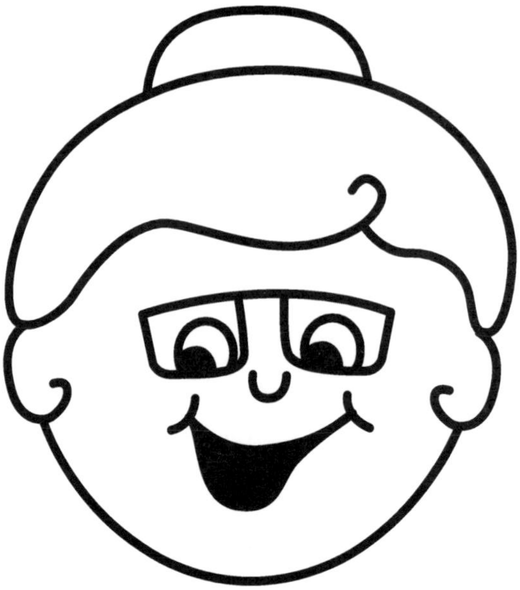

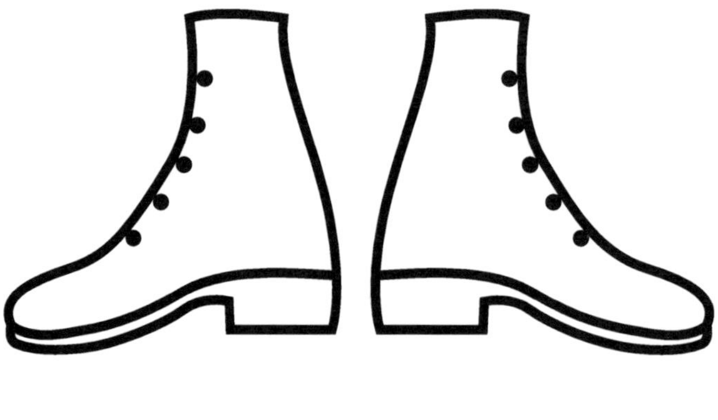

OLD LADY ANIMAL PATTERNS

Horse

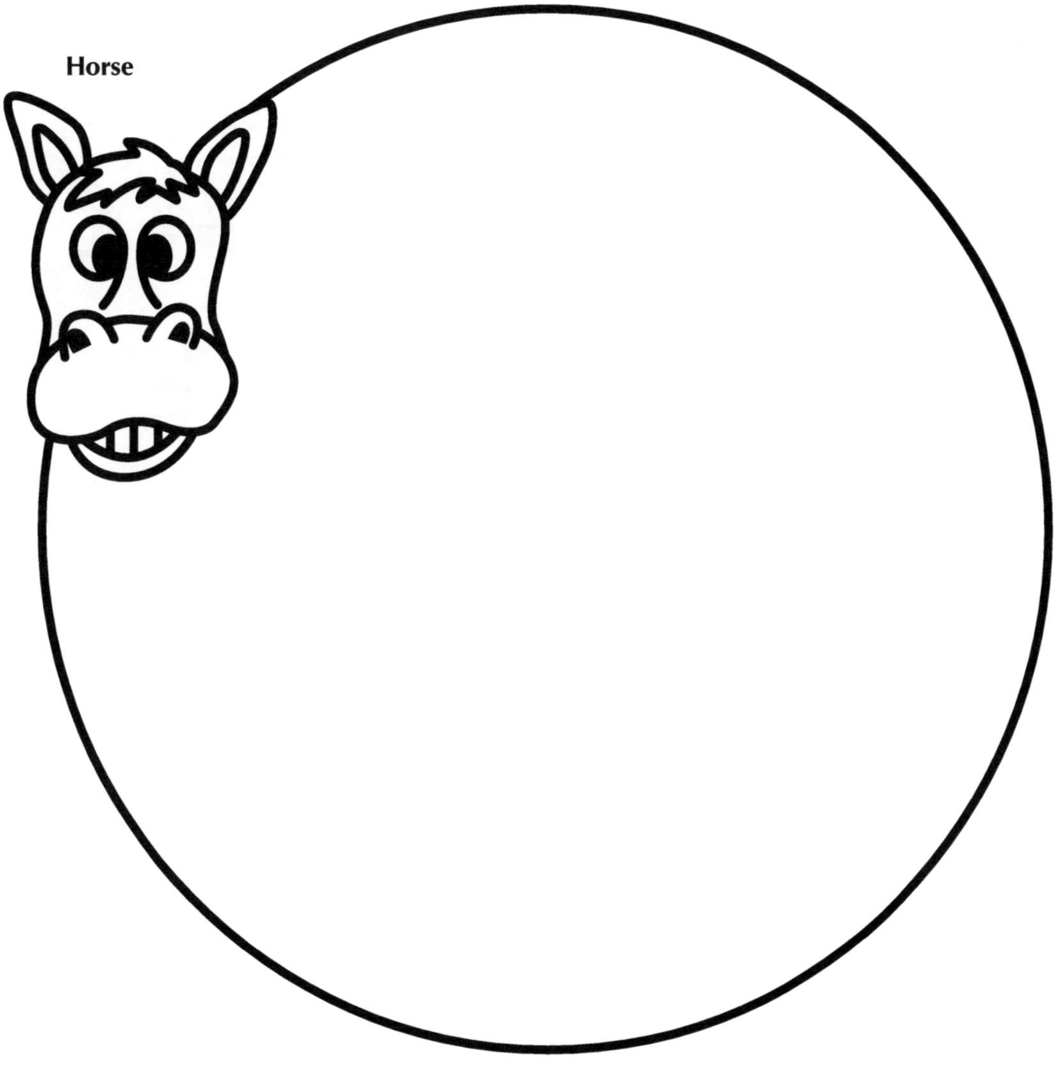

OLD LADY ANIMAL PATTERNS

Cow

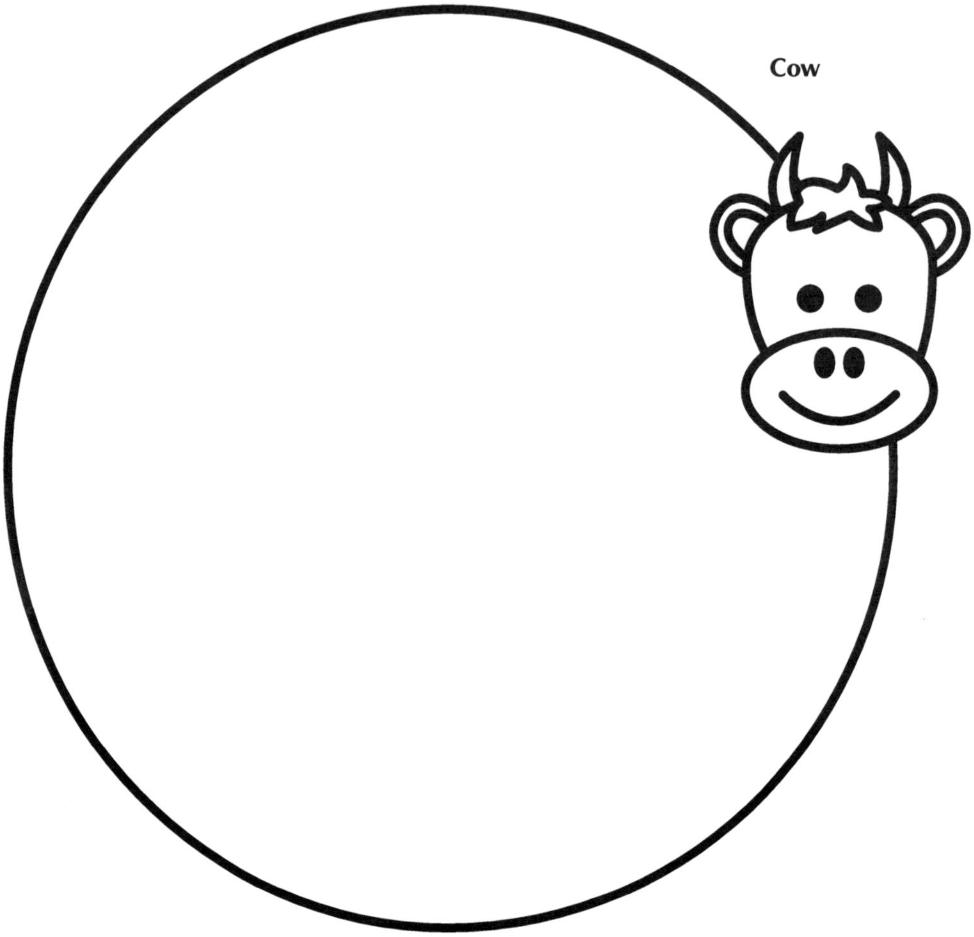

OLD LADY ANIMAL PATTERNS

Cat

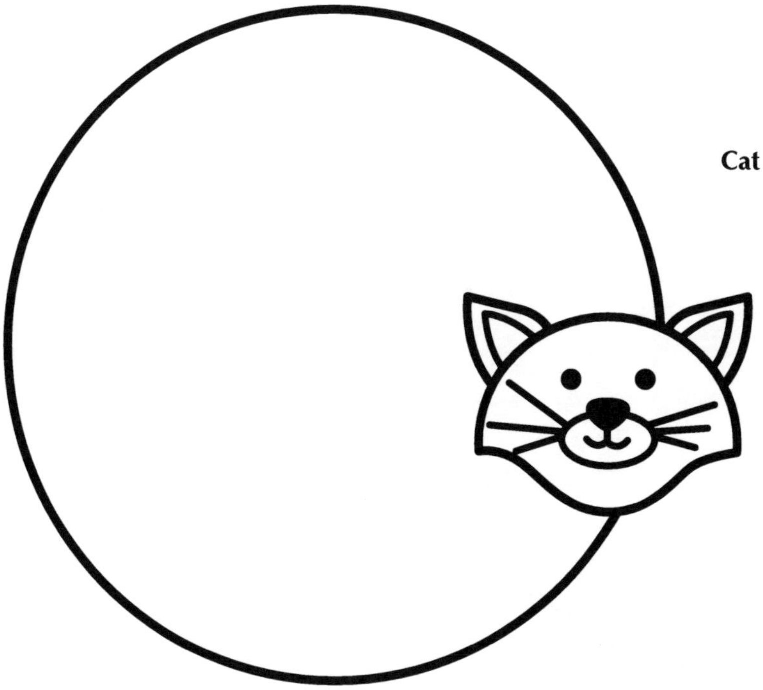

Dog

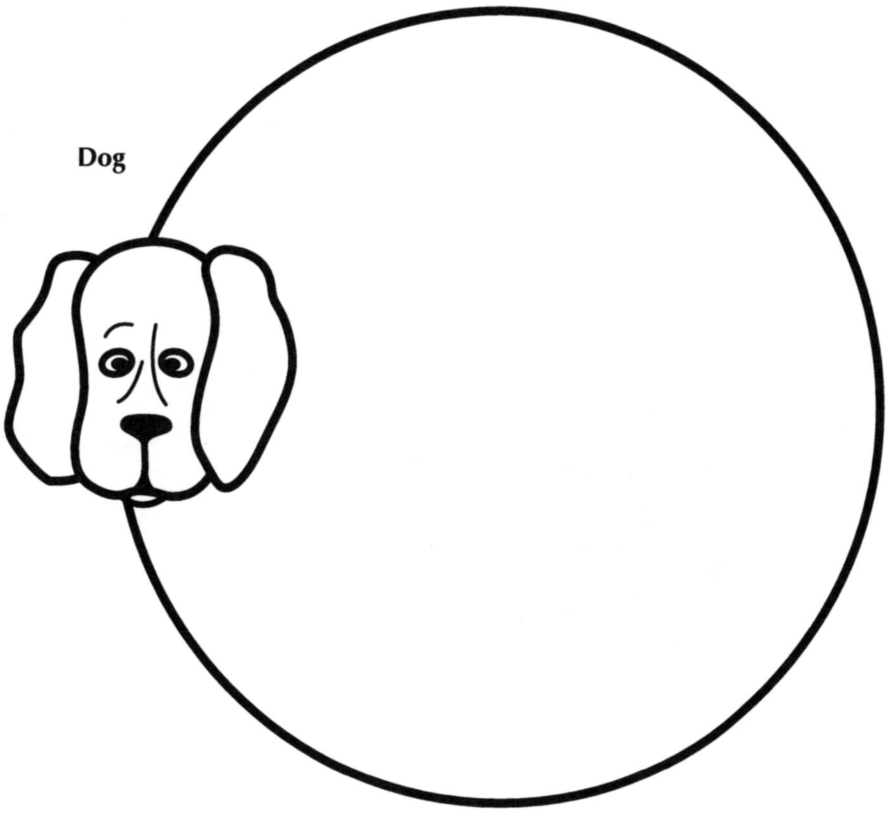

OLD LADY ANIMAL PATTERNS

Bird

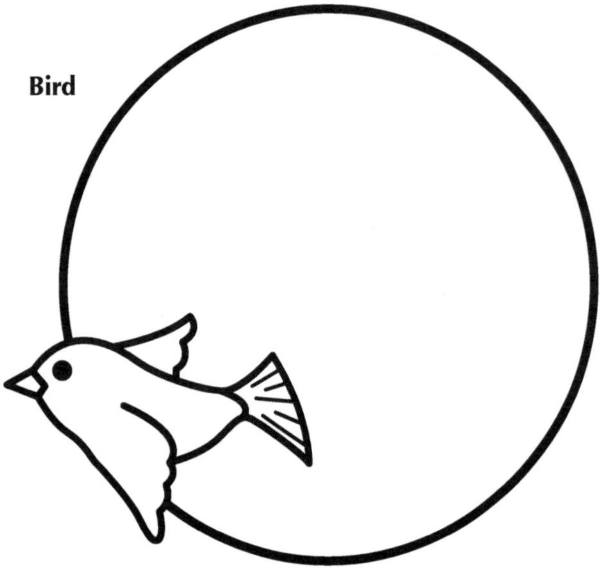

Spider

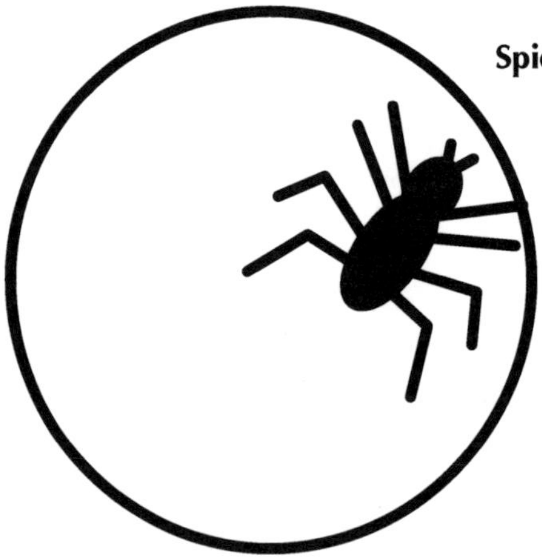

Fly

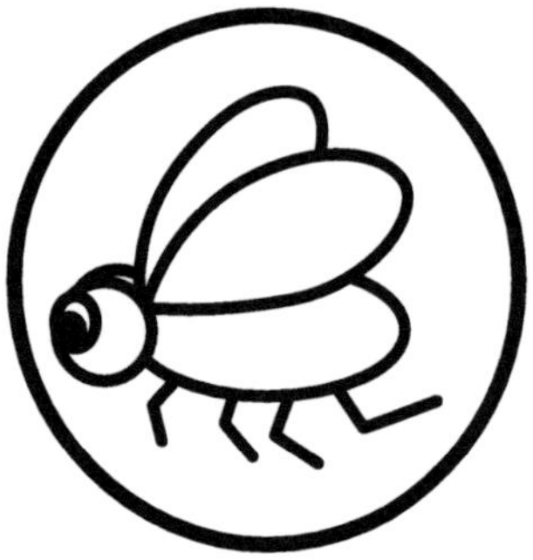

GINGERBREAD PERSON STICK PUPPET

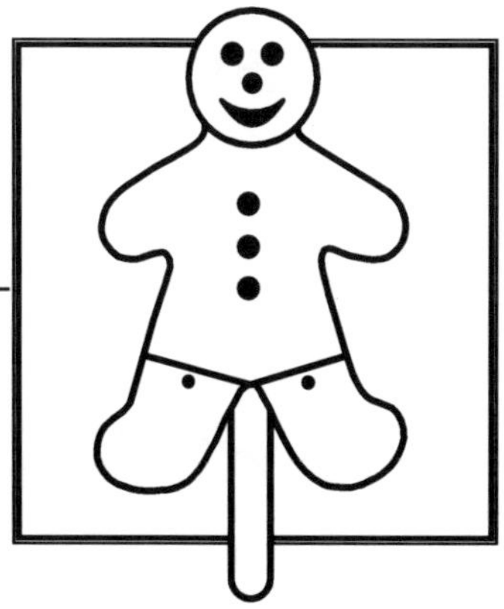

MATERIALS

- Scissors
- Glue
- Single hole punch
- 2 brass fasteners
- 2 google eyes
- Craft stick

DIRECTIONS

1. Photocopy the *Gingerbread Person Patterns* on page 310. Enlarge or reduce the patterns as necessary.
2. Cut out the patterns.
3. Glue the head and body of the gingerbread person together.
4. Punch 1 hole in the top of each leg and 2 holes, slightly spaced, at the bottom of the body.
5. Insert the brass fasteners in the holes in the legs and attach the legs.
6. Glue the facial features on the face and the buttons on the body.
7. Glue the gingerbread person onto the craft stick.
8. Have the model gingerbread person stick puppet and sets of gingerbread person cutouts (1 per child) ready for use in the activity.

GINGERBREAD PERSON PATTERNS

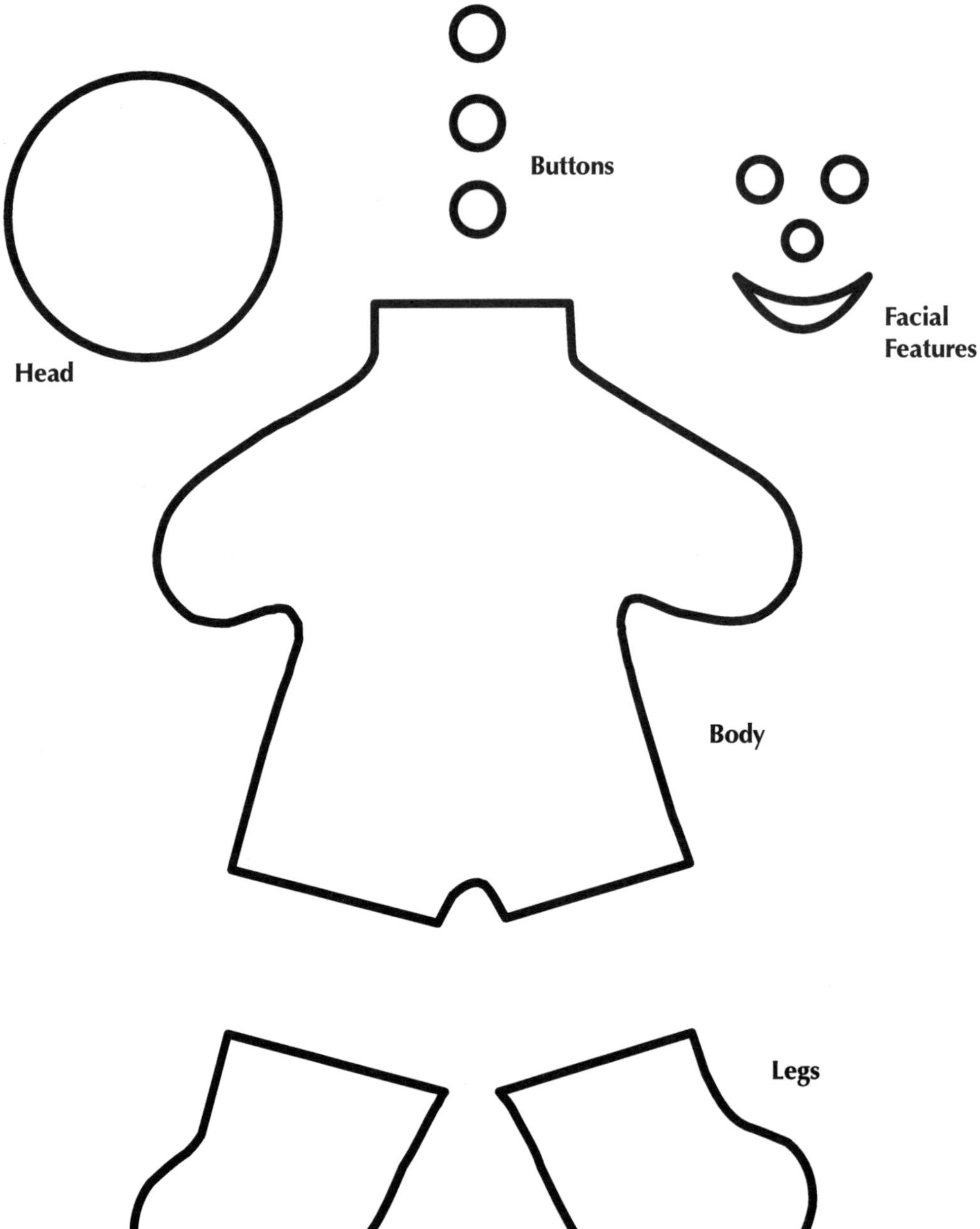

LANGUAGE INTERVENTION PLANNING WORKSHEET

Session type (check one): ☐ Individual ☐ Group

Date(s): ____________________

Child(ren): ____________________

Target for the week: ____________________

Level of support (check one): ☐ Forced choice ☐ Cloze task ☐ Preparatory set

Materials I already have:	**Materials I need to obtain:**
____________	____________
____________	____________
____________	____________
____________	____________
____________	____________

Pretreatment checklist:

- Organized scripts ☐
- Obtained book ☐
- Obtained supplemental book(s) (optional) ☐
- Obtained materials ☐
- Sent family letters ☐
- Prepared data sheets ☐

Notes from previous session/considerations for upcoming sessions:

____

____

____

____

DATA SHEET

Case History:

Date: ______________________

Child: ______________________ **School:** ______________________

Educator: ______________________ **Cycle:** __________ **Week:** __________

Type of session (check one): ☐ Group ☐ Individual

Target (check one):

☐ R3S ☐ IR past tense ☐ R past tense
☐ Copula *be* ☐ R Plurals ☐ Possessives
☐ Pronouns ☐ Auxiliary *be* ☐ Other _______

FOCUSED STIMULATION

Observed child productions of target morpheme(s) (+/-) if they occurred

(If preferred, write in the actual child productions in addition to using +/-)

% correct= __________ (/)

ELICITED PRODUCTION

Level of support (check one): ☐ Forced choice ☐ Cloze task ☐ Preparatory set

Observed child productions of target morpheme(s) (+/-)

% correct= __________ (/)

EXAMPLE COMPLETED DATA SHEET

Case History: Jane is a 4-year, 3-month-old female who has severe morphological deficits (she uses the following morphemes with less than 30% accuracy, as measured on a spontaneous language sample: copula *be*, regular past tense *-ed*, regular third person singular *-s*, and regular plural *-s*). She receives language intervention two times per week, once in an individual session and once in a group session. Her educator records her progress by keeping track of her morphological uses during her individual session in order to keep track of the level of support needed. The following data sheet was used to record Jane's performance during her individual session in Cycle 2, week 2, at which time the regular past tense morpheme was being targeted.

Date: 7/7/2000

Child: Jane Johnson **School:** Anywhere Preschool

Educator: Lilly Language **Cycle:** 2 **Week:** 2

Type of session (check one): ☐ Group ☑ Individual

Target (check one):
☐ R3S ☐ IR past tense (ran) ☑ R past tense
☐ Copula *be* ☐ R Plurals ☐ Possessives
☐ Pronouns ☐ Auxiliary *be* ☐ Other _______

FOCUSED STIMULATION

Observed child productions of target morpheme(s) (+/-) if they occurred

+jumped	–walk								
–jump	+walked								

(As illustrated, the educator may choose to write in the actual child productions in addition to using +/-)

% correct= 50% (10 / 20)

ELICITED PRODUCTION

Level of support (check one): ☐ Forced choice ☑ Cloze task ☐ Preparatory set

Observed child productions of target morpheme(s) (+/-)

+stepped	+stirred	+walked	+colored	+glued	+glued	+glued	+stapled	+glued	+colored
+colored	–stir	–stir	–stir	–stir	+glued	–staple	–glue	+colored	+colored
–rip	–rip	–stir	–walk	+glued					

% correct= 60% (15 / 25)

BIBLIOGRAPHY

Cycle 1: Water Theme

At the Beach (1987)
by Anne Rockwell and Harlow Rockwell
New York: Aladdin

Bubble Bubble (1973)
by Mercer Mayer
Mahwah, NJ: Troll

Bubble Trouble (1994)
by Mary Packard, illustrated by Elena Kucharik
New York: Scholastic

Clifford Counts Bubbles (1992)
by Norman Bridwell
New York: Scholastic

Curious George Goes to the Beach (1999)
by Margret Rey and H.A. Rey
Boston: Houghton Mifflin

For Sand Castles or Seashells (1990)
by Gail Hartman, illustrated by Ellen Weiss
New York: Bradbury Press

Let's Have a Tea Party (1996)
by Emilie Barnes, illustrated by Michal Sparks and Sue Junker
Eugene, OR: Harvest House

Miss Spider's Tea Party (1994)
by David Kirk
New York: Scholastic

This Is Your Garden (1998)
by Maggie Smith
New York: Crown

The Tiny Seed (1987)
by Eric Carle
New York: Simon and Schuster

Cycle 2: Animal Theme

Brown Bear, Brown Bear, What Do You See? (1992)
by Bill Martin Jr., illustrated by Eric Carle
New York: Henry Holt

Franklin Goes to School (1995)
by Paulette Bourgeois, illustrated by Brenda Clark
New York: Scholastic

Froggy Gets Dressed (1997)
by Jonathan London, illustrated by Frank Remkiewicz
New York: Viking

The Grouchy Ladybug (1996)
by Eric Carle
New York: HarperCollins

Have You Seen My Cat? (1987)
by Eric Carle
New York: Little Simon

Mouse Creeps (1997)
by Peter Harris, illustrated by Reg Cartwright
New York: Dial Books

One Fish, Two Fish, Red Fish, Blue Fish (1988)
by Dr. Seuss
New York: Beginner Books

Polar Bear, Polar Bear, What Do You Hear? (1991)
by Bill Martin Jr., illustrated by Eric Carle
New York: Henry Holt

The Rainbow Fish (1992)
by Marcus Pfister
New York: North-South Books

Swimmy (1991)
by Leo Lionni
New York: Random House

The Tale of Tom Kitten (1994)
abridged by Marian Hoffman
Baltimore: Ottenheimer

The Very Lonely Firefly (1995)
by Eric Carle
New York: Philomel Books

The Very Quiet Cricket (1990)
by Eric Carle
New York: Philomel Books

Cycle 3: Food Theme

The Gingerbread Man (1985)
illustrated by Karen Schmidt
New York: Scholastic

Golly Gump Swallowed a Fly (1981)
by Joanna Cole, illustrated by Bari Weissman
Cleveland, OH: Parents Magazine Press

If You Give a Moose a Muffin (1991)
by Laura Joffe Numeroff, illustrated by Felicia Bond
New York: HarperCollins

If You Give a Mouse a Cookie (1985)
by Laura Joffe Numeroff, illustrated by Felicia Bond
New York: HarperCollins

If You Give a Pig a Pancake (1998)
by Laura Joffe Numeroff, illustrated by Felicia Bond
New York: HarperCollins

The Runaway Pancake (1980)
by P.C. Asbjorsen and Jorgen Moe, illustrated by Otto Svend, translated by Joan Tate
New York: Larousse

There Was an Old Lady Who Swallowed a Fly (1997)
illustrated by Pam Adams
Swindon, UK: Child's Play

The Very Hungry Caterpillar (1987)
by Eric Carle
New York: Philomel Books

What's for Lunch (1982)
by Eric Carle
New York: Philomel Books

Whiff, Sniff, Nibble, and Chew: The Gingerbread Boy Retold (1984)
by Charlotte Pomerantz, illustrated by Monica Incisa
New York: HarperCollins

REFERENCES

Adams, P. (1997). *There was an old lady who swallowed a fly.* Swindon, UK: Child's Play.

Bedore, L.M., and Leonard, L.B. (1998). Specific language impairment and grammatical morphemes: A discriminant function analysis. *Journal of Speech, Language, and Hearing Research, 41,* 1185–1192.

Brown, R. (1973). *A first language: The early stages.* Cambridge, MA: Harvard University Press.

Camarata, S., Nelson, K.E., and Camarata, M. (1994). A comparison of conversation based to imitation based procedures for training grammatical structures in specifically language impaired children. *Journal of Speech and Hearing Research, 37,* 1414–1423.

Carle, E. (1987). *The very hungry caterpillar.* New York: Philomel Books.

Carrow, E., and Woolfolk, W. (1999). Comprehensive Assessment of Spoken Language (CASL). Circle Pines, MN: American Guidance Service.

Cleave, P.L., and Fey, M.E. (1997). Two approaches to the facilitation of grammar in children with language impairments: Rationale and description. *American Journal of Speech-Language Pathology, 6,* 22–32.

Crais, E.R. (1991). Moving from "parent involvement" to family-centered services. *American Journal of Speech-Language Pathology, 1,* 5–8.

Donahue-Kilburg, G. (1992). *Family-centered early intervention for communication disorders: Prevention and treatment.* Gaithersburg, MD: Aspen.

Donahue-Kilburg, G. (1993). Family-centered approach to promoting communication wellness. *Asha, 35,* 45–62.

Fey, M., Cleave, P., Long, S., and Hughes, D. (1993). Two approaches to the facilitation of grammar in children with language impairments: An experimental evaluation. *Journal of Speech and Hearing Research, 36,* 141–154.

Goffman, L., and Leonard, J. (2000). Growth of language skills in preschool children with specific language impairment: Implications for assessment and intervention. *American Journal of Speech-Language Pathology, 9,* 151–161.

Haas, A., and Owens, R. (1985). *Preschoolers' pronoun strategies: You and me make us.* Paper presented at the American Speech-Language-Hearing Association annual convention.

Hodson, B.W., and Paden, E.P. (1983). *Targeting intelligible speech.* Austin, TX: Pro-Ed.

Hodson, B.W., and Paden, E.P. (1991). *Targeting intelligible speech* (2nd ed.). Austin, TX: Pro-Ed.

Leonard, L.B. (1998). *Children with specific language impairment.* Cambridge, MA: MIT Press.

Miller, J., and Chapman, R. (1981). The relation between age and mean length of utterance in morphemes. *Journal of Speech and Hearing Research, 24,* 154–161.

Nelson, K.E. (1989). Strategies for first language teaching. In M.L. Rice and R.L. Schiefelbusch (Eds.), *The teachability of language* (pp. 263–310). Baltimore: Brookes.

Newcomer, P.L., and Hammill, D.D. (1997). Test of Language Development–Primary (TOLD–P) (3rd ed.). Austin, TX: Pro-Ed.

O'Hara Werner, E., and Dawson Kresheck, J. (1983). Structured Photographic Expressive Language Test–Preschool (SPELT–P). DeKalb, IL: Janelle.

O'Hara Werner, E., and Dawson Kresheck, J. (1983). Structured Photographic Expressive Language Test–II (SPELT–II). DeKalb, IL: Janelle.

Rice, M.L. (2000, April). *Variations in the acquisition of grammatical forms: Implications for language intervention.* Keynote presentation at the Treatment Efficacy Conference, Vanderbilt University, Nashville, TN.

Rice, M.L., and Wexler, K. (1996). Toward tense as a clinical marker of specific language impairment in English-speaking children. *Journal of Speech, Language, and Hearing Research, 39,* 1239–1257.

Rice, M.L., Wexler, K., and Cleave, P.L. (1995). Specific language impairment as a period of extended optional infinitive. *Journal of Speech and Hearing Research, 38,* 850–863.

Rice, M., Wexler, K., and Hershberger, S. (1998). Tense over time: The longitudinal course of tense acquisition in children with specific language impairment. *Journal of Speech, Language, and Hearing Research, 41,* 1412–1430.

Semel, E., Wiig, E.H., and Secord, W.A. (1995). Clinical Evaluation of Language Fundamentals (CELF–3) (3rd ed.). San Antonio, TX: Psychological Corporation.

Shipley, K.G., Stone, T.A., and Sue, M.B. (1983). Test for Examining Expressive Morphology (TEEM). Tuscon, AZ: Communication Skill Builders.

Tyler, A.A., Lewis, K.E., Haskill, A., and Tolbert, L.C. (2001). *Efficacy and cross-domain effects of a phonology and a language intervention.* Manuscript submitted for publication.

Tyler, A.A., Haskill, A., and Paul, K. (2001). *Generalization of the morpheme BE.* Manuscript submitted for publication.

Wells, G. (1985). *Language development in the preschool years.* New York: Cambridge University Press.

Wiig, E.H., Secord, W., and Semel, E. (1992). Clinical Evaluation of Language Fundamentals–Preschool (CELF–P). San Antonio, TX: Psychological Corporation.